STUDY GUIDE TO
CHILD AND ADOLESCENT
PSYCHIATRY

A Companion to
Dulcan's Textbook of
Child and Adolescent Psychiatry

STUDY GUIDE TO
CHILD AND ADOLESCENT
PSYCHIATRY

A Companion to
Dulcan's Textbook of
Child and Adolescent Psychiatry

Hong Shen, M.D.
Clinical Associate Professor of Psychiatry, Department of Psychiatry and Behavioral Sciences
University of California, Davis School of Medicine
Sacramento, California

Robert E. Hales, M.D., M.B.A.
Joe P. Tupin Chair, Department of Psychiatry and Behavioral Sciences
Interim Director, M.I.N.D. Institute
University of California, Davis School of Medicine
Sacramento, California

Narriman C. Shahrokh
Chief Administrative Officer, Department of Psychiatry and Behavioral Sciences
University of California, Davis School of Medicine
Sacramento, California

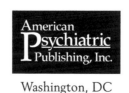

American Psychiatric Publishing, Inc.

Washington, DC
London, England

Note: The authors have worked to ensure that all information in this publication is accurate at the time of publication and consistent with general psychiatric and medical standards, and that information concerning drug dosages, schedules, and routes of administration is accurate at the time of publication and consistent with standards set by the U.S. Food and Drug Administration and the general medical community. As medical research and practice continue to advance, however, therapeutic standards may change. Moreover, specific situations may require a specific therapeutic response not included in this publication. For these reasons and because human and mechanical errors sometimes occur, we recommend that readers follow the advice of physicians directly involved in their care or the care of a member of their family.

Publications of American Psychiatric Publishing, Inc. (APPI), represent the views and opinions of the individual authors and do not necessarily represent the policies and opinions of APPI or the American Psychiatric Association.

If you would like to buy between 25 and 99 copies of this or any other APPI title, you are eligible for a 20% discount; please contact APPI Customer Service at appi@psych.org or 800-368-5777. If you wish to buy 100 or more copies of the same title, please email us at bulksales@psych.org for a price quote.

Manufactured in the United States of America on acid-free paper
13 12 11 10 09   5 4 3 2 1

ISBN 978-1-58562-353-2
First Edition

Typeset in Revival BT and Adobe's The Mix

American Psychiatric Publishing, Inc.
1000 Wilson Boulevard
Arlington, VA 22209-3901
www.appi.org

Contents

Preface..xv

Questions

CHAPTER 1
Assessing Infants and Toddlers 1

CHAPTER 2
Assessing the Preschool-Age Child 2

CHAPTER 3
Assessing the Elementary School–Age Child 4

CHAPTER 4
Assessing Adolescents 5

CHAPTER 5
Classification of Psychiatric Disorders..7

CHAPTER 6
The Process of Assessment and Diagnosis 9

CHAPTER 7
Diagnostic Interviews... 11

CHAPTER 8
Rating Scales 13

CHAPTER 9
Pediatric Evaluation and Laboratory Testing 14

CHAPTER 10
Neurological Examination, Electroencephalography, and Neuroimaging.............. 16

CHAPTER 11
Psychological and Neuropsychological Testing 18

CHAPTER 12
Intellectual Disability (Mental Retardation) 20

CHAPTER 13
Autism Spectrum Disorders 22

CHAPTER 14
Developmental Disorders of Learning, Communication, and Motor Skills. 23

CHAPTER 15
Attention-Deficit/Hyperactivity Disorder. 25

CHAPTER 16
Oppositional Defiant Disorder and Conduct Disorder 27

CHAPTER 17
Substance Abuse and Addictions 28

CHAPTER 18
Depression and Dysthymia 30

CHAPTER 19
Bipolar Disorder 32

CHAPTER 20
Generalized Anxiety Disorder, Specific Phobia, Panic Disorder,
Social Phobia, and Selective Mutism 34

CHAPTER 21
Separation Anxiety Disorder and School Refusal 36

CHAPTER 22
Posttraumatic Stress Disorder 38

CHAPTER 23
Obsessive-Compulsive Disorder 39

CHAPTER 24
Early-Onset Schizophrenia 41

CHAPTER 25
Obesity 43

CHAPTER 26
Anorexia Nervosa and Bulimia Nervosa 45

CHAPTER 27
Tic Disorders 47

CHAPTER 28
Elimination Disorders. 48

C H A P T E R 2 9
Sleep Disorders. 49

C H A P T E R 3 0
Evidence-Based Practices. 51

C H A P T E R 3 1
Child Abuse and Neglect 52

C H A P T E R 3 2
HIV and AIDS 53

C H A P T E R 3 3
Bereavement and Traumatic Grief. 54

C H A P T E R 3 4
Ethnic, Cultural, and Religious Issues 56

C H A P T E R 3 5
Youth Suicide 58

C H A P T E R 3 6
Gender Identity and Sexual Orientation 60

C H A P T E R 3 7
Aggression and Violence 62

C H A P T E R 3 8
Genetics: Fundamentals Relevant to Child and Adolescent Psychiatry. 64

C H A P T E R 3 9
Psychiatric Emergencies. 66

C H A P T E R 4 0
Family Transitions: Challenges and Resilience 68

C H A P T E R 4 1
Psychiatric Aspects of Chronic Physical Disorders 70

C H A P T E R 4 2
Children of Parents With Psychiatric and Substance Abuse Disorders 72

C H A P T E R 4 3
Legal and Ethical Issues 74

C H A P T E R 4 4
Telepsychiatry. 75

CHAPTER 45
Principles of Psychopharmacology 76

CHAPTER 46
Medications Used for Attention-Deficit/Hyperactivity Disorder 78

CHAPTER 47
Antidepressants 79

CHAPTER 48
Mood Stabilizers 81

CHAPTER 49
Antipsychotic Medications 83

CHAPTER 50
Alpha-Adrenergics, Beta-Blockers, Benzodiazepines, Buspirone, and Desmopressin 85

CHAPTER 51
Medications Used for Sleep 87

CHAPTER 52
Electroconvulsive Therapy, Transcranial Magnetic Stimulation,
and Deep Brain Stimulation 88

CHAPTER 53
Individual Psychotherapy 90

CHAPTER 54
Parent Counseling, Psychoeducation, and Parent Support Groups 91

CHAPTER 55
Behavioral Parent Training 93

CHAPTER 56
Family Therapy 94

CHAPTER 57
Interpersonal Psychotherapy for Depressed Adolescents 95

CHAPTER 58
Cognitive-Behavioral Treatment for Anxiety Disorders 97

CHAPTER 59
Cognitive-Behavioral Therapy for Depression 99

CHAPTER 60
Motivational Interviewing 101

CHAPTER 61
Systems of Care, Wraparound Services, and Home-Based Services 102

CHAPTER 62
Milieu Treatment: Inpatient, Partial Hospitalization, and Residential Programs 104

CHAPTER 63
School-Based Interventions 106

CHAPTER 64
Collaborating With Primary Care 108

CHAPTER 65
Juvenile Justice 110

Answer Guide

CHAPTER 1
Assessing Infants and Toddlers 111

CHAPTER 2
Assessing the Preschool-Age Child 114

CHAPTER 3
Assessing the Elementary School–Age Child 118

CHAPTER 4
Assessing Adolescents 121

CHAPTER 5
Classification of Psychiatric Disorders 125

CHAPTER 6
The Process of Assessment and Diagnosis 128

CHAPTER 7
Diagnostic Interviews 131

CHAPTER 8
Rating Scales 134

CHAPTER 9
Pediatric Evaluation and Laboratory Testing 138

CHAPTER 10
Neurological Examination, Electroencephalography, and Neuroimaging.............. 143

CHAPTER 11
Psychological and Neuropsychological Testing................................... 146

CHAPTER 12
Intellectual Disability (Mental Retardation) 149

CHAPTER 13
Autism Spectrum Disorders 153

CHAPTER 14
Developmental Disorders of Learning, Communication, and Motor Skills.............. 157

CHAPTER 15
Attention-Deficit/Hyperactivity Disorder...................................... 160

CHAPTER 16
Oppositional Defiant Disorder and Conduct Disorder 165

CHAPTER 17
Substance Abuse and Addictions 168

CHAPTER 18
Depression and Dysthymia 171

CHAPTER 19
Bipolar Disorder 175

CHAPTER 20
Generalized Anxiety Disorder, Specific Phobia, Panic Disorder,
Social Phobia, and Selective Mutism 178

CHAPTER 21
Separation Anxiety Disorder and School Refusal 183

CHAPTER 22
Posttraumatic Stress Disorder 187

CHAPTER 23
Obsessive-Compulsive Disorder 190

CHAPTER 24
Early-Onset Schizophrenia 194

CHAPTER 25
Obesity 199

CHAPTER 26
Anorexia Nervosa and Bulimia Nervosa 202

CHAPTER 27
Tic Disorders 205

CHAPTER 28
Elimination Disorders. 209

CHAPTER 29
Sleep Disorders 212

CHAPTER 30
Evidence-Based Practices. 216

CHAPTER 31
Child Abuse and Neglect 219

CHAPTER 32
HIV and AIDS 222

CHAPTER 33
Bereavement and Traumatic Grief. 225

CHAPTER 34
Ethnic, Cultural, and Religious Issues 229

CHAPTER 35
Youth Suicide 232

CHAPTER 36
Gender Identity and Sexual Orientation 236

CHAPTER 37
Aggression and Violence 239

CHAPTER 38
Genetics: Fundamentals Relevant to Child and Adolescent Psychiatry. 242

CHAPTER 39
Psychiatric Emergencies. 245

CHAPTER 40
Family Transitions: Challenges and Resilience 248

CHAPTER 41
Psychiatric Aspects of Chronic Physical Disorders 251

CHAPTER 42
Children of Parents With Psychiatric and Substance Abuse Disorders 255

CHAPTER 43
Legal and Ethical Issues 258

CHAPTER 44
Telepsychiatry 261

CHAPTER 45
Principles of Psychopharmacology 264

CHAPTER 46
Medications Used for Attention-Deficit/Hyperactivity Disorder 267

CHAPTER 47
Antidepressants 271

CHAPTER 48
Mood Stabilizers 274

CHAPTER 49
Antipsychotic Medications 278

CHAPTER 50
Alpha-Adrenergics, Beta-Blockers, Benzodiazepines, Buspirone, and Desmopressin 281

CHAPTER 51
Medications Used for Sleep 284

CHAPTER 52
Electroconvulsive Therapy, Transcranial Magnetic Stimulation,
and Deep Brain Stimulation 287

CHAPTER 53
Individual Psychotherapy 291

CHAPTER 54
Parent Counseling, Psychoeducation, and Parent Support Groups 294

CHAPTER 55
Behavioral Parent Training 297

CHAPTER 56
Family Therapy.. 300

CHAPTER 57
Interpersonal Psychotherapy for Depressed Adolescents 304

CHAPTER 58
Cognitive-Behavioral Treatment for Anxiety Disorders............................. 307

CHAPTER 59
Cognitive-Behavioral Therapy for Depression...................................... 312

CHAPTER 60
Motivational Interviewing 315

CHAPTER 61
Systems of Care, Wraparound Services, and Home-Based Services 318

CHAPTER 62
Milieu Treatment: Inpatient, Partial Hospitalization, and Residential Programs 322

CHAPTER 63
School-Based Interventions 326

CHAPTER 64
Collaborating With Primary Care 329

CHAPTER 65
Juvenile Justice.. 332

Preface

The purpose of this study guide is to provide individuals who have purchased *Dulcan's Textbook of Child and Adolescent Psychiatry* an opportunity to evaluate their understanding of the material contained in the textbook. Whenever possible, the selected questions emphasize the major points of each chapter. In addition, every effort is made to select those questions of most relevance to psychiatrists who see patients in a variety of clinical practice settings.

We encourage the readers of the textbook to answer the questions after reading each chapter. The format for the questions is similar to what candidates would expect to encounter when taking Part I of the American Board of Psychiatry and Neurology initial certification examination or the maintenance-of-certification examination in psychiatry that is required every 10 years. At the end of the study guide, the questions are repeated along with detailed answers. The answer section includes an explanation of the correct response for each question, as well as an explanation, in most cases, for why the other responses were incorrect.

An online version is available in addition to the printed study guide. Psychiatrists who wish to earn continuing medical education credits may purchase the online version and obtain CME credit by completing it.

We hope you will find the study guide a useful addition to *Dulcan's Textbook of Child and Adolescent Psychiatry*. Our goal is to have an assessment instrument that is helpful for your understanding of the material and for clarification of important concepts. Although the questions are reviewed numerous times, both by the authors and by editors at American Psychiatric Publishing, Inc., occasionally an incorrect response may be included. If this is the case, we would appreciate your notifying the publisher of the error so it can be corrected in the online version of the self-assessment examination. If you have other suggestions concerning this study guide, please e-mail Dr. Hales at rehales@ucdavis.edu.

Best of luck with your self-examination.

Hong Shen, M.D.
Robert E. Hales, M.D., M.B.A.
Narriman C. Shahrokh

Page numbers in the Answer Guide refer to
Dulcan's Textbook of Child and Adolescent Psychiatry.
Visit **www.appi.org** for more information about this textbook.

| | | |

Purchase the online version of this Study Guide at

www.psychiatryonline.com; click "Subscribe/Renew"

and receive instant scoring and CME credits.

Chapter 1

Assessing Infants and Toddlers

Select the single best response for each question.

1.1   Infant psychiatry focuses on which of the following age groups?

    A. From birth to first birthday.
    B. From birth through age 3 years.
    C. From birth to preschool years.
    D. From conception to age 3 years.
    E. From conception to preschool years.

1.2   Which of the following is the strongest outcome predictor of early childhood development?

    A. Presence or absence of pregnancy complications.
    B. Birth weight.
    C. Child's temperament.
    D. Parental relationship.
    E. Primary caregiving relationship.

1.3   Which of the following assessment or diagnostic tools uses the DSM-IV multiaxial system?

    A. Diagnostic Criteria: Zero to Three, Revised (DC:0–3R).
    B. Child Behavior Checklist 1½–5.
    C. Infant-Toddler Social and Emotional Assessment (ITSEA).
    D. Ages and Stages Questionnaires: Social-Emotional.
    E. None of the above.

1.4   Which of the following is *not* considered a key element of the infant/toddler assessment?

    A. History of presenting problem.
    B. Medical history.
    C. Developmental history.
    D. IQ.
    E. Family history.

1.5   Which of the following is the only diagnostic interview with published data to support its reliability for assessing infants and toddlers?

    A. Preschool Age Psychiatric Assessment (PAPA).
    B. Diagnostic Infant Preschool Structured Interview.
    C. Crowell procedure.
    D. Beck Depression Inventory.
    E. Parenting Stress Index.

C h a p t e r 2

Assessing the Preschool-Age Child

Select the single best response for each question.

2.1 The significant developmental differences between preschool- and school-age children require a tailored approach to obtaining a history and mental status exam. Which of the following principles should be kept in mind when evaluating a preschool-age child?

    A. The most meaningful evaluation occurs when the child is evaluated without the primary caregiver.
    B. The mental status examination should be conducted in the context of play.
    C. The preschooler should be evaluated in one session to avoid conflicting results.
    D. It is desirable to include only the primary caregiver when evaluating the child.
    E. All of the above.

2.2 The Washington University School of Medicine Infant/Preschool Mental Health (WUSM IPMH) clinic uses a standardized format for evaluating preschool-age children. Which of the following statements correctly describes this evaluation?

    A. The assessment is conducted in one 3-hour session.
    B. Free play is observed with the primary caregiver.
    C. A semistructured observation with secondary caregivers is included.
    D. Emotional, psychological, family, and developmental history is obtained only from the mother.
    E. None of the above.

2.3 Which of the following actions should be taken by parents to prepare their preschooler for the play evaluation?

    A. Parents should provide honest information to the child about the purpose of the evaluation.
    B. Parents should not disclose to their child that they have already met with the examiner.
    C. Parents should avoid discussing with the child that the examination will involve play.
    D. It is best to inform the child about the examination over several days to a week so he/she may ask questions.
    E. Parents should not prepare their child for the examination.

2.4 Which of the following statements regarding conduct of the free-play assessment with the preschooler is *true*?

    A. A brief separation between the parent and child midway through the free-play session is useful.
    B. The clinician should avoid disclosing to the child what was learned about his or her problems from the meeting with the parents.
    C. When the parent asks questions of the therapist during the play session, the therapist should freely answer the questions in order to reduce the parents' anxiety.
    D. The examiner should not respond to the child's bids to engage in play.
    E. All of the above.

2.5   Several standardized semistructured interviews may be useful in the dyadic assessment of parent and child. Which of the following are characteristics of the Parent-Child Early Relational Assessment (PCERA)?

    A. The parent blows bubbles to elicit affect from the child.
    B. Tasks of escalating difficulty are performed by the child and parent and videotaped for further review.
    C. The parent and child perform a structured task in which block designs are made from sample cards.
    D. None of the above.
    E. All of the above.

Chapter 3

Assessing the Elementary School–Age Child

Select the single best response for each question.

3.1   The key developmental milestones for the school-age child are related to

   A. Separation and individuation.
   B. Initiation and rapprochement.
   C. Object constancy and individual consolidation.
   D. Peer identity and social identity formation.
   E. Intimacy and generativity.

3.2   Which of the following is key to a successful evaluation?

   A. Seeing the child first.
   B. Seeing the parent(s) first.
   C. Seeing the child and parent(s) together.
   D. Seeing the referral professional first.
   E. Establishing a collaborative relationship between the clinician and the child and his or her family.

3.3   Key procedural information that should be covered in the first evaluation session includes all of the following *except*

   A. Office/departmental procedures.
   B. Plan/process of the evaluation.
   C. Communication with school.
   D. Confidentiality.
   E. Safety plans.

3.4   For the clinician, appropriate steps in the evaluation of a child whose parents are divorced include all of the following *except*

   A. Attempt to include both parents in gathering information.
   B. Agree to complete a custody evaluation.
   C. Clarify which parent has primary custody and request a copy of the custody agreement.
   D. Clarify health insurance responsibility.
   E. Clarify the role of the clinician.

3.5   Common presenting problems in school-age children include all of the following *except*

   A. Sexualized behavior.
   B. Academic difficulties.
   C. Peer difficulties.
   D. School refusal.
   E. Social anxiety.

Chapter 4

Assessing Adolescents

Select the single best response for each question.

4.1 Which of the following statements concerning the assessment of adolescents is *true?*

    A. Because mothers and fathers may have divergent views about the adolescent's problems, only one parent should be interviewed.

    B. Involve as few informants as possible in collecting information to minimize conflicting opinions.

    C. Understanding how the adolescent was referred for treatment is not important.

    D. Prior medical records from primary care physicians should be obtained as part of the assessment.

    E. Data from rating scales or psychological testing are rarely helpful in establishing the correct diagnosis.

4.2 In the initial assessment of an adolescent, which of the following strategies is usually most productive?

    A. Interview one parent, then the adolescent, then the other parent.

    B. Interview the adolescent alone first, then the parent or parents.

    C. Interview both parents, then the adolescent.

    D. Interview the parents together with the adolescent.

    E. None of the above.

4.3 What information obtained from adolescents should be shared with the parents?

    A. All details obtained from the adolescent should be shared with the parents.

    B. No information obtained from the adolescent should be shared with the parents.

    C. Safety issues involving the adolescent, such as suicidal behavior, should be shared with the parents.

    D. None of the above.

    E. All of the above.

4.4 An evidence-based approach that has been successfully used for interviewing adolescents is

    A. Psychodynamic interviewing.

    B. Dialectical behavioral interviewing.

    C. Cognitive-behavioral interviewing.

    D. Interpersonal interviewing.

    E. Motivational interviewing.

4.5 Goals for the initial parent interview include all of the following *except*

    A. Data collection.

    B. Sharing differential diagnostic possibilities.

    C. Understanding the parent's point of view.

    D. Establishing a relationship with the parents.

    E. None of the above.

4.6   A respondent-based interview that is highly structured and designed to be administered by trained lay interviewers is

        A. Diagnostic Interview Schedule for Children, Version IV (DISC-IV).
        B. Schedule for Affective Disorders and Schizophrenia for School-Age Children (K-SADS).
        C. Child Adolescent Psychiatric Assessment (CAPA).
        D. Child Behavior Checklist (CBCL).
        E. Behavior Assessment System for Children (BASC).

C h a p t e r   5

Classification of Psychiatric Disorders

Select the single best response for each question.

5.1 DSM-I (American Psychiatric Association 1952) categories relating specifically to childhood or adolescence included all of the following *except*

    A. Chronic brain syndrome associated with birth trauma.
    B. Schizophrenia reaction, childhood type.
    C. Special symptom reactions such as learning disturbance, enuresis, and somnambulism.
    D. Adjustment reactions.
    E. Hyperkinetic reaction of childhood.

5.2 All of the following statements regarding DSM-II (American Psychiatric Association 1968) are correct *except*

    A. It was intended to coincide with the *International Classification of Diseases*, 8th Revision (ICD-8).
    B. The developers tried to avoid terms that implied either the nature of a disorder or its cause.
    C. It reflected the growing importance of biological theories and research findings.
    D. It emphasized psychoanalytic theory.
    E. Descriptive phenomenology assumed a larger role.

5.3 All of the following statements regarding DSM-III (American Psychiatric Association 1980) are correct *except*

    A. It was highly controversial when introduced.
    B. Assumed etiology was included for most disorders.
    C. It was modeled on the Feighner criteria.
    D. It provided specific phenomenological diagnostic criteria for each disorder, in contrast to the global clinical impression of DSM-IV (American Psychiatric Association 1994).
    E. Each diagnosis had inclusion and exclusion criteria, and a five-part multiaxial system was introduced.

5.4 All of the following statements about DSM-IV (American Psychiatric Association 1994) are correct *except*

    A. It was a reconceptualization of its predecessor.
    B. There was greater coordination and agreement with the ICD development process.
    C. For most DSM-IV disorders, a single criteria set was provided that applies to children, adolescents, and adults.
    D. A number of disorders were moved from Axis II to Axis I, and only personality disorders and mental retardation remained on Axis II.
    E. The category "attention-deficit and disruptive behavior disorders" replaced the DSM-III-R (American Psychiatric Association 1987) category of disruptive behavior disorders.

5.5   Other diagnostic systems have been developed for populations of patients or professionals who have not been well served by either the DSM or ICD models. All of the following statements are correct *except*

    A. The *Diagnostic and Statistical Manual for Primary Care* (DSM-PC) was developed collaboratively by the American Academy of Pediatrics and the American Psychiatric Association.

    B. DSM-PC was designed to be used by pediatricians and faculty physicians to classify emotional and behavioral problems.

    C. DSM-PC includes a simplified single cluster approach.

    D. The Diagnostic Classification on Infancy and Early Childhood (DC:0–3) was revised in 2005.

    E. The goals of DC:0–3 were to increase the recognition of mental health and developmental challenges in young children.

Chapter 6

The Process of Assessment and Diagnosis

Select the single best response for each question.

6.1 Child assessment differs from adult assessment in a number of ways. Which of the following describes aspects of the child assessment that are different from the adult assessment?

    A. Multiple sources constitute the field for data collection with children.
    B. Child assessments frequently require information from the school.
    C. For younger children, verbal communication is much less important than play.
    D. Children rarely seek out an evaluation.
    E. All of the above.

6.2 In conducting the parent interview, clinicians should *not*

    A. Request information about the child's interests, activities, or strengths.
    B. Ask what preparation the parents have given the child for the evaluation.
    C. Ask parents for their understanding of the problem.
    D. Explain that the evaluation will invariably lead to treatment by the clinician.
    E. Discuss confidentiality of sessions between the child and the clinician.

6.3 Which of the following is the most important source of an outside report the clinicians should obtain (with permission) when assessing a child?

    A. Friends.
    B. Teachers.
    C. Siblings.
    D. Noncaregiving relatives.
    E. Group activities.

6.4 In constructing a case formulation, Ebert et al. (2000) suggested that the clinician examine child and family factors along a time axis and categorize them as predisposing, precipitating, perpetuating, or prognostic. According to this approach, parents going through a divorce would be considered what type of factor?

    A. Predisposing.
    B. Precipitating.
    C. Perpetuating.
    D. Prognostic.
    E. None of the above.

6.5   The major purpose of the parental feedback interview is

    A. To develop a concrete treatment plan to help their child.
    B. To gather additional information about the relationship between the child and parents.
    C. To test hypotheses concerning the case formulation.
    D. To inform the parents and child what has been found and what the clinician would recommend to address the issues that led to the assessment.
    E. To provide referral sources to the parents for either further assessment or treatment of their child.

Chapter 7

Diagnostic Interviews

Select the single best response for each question.

7.1   The process of making a psychiatric diagnosis is fraught with numerous potential biases. Which of the following clinician practices is *least* likely to result in a biased diagnosis?

    A. Making diagnoses before all relevant information is collected.
    B. Collecting information selectively.
    C. Neglecting to be systematic in collecting and/or organizing information.
    D. Preventing the clinician's particular expertise from influencing diagnosis assignment.
    E. Assuming correlation between symptoms and illness.

7.2   Various diagnostic tools have been developed to enhance the reliability of the information gathered and the diagnosis assignment. Which of the following statements is *false*?

    A. Clinicians and researchers commonly use diagnostic interviews and questionnaires.
    B. Patients, parents, and teachers usually complete questionnaires.
    C. Structured diagnostic interviews are primarily used by clinicians in daily clinical practice.
    D. The instruments vary as to whether they are administered by clinicians or trained nonclinical interviewers.
    E. Structured interviews specific for children and adolescents have been developed.

7.3   The term *face validity* refers to

    A. How well a category as defined appears to describe a recognized illness.
    B. How well the category predicts a pertinent aspect of care, such as treatment needs or prognosis.
    C. Whether the category has meaning in terms of what it is designed to describe.
    D. How often different interviews assign the same diagnosis.
    E. How consistently respondents report the same symptoms over time.

7.4   "The percentage of individuals in a sample who do not have the disorder and are accurately identified by the interview as not having the disorder" defines which of the following terms?

    A. Sensitivity.
    B. Specificity.
    C. Predictive value positive.
    D. Predictive value negative.
    E. None of the above.

7.5   Interviews are usually described as either structured or semistructured, depending on how much freedom the interviewer has to ask questions and interpret the responses. *Semistructured* interviews are designed for clinical research and allow the interviewer some leeway in wording questions and interpreting responses. All of the following instruments are semistructured *except*

   A. Schedule for Affective Disorders and Schizophrenia for School-Aged Children—Present and Lifetime (K-SADS-PL).
   B. Washington University Schedule for Affective Disorders and Schizophrenia for School-Aged Children (WASH-U-KSADS).
   C. Schedule for Affective Disorders and Schizophrenia for School-Aged Children—Epidemiological (K-SADS-E).
   D. Anxiety Disorders Interview Schedule for DSM-IV: Child and Parent Version (ADIS-CP).
   E. National Institute of Mental Health Diagnostic Interview Schedule for Children Version IV (NIMH DISC-IV).

Chapter 8

Rating Scales

Select the single best response for each question.

8.1   Which of the following terms is used to describe whether a scale is stable over time?

    A. Internal reliability.
    B. Interrater reliability.
    C. Test-retest reliability.
    D. Reliability.
    E. Psychometric properties.

8.2   Which of the following types of concurrent validity is defined as the extent of correlation of related variables?

    A. Content validity.
    B. Face validity.
    C. Criterion validity.
    D. Discriminative validity.
    E. Convergent validity.

8.3   A "broad-band" rating scale that includes multiple versions for different reporters and age groups and that can be scored using factors that approximate DSM-IV-TR (American Psychiatric Association 2000) diagnostic criteria is

    A. The Behavior Assessment System for Children, 2nd Edition (BASC-2).
    B. The Child Behavior Checklist (CBCL).
    C. The Child Symptom Inventories (CSI).
    D. The Eyberg Child Behavior Inventory (ECBI).
    E. The Sutter-Eyberg Student Behavior Inventory-Revised (SESBI-R).

8.4   Of the following rating scales, which assesses the same aspects of depression with adolescents that it assesses with adults and additionally discriminates depressed teens from those with anxiety and conduct disorders?

    A. Children's Depression Inventory (CDI).
    B. Children's Depression Rating Scale-Revised (CDRS-R).
    C. Reynolds Adolescent Depression Scale (RADS).
    D. Beck Depression Inventory-II (BDI-II).
    E. Reynolds Child Depression Scale (RCDS).

8.5   A friend contacts you and expresses concern that her 8-year-old son may have attention-deficit/hyperactivity disorder (ADHD). She asks if there is a good rating scale available at no cost that a parent can use. You tell her to search online for the following:

    A. Vanderbilt ADHD Parent Rating Scale (VADPRS).
    B. Conners' Rating Scale–Revised (CRS-R).
    C. ADHD Rating Scale–IV (ADHD-RS-IV).
    D. Social Communication Questionnaire (SCQ).
    E. Vineland Adaptive Behavior Scales, 2nd Edition (VABS-II).

Chapter 9

Pediatric Evaluation and Laboratory Testing

Select the single best response for each question.

9.1   A comprehensive medical history, the use of collateral informants, and close collaboration with the pediatric provider are essential in the evaluation of children and adolescents who present with psychiatric and behavioral symptoms. All of the following statements are correct *except*

   A. The presence of regular pediatric visits, well-child visits, and immunizations as scheduled should be established.
   B. History gathering begins with the child's delivery.
   C. A history of labor and delivery, including gestational age, Apgar scores, nature of delivery, and complications, should be reviewed.
   D. History gathering should include the family pedigree and family medical and psychiatric history.
   E. Family history of sudden cardiac death and hypercholesterolemia may need to be elicited.

9.2   Assessing a child's development is an integral component of the overall medical evaluation. All of the following statements are accurate *except*

   A. The Denver Development Screening Tool (DDST) is used for children up to 6 years of age.
   B. The medical history for the 6- to 11-year-old child focuses on growth, development, and skills acquisition.
   C. During the period between 6 and 11 years of age, the head grows rapidly.
   D. Adolescent physical development is characterized by physical growth and sexual development.
   E. The peak of growth in male adolescents comes 2–3 years later than that in females.

9.3   Which of the following syndromes has a recognizable behavioral phenotype?

   A. Fragile X syndrome.
   B. Prader-Willi syndrome.
   C. Angelman's syndrome.
   D. Turner syndrome.
   E. All of the above.

9.4   All of the following baseline laboratory assessments should be obtained when children and adolescents present with behavioral symptoms whose history or physical findings suggest an organic etiology *except*

   A. Complete blood count.
   B. Renal function tests.
   C. Hepatic function tests.
   D. Thyroid function tests.
   E. Lipid profile.

9.5   Which of the following statements regarding cardiac risk and assessment of children and adolescents is *false?*

      A. Cardiac evaluation and testing are suggested if positive for a family or medical history of sudden cardiac death, symptoms of palpitation, fainting, chest pain, exercise intolerance, arrhythmia, syncope, and hypertension.

      B. Electrocardiograms (ECGs) are often used in psychiatric practice for monitoring the effects of drugs known to adversely affect cardiac function.

      C. An ECG should be obtained prior to initiation of certain psychotropic medications.

      D. Lithium can potentially cause benign reversible T-wave changes and impair SA nodal function.

      E. Current recommendations advocate routine ECGs before initiating stimulant treatment.

Chapter 10

Neurological Examination, Electroencephalography, and Neuroimaging

Select the single best response for each question.

10.1 Which of the following are characteristic of upper motor neuron lesions?

    A. Bilateral distribution.
    B. Flaccid paralysis.
    C. Hypotonia.
    D. Decreased or absent deep tendon reflexes.
    E. Babinski reflex positive.

10.2 Which part of the neurological examination is the least objective in the nonverbal and/or young patient?

    A. Motor examination.
    B. Sensory examination.
    C. Coordination assessment.
    D. Gait examination.
    E. Cranial nerve assessment.

10.3 Which part of the neurological examination may be accomplished by holding toys so that the patient has to reach across the midline to reach them?

    A. Motor examination.
    B. Sensory examination.
    C. Coordination assessment.
    D. Gait assessment.
    E. Cranial nerve assessment.

10.4 Which of the following EEG rhythms are the predominant pattern when children are awake with their eyes closed?

    A. Delta.
    B. Theta.
    C. Alpha.
    D. Beta.
    E. None of the above.

10.5 Which of the following EEG findings commonly reflect primary generalized epilepsy and may be elicited by hyperventilation or photic stimulation?

    A. Spike and slow-wave discharges.
    B. Sharp and slow-wave complex discharges.
    C. Focal epileptiform discharges.
    D. Periodic lateralized epileptiform discharges.
    E. Rhythmic slowing.

Chapter 11

Psychological and Neuropsychological Testing

Select the single best response for each question.

11.1 According to the American Education Research Association, clinically relevant requirements for the ethical administration and interpretation of tests include all of the following *except*

   A. Test publishers have a number of responsibilities.
   B. Test users must be qualified in the area in which they are conducting an assessment.
   C. Testing must be guided by the best interests of the patient.
   D. Decisions must be based on test data that are current.
   E. Tests must be ready for readministration within 1 year.

11.2 A psychological test must be appropriately constructed and standardized. Interpretation is based on some type of standardized score, which in turn is based on the standard deviation (SD), or dispersion, of test scores for the sample. Correct statements regarding the SD include all of the following *except*

   A. About 68% of scores fall within one standard deviation of the mean.
   B. 80% of scores fall within two standard deviations.
   C. For most tests, the mean of standardized scores is low.
   D. Some tests are constructed with a mean of 50.
   E. Some tests are constructed with a mean of 0.

11.3 Which of the following is the correct definition of reliability?

   A. The degree to which the test measures what it claims to measure.
   B. The degree to which the questions and tasks are representative of the universe of behavior the test was designed to sample.
   C. A test that, if repeated or if administered by another examiner, would yield approximately the same score.
   D. The extent to which a test estimates a person's performance on some outcome measure or criterion.
   E. A theoretical, intangible quality or trait in which individuals differ.

11.4 All of the following are IQ tests *except*

   A. Stanford-Binet.
   B. Wechsler Intelligence Scale for Children.
   C. Differential Ability Scales.
   D. Bayley-III.
   E. Kaufman.

11.5   Assessment of intellectual deficiency (mental retardation) must include which of the following measures?

    A. The Iowa Tests of Basic Achievement.
    B. Standard Achievement Test.
    C. Woodcock-Johnson Tests of Achievement.
    D. Halstead-Reitan Test Battery.
    E. Test of adaptive functioning.

Chapter 12

Intellectual Disability (Mental Retardation)

Select the single best response for each question.

12.1 In 1992, the American Association on Mental Retardation (AAMR), now the American Association on Intellectual Disability and Developmental Disabilities (AAIDD), proposed a new classification system for intellectual disability based on intensity of supports needed as opposed to the traditional system of classification by IQ score. For the new proposed classification, where would someone be classified if he or she requires additional support to navigate through everyday situations?

    A. Intermittent support.
    B. Limited support.
    C. Extensive support.
    D. Pervasive support.
    E. None of the above.

12.2 Which of the following predisposing factors is associated with the highest percentage of cases of intellectual disability?

    A. Environmental influences.
    B. Pregnancy and perinatal complications.
    C. Acquired medical conditions.
    D. Heredity.
    E. Chromosomal changes and exposure to toxins during prenatal development.

12.3 Which of the following risk factors for intellectual disability of unknown etiology is the strongest predictor of disability?

    A. Lower level of maternal education.
    B. Children born to older women.
    C. Low birth weight.
    D. Males.
    E. Multiple births.

12.4 Which of the following genetic causes of intellectual disability is associated with a deletion at 22q11.2?

    A. Angelman syndrome.
    B. Williams syndrome.
    C. Prader-Willi syndrome.
    D. Velocardiofacial syndrome (VCFS).
    E. Rett syndrome.

12.5   Which of the following atypical antipsychotic medications has the most scientific evidence to support its use in treating children with extreme irritability, aggression, or self-injury in the setting of intellectual disability?

   A. Aripiprazole.
   B. Olanzapine.
   C. Quetiapine.
   D. Risperidone.
   E. Ziprasidone.

Chapter 13

Autism Spectrum Disorders

Select the single best response for each question.

13.1   In which of the following DSM editions did autism become an official and codified diagnosis?

    A. DSM-I.
    B. DSM-II.
    C. DSM-III.
    D. DSM-III-R.
    E. DSM-IV.

13.2   A DSM-IV-TR (American Psychiatric Association 2000) diagnosis of autism requires all of the following *except*

    A. Qualitative impairments in social interaction.
    B. Qualitative impairments in communication.
    C. Restricted repetitive and stereotyped patterns of behavior, interests, and activities.
    D. Delays or abnormal functioning in at least one of above areas prior to age 3 years.
    E. Low IQ.

13.3   Evaluation instruments designed for autism include all of the following *except*

    A. Checklist for Autism in Toddlers (CHAT).
    B. Autism Diagnostic Interview—Revised (ADI-R).
    C. Autism Diagnostic Observation Schedule—Generic (ADOS-G).
    D. Childhood Autism Rating Scale (CARS).
    E. Vineland Adaptive Behavior Scales (VABS).

13.4   DSM-IV-TR (American Psychiatric Association 2000) pervasive development disorders (PDDs) include all of the following *except*

    A. Asperger's disorder.
    B. PDD not otherwise specified (NOS).
    C. Rett's disorder.
    D. Childhood disintegrative disorder (CDD).
    E. Fragile X syndrome.

13.5   Based on a 2001 study funded by the National Academy of Sciences, recommended targets for educational intervention in children with autism spectrum disorders include all of the following *except*

    A. Functional spontaneous communication.
    B. Social skills.
    C. Play skills.
    D. Cognitive development.
    E. Self-care skills.

Chapter 14

Developmental Disorders of Learning, Communication, and Motor Skills

Select the single best response for each question.

14.1   Which of the following is the most common learning disorder?

   A. Expressive language disorder.
   B. Receptive language disorder.
   C. Disorder of written expression.
   D. Reading disorder.
   E. Mathematics disorder.

14.2   "The ability to use working memory to retain sounds and then words" defines which of the following basic building blocks of reading?

   A. Phonological awareness.
   B. Rapid naming.
   C. Phonological memory.
   D. Word recognition.
   E. Spelling.

14.3   Which of the following core cognitive processes is required for adequate reading comprehension?

   A. Language skills.
   B. Listening comprehension.
   C. Working memory.
   D. Inference.
   E. All of the above.

14.4   Which of the following terms is used to describe problems that ensue when the brain fails to recognize and interpret a sound?

   A. Phonological disorder.
   B. Auditory processing disorder (APD).
   C. Fluency disorder.
   D. Expressive language disorder.
   E. Oral expression disorder.

14.5 Which of the following statements concerning mathematics disability is *true?*

    A. Research in dyslexia lags behind dyscalculia.
    B. Several core deficits have been identified in the mathematics arena.
    C. The prevalence of a math disability is estimated to be 10%–12%.
    D. There is no evidence to support the heritability of math difficulties.
    E. Federal guidelines break down mathematics disorder into the ability to perform calculations and problem solving.

C h a p t e r   1 5

Attention-Deficit/ Hyperactivity Disorder

Select the single best response for each question.

15.1   All of the following are accurate statements regarding comorbidity with attention-deficit/hyperactivity disorder (ADHD) *except*

    A. Both oppositional defiant disorder (ODD) and conduct disorder are comorbidly present in at least 25% of children with ADHD.

    B. Learning and language disorders are comorbidly present in up to 25% of children with ADHD.

    C. Many children with ADHD have two or more comorbid disorders.

    D. Family studies suggest that ADHD with ODD/conduct disorder and ADHD alone are separate genetic subtypes.

    E. Compared with those with ADHD alone, those with comorbid anxiety are less likely to respond to psychosocial interventions.

15.2   All of the following statements concerning the etiology and risk factors of attention-deficit/hyperactivity disorder (ADHD) are correct *except*

    A. If a child has ADHD, there is a 10%–35% chance of first-degree relatives having the disorder.

    B. If a parent has ADHD, there is a 57% chance the child will develop ADHD.

    C. The rate of ADHD in biological relatives is 18% compared with 6% in the adopted relatives.

    D. About 50% of the variance in ADHD traits is found to be attributable to genetics.

    E. Nongenetic risk factors include perinatal stress, low birth weight, traumatic brain injury, and maternal smoking during pregnancy.

15.3   All of the following statements regarding the pathophysiology of attention-deficit/hyperactivity disorder (ADHD) are correct *except*

    A. Hippocampal volume is increased bilaterally in a large sample of children with ADHD relative to control subjects.

    B. Children with ADHD show larger volumes of the dorsolateral prefrontal cortex (DLPFC), anterior cingulate, and caudate regions compared with control subjects.

    C. Compared with children with ADHD, control subjects have increased activation in the prefrontal cortex (PFC) bilaterally when performing response inhibition tasks.

    D. The parents of ADHD children (who had ADHD themselves) show decreased activity in the frontostriatal areas and anterior cingulate cortex (ACC).

    E. ADHD may be seen as a disorder of both frontostriatal and frontocerebellar circuitry.

15.4 Research findings concerning the course and prognosis of attention-deficit/hyperactivity disorder (ADHD) include all of the following *except*

    A. More than 60% of children with ADHD continue to suffer from the disorder during teenage years.

    B. At a 3-year follow-up, the NIMH Multimodal Treatment Study of ADHD (MTA) found that 20% of the sample no longer met criteria for ADHD.

    C. Follow-up studies in the adult population showed variable rates of ADHD depending on informants and presence or absence of comorbidity.

    D. Adults with a childhood history of ADHD show higher rates of antisocial behavior, injuries and accidents, and employment and marital difficulties.

    E. Adults with a childhood history of ADHD have higher rates of substance use disorders.

15.5 All of the following statements regarding attention-deficit/hyperactivity disorder (ADHD) treatment are correct *except*

    A. Pharmacological treatment of ADHD is the best-studied intervention in child and adolescent psychiatry.

    B. Pharmacological intervention for ADHD is more effective than behavioral treatment alone.

    C. Comorbid anxiety has been found to predict a poorer response to behavioral treatment.

    D. According to recent American Academy of Child and Adolescent Psychiatry and Texas Children's Medication Algorithm Project (CMAP) guidelines, U.S. Food and Drug Administration (FDA)–approved agents should be the initial choice of medications.

    E. The long-acting agents have similar safety and efficacy profiles compared with the immediate-release forms.

Chapter 16

Oppositional Defiant Disorder and Conduct Disorder

Select the single best response for each question.

16.1   The most common comorbid disorder found with oppositional defiant disorder (ODD) is

    A. Separation anxiety disorder.
    B. Obsessive-compulsive disorder (OCD).
    C. Attention-deficit/hyperactivity disorder (ADHD).
    D. Major depressive disorder.
    E. Dysthymic disorder.

16.2   Which of the following family attributes are correlated with higher rates of oppositional behaviors?

    A. Parental discord.
    B. Domestic violence.
    C. Low family cohesion.
    D. Child abuse.
    E. All of the above.

16.3   Oppositional defiant disorder (ODD) is most predictive of the later occurrence of which of the following disorders?

    A. Antisocial personality disorder.
    B. Conduct disorder.
    C. Obsessive-compulsive disorder.
    D. Substance use disorder.
    E. Mood disorder.

16.4   Which of the following psychotherapeutic interventions have been shown to have the greatest efficacy in treating oppositional defiant disorder (ODD)?

    A. Cognitive-behavioral therapy.
    B. Family therapy.
    C. Parent management training.
    D. Psychodynamic psychotherapy.
    E. None of the above.

16.5   Conduct disorder is more prevalent in which of the following populations?

    A. Boys.
    B. Rural communities.
    C. Higher socioeconomic status families.
    D. Suburbs.
    E. Neighborhoods with low rates of crime.

Chapter 17

Substance Abuse and Addictions

Select the single best response for each question.

17.1 All of the following statements regarding the definition and diagnosis of substance abuse or dependence are correct *except*

    A. Substance use per se is sufficient for a diagnosis of abuse or dependence.

    B. *Misuse* can be defined as use for a purpose not consistent with medical guidelines.

    C. Recurrent substance use in adolescents rarely leads to impaired functioning.

    D. The diagnosis of substance abuse requires evidence of a maladaptive pattern of substance use with clinically significant levels of impairment or distress.

    E. A substance dependence diagnosis requires that additional criteria, such as withdrawal, tolerance, and loss of control over use, be met.

17.2 Regarding the comorbidity of substance use disorder (SUD), all of the following statements are correct *except*

    A. In addiction treatment programs, more than 50% of adolescents with co-occurring mental illness have three or more co-occurring psychiatric disorders.

    B. The most common comorbid conditions are conduct problems, attention-deficit/hyperactivity disorder (ADHD), mood disorders, and trauma-related symptoms.

    C. Some studies of youth with SUD show that females exhibit more internalizing symptoms than males.

    D. Except for depression, the early symptoms of most psychiatric disorders generally emerge prior to the onset of substance use.

    E. The specific type of a comorbid psychiatric diagnosis predicts relapse risk.

17.3 The "gateway" substances with which most adolescents start are

    A. Tobacco and alcohol.

    B. Inhalants.

    C. Marijuana and alcohol.

    D. Amphetamines.

    E. Over-the-counter cough and cold medicines.

17.4 All of the following statements regarding the validity of adolescent self-report of substance use are true *except*

    A. A majority of adolescents in drug clinics or schools provide temporally consistent reports.

    B. An "intake-discharge effect" is often observed, wherein the level of use reported at discharge is much lower than that endorsed at admission to a treatment program.

    C. The use of a structured interview may support or validate the self-report.

    D. Urine drug screen (UDS) is associated with greater drug use disclosures.

    E. The engagement and skillfulness of the assessment interviewer predict more valid self-report responses.

17.5 The pretreatment factors that are associated with poorer outcomes of substance use and relapse include all of the following *except*

A. Co-occurring psychopathology.
B. Higher severity of substance use.
C. Nonwhite race.
D. Criminality.
E. Lower educational status.

Chapter 18

Depression and Dysthymia

Select the single best response for each question.

18.1   Which of the following epidemiological findings concerning depression in children and adolescents is *true?*

    A. The prevalence of major depressive disorder is approximately 4%–8% in children.

    B. The male-to-female ratio for depression in children is 1:2.

    C. The cumulative prevalence of depression by age 18 is approximately 10% in community samples.

    D. The risk for depression remains constant after puberty.

    E. Approximately 5%–10% of children and adolescents have subsyndromal symptoms of major depressive disorder.

18.2   Although most children and adolescents recover from their first depressive episode, longitudinal studies of clinical and community samples of depressed youth have shown that the probability of recurrence after 5 years is

    A. 10%.

    B. 20%.

    C. 30%.

    D. 50%.

    E. 70%.

18.3   You elect to treat a depressed adolescent with psychotherapy. Which of the following psychotherapies has been shown to be efficacious in randomized controlled clinical trials?

    A. Systemic behavioral family therapy.

    B. Long-term psychodynamic psychotherapy.

    C. Brief psychodynamic psychotherapy.

    D. Interpersonal psychotherapy.

    E. None of the above.

18.4   A meta-analysis of all published and unpublished pharmacological, randomized controlled trials (RCTs) for major depressive disorder (MDD) in youth showed a benefit of selective serotonin reuptake inhibitor (SSRI) antidepressants over placebo, yielding a risk difference of

    A. 11%.

    B. 19%.

    C. 24%.

    D. 30%.

    E. 35%.

18.5 You wish to start your patient, a 13-year-old girl with depression, on a selective serotonin reuptake inhibitor (SSRI), but her parents express concern about the U.S. Food and Drug Administration (FDA) "black box" warning of an increased risk of suicide in youths receiving SSRIs. Being familiar with results from a meta-analysis that reanalyzed the FDA findings (Hammad et al. 2006) and a study that used more appropriate statistical analyses (Bridge et al. 2007), you respond by providing the following information:

A. Only about 5 in 100 youth exposed to antidepressants had a new or worsening spontaneously reported suicidal ideation or behavior.

B. Pharmacoepidemiological studies support a positive relationship between SSRI use and the reduction in the adolescent and young adult suicide rate.

C. The number needed to harm (NNH) that can be attributed to the active treatment for antidepressants was 10.

D. Evaluation of suicidal ideation and attempts ascertained through rating scales in 17 studies showed a modest increase in the onset and worsening of suicidality.

E. After the black box warning was imposed, the prescription of antidepressants declined and the rates of suicide increased.

Chapter 19

Bipolar Disorder

Select the single best response for each question.

19.1   Which of the following statements regarding the DSM-IV-TR (American Psychiatric Association 2000) definition of bipolar disorder is *false?*

    A. Manic episode must be present in bipolar I disorder.
    B. Depressive episode must be present in bipolar I disorder.
    C. Depressive episode must be present in bipolar II disorder.
    D. Hypomania must be present in bipolar II disorder.
    E. Cyclothymia presents with cycles of subsyndromal mania and depression.

19.2   In bipolar disorder, what episode frequency defines "rapid cycling" according to DSM-IV-TR (American Psychiatric Association 2000)?

    A. One per month.
    B. Two or more per year.
    C. Four or more per year.
    D. Six or more per year.
    E. Once per season.

19.3   All of the following statements regarding comorbidity of bipolar disorder are correct *except*

    A. The most common simultaneous comorbidities occurring during mania are attention-deficit/hyperactivity disorder (ADHD), oppositional defiant disorder (ODD), conduct disorder, and anxiety.
    B. ADHD co-occurs with bipolar disorder more in prepubertal children than in adolescents.
    C. The combination of externalizing disorders and bipolar disorder may represent a phenotype specific to adolescents.
    D. About 20% of children with mania have a comorbid pervasive developmental disorder.
    E. Early-onset bipolar disorder appears to increase the rate of substance abuse.

19.4   Functional magnetic resonance imaging (fMRI) studies of children with bipolar disorder suggest perturbations in prefrontal limbic circuitry. Findings from recent studies include all of the following *except*

    A. Children detect greater hostility in emotionally neutral faces.
    B. Children show elevated levels of fear when viewing faces.
    C. Activation of the left amygdala-striatal-ventral prefrontal circuit is increased when rating face hostility.
    D. Activation of the amygdala during emotional changes is decreased.
    E. Probability of misinterpreting facial expression is increased.

19.5 All of the following statements regarding the onset, course, and prognosis of bipolar disorder are correct *except*

    A. Bipolar disorder often begins with depression or dysthymia.

    B. Early-onset bipolar disorder is characterized by slow response to treatment and persistent mood fluctuations.

    C. Bipolar disorder NOS has a faster response to treatment than bipolar I disorder or bipolar II disorder.

    D. About one-quarter of children with bipolar disorder NOS converted to bipolar I disorder or bipolar II disorder based on a 2-year follow-up study.

    E. Poor prognostic indicators may include nonadherence to prescribed medications, low socioeconomic status (SES), low maternal warmth, psychosis, comorbid anxiety, and rapid cycling.

19.6 Which of the following medications has been approved by the U.S. Food and Drug Administration (FDA) for the treatment of mania in youth?

    A. Olanzapine.

    B. Divalproex.

    C. Carbamazepine.

    D. Ziprasidone.

    E. Aripiprazole.

Chapter 20

Generalized Anxiety Disorder, Specific Phobia, Panic Disorder, Social Phobia, and Selective Mutism

Select the single best response for each question.

20.1 Which of the following childhood-onset disorders has a chronic waxing and waning course and may remit spontaneously in one-third of lifetime cases?

    A. Generalized anxiety disorder.
    B. Specific phobia.
    C. Panic disorder.
    D. Social phobia.
    E. Selective mutism.

20.2 In regard to common biological influences on the development of childhood anxiety, which of the following statements is *true*?

    A. Children with anxiety disorders show less autonomic reactivity in response to stress.
    B. State anxiety has demonstrated more evidence for genetic influences when compared with trait anxiety.
    C. Behavioral inhibition in children is associated with the development of anxiety.
    D. Children at risk for anxiety disorders are less likely to have irregularities in sleeping and eating patterns.
    E. Longitudinal studies have failed to demonstrate a link between anxiety sensitivity and the development of panic disorder.

20.3 Which of the following parenting behaviors is associated with higher levels of anxiety in children?

    A. High levels of parental control.
    B. High levels of parental warmth.
    C. High levels of parental sensitivity.
    D. Lower levels of parental rejection.
    E. Lower levels of parental criticism.

20.4 Which of the following psychotherapies has received the most empirical support from randomized controlled studies for efficacy in the treatment of anxiety disorders in children and adolescents?

    A. Interpersonal psychotherapy (IPT).
    B. Cognitive-behavioral therapy (CBT).
    C. Dialectical behavioral therapy.
    D. Psychodynamic psychotherapy.
    E. Supportive psychotherapy.

20.5 Which of the following agents is considered the first-line treatment for anxiety disorders in children?

    A. Serotonin-norepinephrine reuptake inhibitors (SNRIs).
    B. Atypical antipsychotics.
    C. Tricyclic antidepressants.
    D. Benzodiazepines.
    E. Selective serotonin reuptake inhibitors (SSRIs).

Chapter 21

Separation Anxiety Disorder and School Refusal

Select the single best response for each question.

21.1   All of the following statements regarding separation anxiety disorder (SAD) are correct *except*

    A. SAD is the only anxiety disorder in DSM-IV-TR (American Psychiatric Association 2000) that is included under the category of disorders usually first diagnosed in infancy, childhood, or adolescence.

    B. Separation anxiety can be a developmentally appropriate response.

    C. Separation anxiety typically declines between 7 and 9 years of age.

    D. SAD only occurs when the child shows developmentally inappropriate and excessive anxiety associated with separation from a primary caregiver.

    E. A child may experience anxiety prior to, during, and/or in anticipation of the separation.

21.2   Which of the following statements regarding the epidemiology and comorbidity of separation anxiety disorder (SAD) is *false?*

    A. Prevalence rates of SAD range between 3% and 5%.

    B. Several studies show higher prevalence rates of SAD in girls than in boys.

    C. Fifty percent of a community sample of 8-year-old children exhibited subclinical levels of separation anxiety.

    D. Children with SAD are more likely to have a comorbid mood disorder compared with children with generalized anxiety disorder (GAD) or social phobia (SP).

    E. Children with SAD are more likely to have a sleep terror disorder compared with children with GAD or SP.

21.3   According to the American Academy of Child and Adolescent Psychiatry (AACAP) practice parameter (2007), effective treatment of children with separation anxiety disorder (SAD) often includes all of the following *except*

    A. Psychoeducation.

    B. School consultation.

    C. Cognitive-behavioral therapy (CBT).

    D. Selective serotonin reuptake inhibitors (SSRIs).

    E. Psychoanalytical psychotherapy.

21.4   All of the following statements regarding school refusal are correct *except*

    A. It is an anxiety disorder listed in DSM-IV-TR (American Psychiatric Association 2000).

    B. It is associated with separation anxiety disorder (SAD), generalized anxiety disorder (GAD), social phobia (SP), depression, and oppositional defiant disorder (ODD).

    C. It presents as having trouble attending school.

    D. Separation anxiety and school phobia have also been used to describe school refusal.

    E. School refusal does not usually include children who do not attend school because of truancy, antisocial behaviors, or conduct disorders.

21.5 All of the following statements regarding evaluation of school refusal are correct *except*

    A. Evaluation should follow consensus guidelines.
    B. Multimodal assessment with multiple informants should be used.
    C. Comprehensive evaluation may include clinical interviews, semistructured diagnostic interview, examining contributing factors.
    D. Psychoeducational and language evaluations can be helpful.
    E. The School Refusal Assessment Scale can be used.

Chapter 22

Posttraumatic Stress Disorder

Select the single best response for each question.

22.1 A variety of risk factors have been identified in the development of posttraumatic stress disorder (PTSD) after a disaster. Which of the following is one of those risk factors?

    A. Experiencing sleep disturbance immediately after the event.

    B. The presence of a predisaster personality disorder.

    C. Increased media viewing of the disaster.

    D. Having an immediate evacuation.

    E. None of the above.

22.2 In childhood samples, the psychiatric disorders most often comorbid with posttraumatic stress disorder (PTSD) are

    A. Attention-deficit/hyperactivity disorder (ADHD) or oppositional/conduct disorders.

    B. Psychotic disorders.

    C. Depressive disorders.

    D. Substance use disorders.

    E. None of the above.

22.3 The most evidence for treatment of childhood posttraumatic stress disorder (PTSD) exists for which of the following treatments?

    A. Brief psychodynamic psychotherapy.

    B. Trauma-focused psychotherapy.

    C. Selective serotonin reuptake inhibitor (SSRI) antidepressants.

    D. Interpersonal psychotherapy.

    E. Atypical antipsychotics.

22.4 Which of the following medications has been found beneficial in treating childhood posttraumatic stress disorder (PTSD)?

    A. Olanzapine.

    B. Lorazepam.

    C. Clonidine.

    D. Monoamine oxidase inhibitors (MAOIs).

    E. All of the above.

22.5 Which of the following newer treatments has been found effective in decreasing posttraumatic stress disorder (PTSD) symptoms in children?

    A. Restricting movement through binding.

    B. Eye movement desensitization and reprocessing (EMDR).

    C. Restricting nutritional intake.

    D. "Rebirthing" techniques.

    E. None of the above.

Chapter 23

Obsessive-Compulsive Disorder

Select the single best response for each question.

23.1 Unique characteristics of pediatric obsessive-compulsive disorder (OCD) relative to adult-onset OCD include all of the following *except*

    A. Pediatric OCD is male predominant.

    B. Pediatric OCD is more familial and has a better prognosis than OCD beginning in adulthood.

    C. Pediatric OCD frequently manifests with obsessions without well-defined compulsions.

    D. Religious and sexual obsessions are overrepresented in adolescents.

    E. Hoarding is seen more often in children than in adolescents and adults.

23.2 Which of the following statements regarding pathophysiology and risk factors of obsessive-compulsive disorder (OCD) is *true*?

    A. Frontal cortico-striatal-thalamic circuits are involved.

    B. Imaging studies detected structural abnormalities in the cingulate cortex, basal ganglia, and thalami.

    C. Magnetic resonance spectroscopy (MRS) studies show a significant reduction in *N*-acetylaspartate (NAA)/choline level in the medial thalami region.

    D. In a single photon emission computed tomography (SPECT) study, early-onset cases showed decreased cerebral blood flow in the right thalamus, left anterior cingulate cortex, and bilateral inferior prefrontal cortex compared with late-onset ones.

    E. All of the above.

23.3 Which of the following statements regarding genetics and environmental factors in obsessive-compulsive disorder (OCD) is *false*?

    A. The concordance rates for monozygotic twins are much higher than those for dizygotic twins.

    B. Childhood-onset OCD demonstrates higher genetic and familial risks.

    C. A genome-wide linkage study found susceptibility loci on several chromosomes.

    D. Studies support the possibility that a single gene is responsible for OCD.

    E. Nonheritable etiological factors of OCD are at least as important as genetic factors.

23.4 Which of the following statements regarding the Children's Yale-Brown Obsessive-Compulsive Scale (CY-BOCS) is *true*?

    A. It is a 10-item anchored ordinal scale (0–4) that rates the clinical severity of the disorder.

    B. The scores include the time occupied, degree of life interference, subjective distress, internal resistance, and degree of control.

    C. It includes a checklist of more than 60 symptoms of obsessions and compulsions.

    D. Scores of 8–15 represent mild cases, 16–23 moderate cases, and ≥24 severe cases.

    E. All of the above.

23.5   Which of the following is the first-line treatment of choice for mild to moderate cases of obsessive-compulsive disorder (OCD) in children?

       A. Behavioral modification.
       B. Family therapy.
       C. Psychoeducation.
       D. Cognitive-behavioral therapy (CBT).
       E. Clomipramine.

23.6   Which of the following are U.S. Food and Drug Administration (FDA)–approved medications for treating pediatric obsessive-compulsive disorder (OCD)?

       A. Clomipramine.
       B. Fluoxetine.
       C. Fluvoxamine.
       D. Sertraline.
       E. All of the above.

Chapter 24

Early-Onset Schizophrenia

Select the single best response for each question.

24.1   All of the following statements regarding early-onset schizophrenia (EOS) are correct *except*

    A. EOS is defined as schizophrenia with onset prior to age 16 years.

    B. Childhood-onset schizophrenia (COS) refers to schizophrenia with onset prior to age 13 years.

    C. EOS is considered to be continuous with adult-onset schizophrenia (AOS).

    D. COS appears to be rare.

    E. EOS, especially COS, appears more often in males.

24.2   All of the following statements regarding the etiology of early-onset schizophrenia (EOS)/childhood-onset schizophrenia (COS) are correct *except*

    A. Schizophrenia is viewed as a heterogeneous disorder with multiple etiologies.

    B. Based on genetic studies, causal relationships between the illness and candidate genes are established.

    C. Youth with COS appear to have a higher rate of cytogenetic abnormalities than adults.

    D. Environmental exposures may mediate disease risk.

    E. Based on imaging studies, age-specific gray matter reduction was found.

24.3   In regard to differences between early-onset schizophrenia (EOS) and adult-onset schizophrenia (AOS), all of the following statements are correct *except*

    A. EOS is diagnosed using the same criteria as for adults.

    B. Negative symptoms appear to be the most specifically associated with EOS.

    C. Catatonia occurs more frequently in EOS.

    D. Thought disorder in EOS is generally characterized by loose associations and illogical thinking.

    E. The majority of youth with EOS have histories of premorbid problems.

24.4   All of the following statements regarding differential diagnosis of early-onset schizophrenia (EOS) are correct *except*

    A. Both psychotic and nonpsychotic disorders can present with psychosis.

    B. Psychosis caused by medical conditions is often associated with delirium.

    C. Both legal and illegal drugs can provoke psychosis.

    D. Research supports that prolonged episodes of substance abuse are the environmental stimulus for the expression of schizophrenia.

    E. Most children reporting apparent psychotic symptoms do not have a true psychotic disorder.

24.5 All of the following statements regarding the treatment of early-onset schizophrenia (EOS) are correct *except*

  A. A comprehensive integrated approach is required.
  B. Risperidone and aripiprazole have been approved by the U.S. Food and Drug Administration (FDA) for the treatment of adolescents with schizophrenia.
  C. Clozapine was found to be superior in treating youth with treatment-resistant schizophrenia.
  D. To avoid risks of side effects, rapid increases in dose should be avoided.
  E. There is a strong empirical evidence for psychosocial interventions in EOS.

Chapter 25

Obesity

Select the single best response for each question.

25.1 A child is considered obese when his or her body mass index (BMI) is at or above what percentile?

    A. 80th percentile.
    B. 85th percentile.
    C. 90th percentile.
    D. 95th percentile.
    E. 99th percentile.

25.2 Which of the following genetic syndromes is associated with obesity?

    A. Prader-Willi syndrome.
    B. Laurence-Moon/Bardet-Biedl syndrome.
    C. Borjeson-Forssman-Lehmann syndrome.
    D. Cohen syndrome.
    E. All of the above.

25.3 According to the Barlow and Expert Committee report, all of the following play important roles in hunger, satiety, and fat distribution *except*

    A. γ-Aminobutyric acid (GABA).
    B. Leptin.
    C. Ghrelin.
    D. Adiponectin.
    E. Insulin.

25.4 True statements regarding risk factors for obesity include all of the following *except*

    A. Maternal or gestational diabetes are linked with later development of child obesity.
    B. Birth weight > 97th percentile predicts a higher future body mass index (BMI).
    C. Breast-feeding predicts a higher future BMI.
    D. Early adiposity rebound predicts future overweight.
    E. Up to 80% of overweight adolescents become obese adults.

25.5 According to the Barlow and Expert Committee report, what is the primary goal of obesity treatment?

    A. Weight loss.
    B. Weight maintenance.
    C. Body mass index (BMI) maintenance.
    D. Long-term physical health through permanent healthy lifestyle habits.
    E. Food intake reduction.

25.6 Which of the following pairs of medications has been approved by the U.S. Food and Drug Administration (FDA) for use in youth with obesity?

    A. Topiramate and bupropion.
    B. Metformin and modafinil.
    C. Sibutramine and orlistat.
    D. Methylphenidate and dextroamphetamine.
    E. Adderall and lisdexamfetamine.

Chapter 26

Anorexia Nervosa and Bulimia Nervosa

Select the single best response for each question.

26.1 In a study examining the relative rates of eating disorder diagnoses in an adolescent clinical sample, what was the most common diagnosis?

    A. Anorexia nervosa.

    B. Bulimia nervosa.

    C. Eating disorder not otherwise specified (EDNOS).

    D. Body dissatisfaction disorder.

    E. None of the above.

26.2 In a recent national comorbidity survey, the lifetime prevalence rate of binge-eating disorder (BED) among women was

    A. 0.5%.

    B. 0.9%.

    C. 1.5%.

    D. 2.0%.

    E. 3.5%.

26.3 The mortality rate in young women with anorexia nervosa is how many times higher than in young women in the general population?

    A. 2 times.

    B. 4 times.

    C. 6 times.

    D. 8 times.

    E. 12 times.

26.4 The National Institute for Health and Clinical Excellence (NICE) in the United Kingdom summarized guidelines for adult and adolescent eating disorders based on a comprehensive review of the literature. NICE graded treatment modalities using an A to C grade. Which of the following treatments received an A grade?

    A. Interpersonal psychotherapy for adolescents with anorexia nervosa.

    B. Cognitive-behavioral therapy (CBT) for adults with bulimia nervosa.

    C. Family intervention for adolescent anorexia nervosa.

    D. Selective serotonin reuptake inhibitors (SSRIs) for adults with anorexia nervosa.

    E. Dialectical behavioral therapy for adolescents with bulimia nervosa.

26.5 Which of the following findings have been reported about the efficacy of using medications to treat bulimia nervosa?

    A. In adults with bulimia nervosa, antidepressants are no different than placebo in reducing binge frequency.

    B. Weight and shape concerns in patients with bulimia nervosa are unaffected by medication compared with placebo.

    C. When added to psychological treatments of bulimia nervosa, medications greatly improved treatment outcomes.

    D. Mood disturbance in patients with bulimia nervosa is unaffected by medication compared with placebo.

    E. None of the above.

Chapter 27

Tic Disorders

Select the single best response for each question.

27.1 Characteristics of tics include all of the following *except*

    A. Tics are sudden, quick, and repetitive stereotyped movements occurring in any part of the body.
    B. Tics may wax and wane.
    C. Tics are totally involuntary.
    D. Unlike other movement disorders, tics may occur during sleep.
    E. Tics can be categorized as either simple or complex.

27.2 Comorbid diagnoses common with Tourette's disorder include all of the following *except*

    A. Attention-deficit/hyperactivity disorder (ADHD).
    B. Obsessive-compulsive disorder (OCD).
    C. Anxiety disorder.
    D. Major depression.
    E. Schizophrenia.

27.3 Which of the following statements regarding the neuroanatomy and neurophysiology of tics is *true?*

    A. Association between tics and abnormal functioning in cortico-striatal-thalamo-cortical (CSTC) loop circuits was not found.
    B. Circuits originating in motor and dorsolateral cortex are least important for tics.
    C. Dopamine plays an important role in producing tics.
    D. Disorganizing thalamic discharges lead to decreased activation in the frontal cortex.
    E. None of the above.

27.4 All of the following statements regarding treatment recommendations for tics are correct *except*

    A. Behavioral interventions can reduce the severity and frequency of tics.
    B. Dopamine antagonists are the mainstay of treatment for moderate to severe tics.
    C. Clonidine can be used in the treatment of mild to moderate tics.
    D. Selective serotonin reuptake inhibitors (SSRIs) with cognitive-behavior therapy (CBT) are recommended for patients with obsessive-compulsive disorder (OCD) plus a family history of tic disorders.
    E. Stimulants are indicated in children with tics and Tourette's disorder.

27.5 In regard to the genetics of tic disorders, all of the following statements are correct *except*

    A. Twin and family studies support evidence that Tourette's disorder is fundamentally a genetic condition.
    B. The twin concordance rate for Tourette's is 53%–56% for monozygotic pairs and 8% in dizygotic siblings.
    C. The prevalence of Tourette's disorder in families of European origin in first-degree relatives is between 15% and 53%.
    D. Rates of obsessive-compulsive disorder (OCD) symptoms among relatives of Tourette's probands are 5–10 times the general population prevalence.
    E. There is evidence for genetic susceptibility for chromosomes 2, 3, 4, 5, 6, 8, 13, 14, and 21.

Chapter 28

Elimination Disorders

Select the single best response for each question.

28.1 Which of the following comorbid psychiatric disorders is most common in children with secondary enuresis?

    A. Attention-deficit/hyperactivity disorder (ADHD).
    B. Major depressive disorder.
    C. Generalized anxiety disorder.
    D. Panic disorder.
    E. Social phobia.

28.2 Which of the following medications is most frequently used as a first-line treatment for enuresis?

    A. Imipramine.
    B. Amitriptyline.
    C. Desmopressin acetate (DDAVP).
    D. Selective serotonin reuptake inhibitors (SSRIs).
    E. Atypical antipsychotics.

28.3 In a large longitudinal study, researchers found that the most effective treatment of enuresis, in terms of degree of relapse after the cessation of active treatment, was

    A. Imipramine.
    B. Fluid restriction.
    C. Desmopressin acetate (DDAVP).
    D. Nighttime awakening to urinate.
    E. Bell and pad method of conditioning.

28.4 Which of the following epidemiological findings concerning encopresis is *false*?

    A. Male to female ratio of 3:1.
    B. More prevalent than enuresis.
    C. Prevalence rate in children between 7 and 8 years of age is approximately 1.5%.
    D. Prevalence decreases as children age.
    E. None of the above.

28.5 Which of the following statements concerning encopresis is *true*?

    A. Two subtypes of encopresis are recognized in DSM-IV-TR (American Psychiatric Association 2000): voluntary and involuntary.
    B. Nonretentive encopresis has been more extensively studied than retentive encopresis.
    C. The most accepted treatment of encopresis is imipramine.
    D. The natural history of encopresis is to move toward continence.
    E. None of the above.

C h a p t e r   2 9

Sleep Disorders

Select the single best response for each question.

29.1   The most dramatic developmental changes in sleep architecture and sleep requirements occur during

    A. The first 6 months.
    B. The first year.
    C. The first 5 years.
    D. The first 12 years.
    E. The first 18 years.

29.2   Which of the following questionnaire or scales uses eight subscales that reflect the major domains of behavioral and medical sleep disorders?

    A. The Pediatric Sleep Questionnaire (PSQ).
    B. The Children's Sleep Habits Questionnaire (CSHQ).
    C. The Sleep Disorders Inventory for Students (SDIS).
    D. The Epworth Sleepiness Scale.
    E. A sleep log/sleep diary.

29.3   Which of the following statements correctly describes nocturnal polysomnography (PSG)?

    A. PSG is the gold standard procedure to study sleep-disordered breathing and other types of intrinsic sleep disorders in children.
    B. PSG records electroencephalogram (EEG), electro-oculogram, airflow, respiratory and abnormal efforts, oxygen saturation, end-tidal carbon dioxide (ET CO_2), and limb muscle activity.
    C. PSG is indicated for the diagnosis of obstructive sleep apnea, central apnea, alveolar hypoventilation, snoring, and upper airway resistance syndrome in youth.
    D. PSG is used for diagnosing periodic limb movement disorder (PLMD) and for evaluating nocturnal seizures and parasomnias.
    E. All of the above.

29.4   According to recent studies, attention-deficit/hyperactivity disorder (ADHD) is strongly associated with which of the following sleep disorders?

    A. Kleine-Levin syndrome (KLS).
    B. Narcolepsy.
    C. Obstructive sleep apnea (OSA).
    D. Restless legs syndrome (RLS) and periodic limb movement disorder (PLMD).
    E. Circadian rhythm sleep disorder.

29.5 Many psychiatric disorders are associated with significant comorbid sleep problems. In which of the following disorders are sleep complaints among adolescents most prevalent?

    A. Attention-deficit/hyperactivity disorder (ADHD).
    B. Mood disorders.
    C. Autism spectrum disorders.
    D. Substance abuse disorders.
    E. Anxiety disorders.

29.6 All of the following statements regarding treatment of primary insomnia are correct *except*

    A. Nonpharmacological interventions are the first choice of treatment.
    B. Behavioral interventions can be useful.
    C. Sleeping environment should be controlled.
    D. Cognitive therapy can be used especially for older children and adolescents.
    E. The U.S. Food and Drug Administration (FDA) has approved two agents for use in pediatric insomnia.

Chapter 30

Evidence-Based Practices

Select the single best response for each question.

30.1 Which of the following sources would be likely to offer the most complete information regarding the efficacy of a specific medication in the treatment of adolescents, based on randomized controlled clinical trials?

A. PubMed.

B. PsycINFO, which uses a Medical Index Subject Heading (MeSH).

C. Cochrane Library Systematic Reviews database.

D. Cochrane Library Clinical Trials database.

E. None of the above.

30.2 Clinicians seeking information about a specific disorder and its treatment would do well to apply which of the following search strategies?

A. Start narrow and then go broad.

B. Tailor the search to the question.

C. Reject transparency.

D. Avoid consensus-driven guidelines such as the *Cochrane Handbook for Systematic Reviews of Interventions*.

E. None of the above.

30.3 Which of the following integrates consensus and evidence into prescriptive decision trees?

A. Practice guidelines.

B. Treatment algorithms.

C. Systematic reviews.

D. Expert consensus statements.

E. None of the above.

30.4 Which of the following qualities characterizes organizations that are effective at implementing innovation?

A. Strong leadership.

B. Openness to experimentation.

C. Effective monitoring.

D. Knowledge sharing.

E. All of the above.

30.5 A set of protocols that share common features or mechanisms of action is called

A. Treatment family.

B. Specific protocol.

C. Common practices within a protocol.

D. Core component method.

E. Distillation and matching.

C h a p t e r   3 1

Child Abuse and Neglect

Select the single best response for each question.

31.1 Correct statements regarding the epidemiology of child abuse and neglect include all of the following *except*

 A. Sexual abuse still appears to be underreported.
 B. Between 1993 and 2001, the overall number of victimized children declined.
 C. More children experience physical abuse than experience neglect or sexual abuse.
 D. Young age (under 3 years) and male gender are risk factors for fatalities caused by maltreatment.
 E. Some studies report that up to 25% of girls are sexually abused in some manner before age 18 years.

31.2 Risk factors for child abuse include which of the following?

 A. Single-parent and stepfamilies.
 B. Unstable families and personality disorder in the parents.
 C. Parental mental illness, substance abuse, poverty, minority ethnicity.
 D. Child's prematurity, mental retardation, and physical handicaps.
 E. All of the above.

31.3 Which of the following tests should be the first-line imaging investigation of a suspected brain or head injury?

 A. Magnetic resonance imaging (MRI).
 B. Computed tomography (CT).
 C. Ultrasound.
 D. Functional MRI (fMRI).
 E. Single photon emission computed tomography (SPECT).

31.4 Which of the following findings is considered to be a definitive confirmation of sexual activity in or sexual abuse of a child?

 A. Bruising or scarring of perianal area.
 B. Presence of HIV.
 C. Presence of chlamydia.
 D. Presence of anogenital condylomata acuminata.
 E. Pregnancy or the presence of semen.

31.5 All of the following are guidelines outlined by the American Academy of Pediatrics Committee on Child Abuse and Neglect for performing a physical examination of sexual abuse victims *except*

 A. Careful explanation of every step.
 B. Particular attention given to the examination of the mouth, genitals, perineal region, anus, buttocks, and thighs.
 C. Presence of a supportive adult and a nursing chaperone.
 D. Use of sedation is contraindicated.
 E. Thorough documentation and appropriate agency reporting.

Chapter 32

HIV and AIDS

Select the single best response for each question.

32.1 Which of the following epidemiological findings regarding HIV/AIDS in adolescents/young adults living in the United States is *true*?

    A. The number of adolescents/young adults living with HIV/AIDS in the United States has remained constant since 2000.

    B. In adolescents between the ages of 13 and 19 years, females account for 40% of the cases.

    C. For males, heterosexual contact accounts for 75% of new HIV/AIDS infections.

    D. Latino youth are the minority population most affected by HIV/AIDS.

    E. None of the above.

32.2 The leading cause of new HIV infection in adolescents and young adults in the United States is

    A. Intravenous drug abuse.

    B. Medical procedures.

    C. Blood transfusions.

    D. Sexual intercourse.

    E. None of the above.

32.3 Which of the following mechanisms of HIV-induced neurotoxicity is believed to produce cognitive impairment?

    A. Direct neuronal injury by virus proteins.

    B. Products of macrophage activation.

    C. Neuroreceptor blockade.

    D. Antibody-mediated cellular toxicity.

    E. All of the above.

32.4 Which of the following statements concerning the cognitive effects of HIV infection in children and adolescents is *true*?

    A. Receptive language is significantly more impaired than expressive language.

    B. Impairment is more cortical than subcortical.

    C. Visuomotor skills are frequently spared.

    D. Spatial learning and memory are frequently impaired.

    E. The Folstein Mini-Mental State Examination is more sensitive than the HIV Dementia Scale for detecting cognitive impairment in HIV-infected adults and adolescents.

32.5 In studies of HIV-infected adolescents, which of the following has been reported?

    A. High rates of depression on screening measures.

    B. Significant psychosocial stresses.

    C. Half continue to have unprotected sex.

    D. Approximately 85% had at least one DSM diagnosis.

    E. All of the above.

Chapter 33

Bereavement and Traumatic Grief

Select the single best response for each question.

33.1 According to Worden (1996) and Wolfelt (1996), a typical task facing children who experience uncomplicated bereavement is

   A. Accepting the reality of the death.
   B. Fully experiencing the pain of the death.
   C. Adjusting to an environment and self-identity without the deceased.
   D. Converting the relationship with the deceased from one of interaction to one of memory.
   E. All of the above.

33.2 All of the following statements regarding uncomplicated bereavement are correct *except*

   A. Bereavement is the condition of having had someone close die.
   B. Grief is the intense emotion that one feels upon having someone close die.
   C. Mourning encompasses the religious, ethnic, community, and/or cultural practices associated with bereavement.
   D. In contrast to adults, children often show more constant and prolonged grief.
   E. Uncomplicated bereavement in children resembles depression in many ways.

33.3 There is little empirical information on the interventions for uncomplicated bereavement. Peer support groups have been providing services to bereaved children. All of the following descriptions of the Dougy model are correct *except*

   A. Groups are facilitated by adult volunteers.
   B. Providers conceptualize the group activities as therapeutic interventions.
   C. Providers do not regard child attendees as having pathological responses.
   D. Many providers do not believe in the existence of "traumatic grief" in children.
   E. Peer support is well accepted by families and children.

33.4 All of the following statements regarding the differences between uncomplicated bereavement and childhood traumatic grief (CTG) are correct *except*

   A. The nature of the death is often qualitatively different in cases of CTG.
   B. Not all causes of death lead to CTG.
   C. Core posttraumatic stress disorder (PTSD) symptoms are less typical in uncomplicated bereavement.
   D. In CTG, PTSD symptoms impinge on children's abilities to resolve bereavement tasks.
   E. Children with CTG demonstrate a certain degree of functional impairment.

33.5   All of the following treatment approaches have been used for childhood traumatic grief (CTG). Which one of the approaches has been supported as a randomized clinical trial (RCT) for young children experiencing domestic violence?

    A. Traumatic grief–cognitive-behavioral therapy (TG-CBT).

    B. UCLA traumatic grief program for adolescents.

    C. Grief and trauma intervention for elementary-age children.

    D. Child-parent psychotherapy (CPP) for traumatic grief in early childhood.

    E. None of the above.

Chapter 34

Ethnic, Cultural, and Religious Issues

Select the single best response for each question.

34.1 According to the Committee on Cultural Psychiatry for the Group for the Advancement of Psychiatry, which concept is accurately defined by the description "It encompasses one's identity with a group of people sharing common origins, history, customs, and beliefs"?

    A. Culture.

    B. Ethnicity.

    C. Race.

    D. Cultural psychiatry.

    E. Religion.

34.2 The term *cultural-bound syndromes* was introduced in 1967 and is currently included in Appendix I of DSM-IV-TR (American Psychiatric Association 2000). Which of the following characteristics accurately describes the disorders under this category?

    A. Are discrete and well-defined.

    B. Are accepted as specific disorders in the country of origin.

    C. Occur in response to specific precipitants in that culture.

    D. Occur much more frequently in the home culture than in other cultures.

    E. All of the above.

34.3 Which of these terms is accurately defined by the statement "the biological processes of drug absorption, distribution, metabolism, and excretion?"

    A. Pharmacokinetics.

    B. Pharmacodynamics.

    C. Pharmacogenetics.

    D. Ethnopsychopharmacology.

    E. None of the above.

34.4 There are numerous cytochrome P450 (CYP) liver enzymes responsible for oxidative metabolism of many psychotropic medications. Which of the following CYP enzymes is the least significant in ethnopsychopharmacology?

    A. CYP2D6.

    B. CYP2C19.

    C. CYP2C9.

    D. CYP3A4.

    E. CYP1A2.

34.5 The screening mnemonic FICA (Puchalski and Romer 2000) is a useful tool for beginning a discussion of patients' past religious and spiritual experiences. Which of the following questions is *not* included in the FICA screen?

    A. Is religious faith part of your day-to-day life?
    B. How has faith influenced your life, past and present?
    C. Are you currently part of a religious or spiritual community?
    D. What kind of religion are you practicing?
    E. What are the spiritual needs you would like to have addressed?

Chapter 35

Youth Suicide

Select the single best response for each question.

35.1 All of the following definitions of suicide-related behaviors are correct *except*

A. *Suicide* refers to a fatal, self-inflicted destructive act with explicit or implicit intent to die.

B. *Suicide attempt* refers to a nonfatal, self-inflicted destructive act that leads to injury and that involves an explicit or implicit intent to die.

C. *Suicidal ideation* refers to thoughts of harming or killing oneself.

D. *Suicidality* refers to all suicide-related behaviors and thoughts.

E. *Nonsuicidal self-injurious behavior* refers to any self-inflicted destructive act performed without intent to die.

35.2 Which of the following statements regarding the characteristics of youth suicide is *false?*

A. The rates of suicide increase with age.

B. Suicidal behavior is rare in preschool-aged children.

C. The rate of completed suicide among youth is higher for males than females.

D. Females endorse similar rates of specific ideations and suicide attempt rates compared with males.

E. Increased suicide risk is associated with lower socioeconomic status except for young African American males.

35.3 Which of the following groups of psychiatric disorders is most closely linked to suicidal behavior in youth?

A. Mood disorders.

B. Anxiety disorders.

C. Disruptive behavioral and conduct disorders.

D. Substance use disorders.

E. None of the above.

35.4 A promising approach to treatment of youth suicidality is

A. Safety planning.

B. Means restriction.

C. Dialectical behavior therapy (DBT).

D. Developmental group therapy.

E. All of the above.

35.5 All of the following statements regarding pharmacological approaches to the treatment of youth suicidality are correct *except*

    A. The Treatment of Adolescent Depression Study (TADS) showed a twofold increase in suicide-related adverse events among youth receiving medication compared with placebo groups.

    B. The U.S. Food and Drug Administration's (FDA's) meta-analysis of short-term placebo-controlled trials of selective serotonin reuptake inhibitors (SSRIs) and other antidepressants in youth indicated an increased risk of suicidality in patients taking antidepressants.

    C. The mechanism by which SSRIs might increase risk for suicidal behavior is not known.

    D. The recent decrease in SSRI prescriptions was associated with a marked decrease in youth suicide in the United States.

    E. Recent analysis supports the assertion that many more youth will show a good clinical response to SSRIs than will become suicidal.

Chapter 36

Gender Identity and Sexual Orientation

Select the single best response for each question.

36.1 By which age have most children established their gender identity?

    A. By the age of 2.
    B. By the age of 3.
    C. By the age of 5.
    D. By the age of 8.
    E. By the age of 12.

36.2 All of the following statements regarding epidemiology and comorbidity of gender identity disorder (GID) in children and adolescents are correct *except*

    A. GID in youth is relatively uncommon.
    B. People are less tolerant of cross-gender behavior in boys than in girls.
    C. The number of annual adolescent referrals for GID tripled between 2004 and 2007.
    D. In boys with GID, externalizing comorbid disorders predominate, whereas in girls with GID, there is a mixture of comorbid internalizing and externalizing disorders.
    E. Children and adolescents with GID should be evaluated systematically for comorbid conditions.

36.3 Based on up-to-date research, all of the following statements regarding the etiology of gender identity disorder (GID) are correct *except*

    A. The vast majority of children with GID do not have a disorder of sex development (DSD).
    B. Within-sex variation in sex-dimorphic behavior has a heritable component.
    C. Boys with GID have an elevated rate of right-handedness.
    D. A greater-than-average proportion of boys with GID have older male siblings.
    E. There is no evidence that parents of children with GID disproportionately wished for a child of the opposite sex during the pregnancy.

36.4 Based on up-to-date follow-up studies of both boys and girls with gender identity disorder (GID), which of the following psychosexual outcomes is found?

    A. Persistence of GID with a co-occurring homosexual/bisexual sexual orientation.
    B. Desistence of GID with a co-occurring homosexual/bisexual sexual orientation.
    C. Desistence of GID with a co-occurring heterosexual orientation.
    D. All of the above.
    E. None of the above.

36.5 Homosexuality was delisted from DSM as a mental disorder more than 30 years ago. Mental health professionals should remain current about what is known of people with a minority sexual orientation because

    A. It represents a form of cultural competence in delivering clinical care.

    B. It requires sensitivity in training clinicians.

    C. There may be heightened mental health challenges associated with a minority sexual orientation.

    D. Many youth struggle with their emerging minority sexual orientation.

    E. All of the above.

Chapter 37

Aggression and Violence

Select the single best response for each question.

37.1 Which of the following medical conditions may carry risk for transient or permanent aggressive behavior?

    A. Encephalitis.
    B. Endocrine abnormalities.
    C. Seizure disorders.
    D. Traumatic brain injury (TBI).
    E. All of the above.

37.2 Which of the following statements regarding the neurochemical and hormonal mechanisms and risk factors of aggression and violence is *false*?

    A. An inverse relationship between central serotonin (5-hydroxytryptophan [5-HT]) function and impulsive aggression has been established in children.
    B. Blunted prolactin response to fenfluramine at ages 7–11 years predicts aggressive outcome in adolescence.
    C. Higher 5-HT responsivity in childhood might be a protective factor.
    D. Aggression has been linked with both elevated peripheral cortisol and reduced cortisol.
    E. Testosterone concentration and aggressive behavior are correlated in boys only after puberty.

37.3 All of the following statements regarding genetic factors in aggression and violence are correct *except*

    A. The variability in heritability across studies indicates that genes account for only a portion of the variance.
    B. The candidate genes most consistently linked to aggression are the monoamine oxidase A (MAOA) and serotonin (5-hydroxytryptophan [5-HT]) transporter (5-HTT) genes.
    C. A rare mutation in the MAOA gene has been associated with impulsively violent behavior.
    D. Youth with one or more 5-HTT long variants show high levels of externalizing behavior.
    E. Two polymorphisms of the tryptophan hydroxylase gene are associated with increased irritability and assaultiveness.

37.4 Which of the following are characteristics of successful intervention programs for aggression and violence?

    A. Multimodal intervention.
    B. Consistently delivered interventions on a daily to weekly basis.
    C. School/family collaboration.
    D. Application of individual management techniques.
    E. All of the above.

37.5 Which of the following medications is the best studied, and has been approved by the U.S. Food and Drug Administration (FDA) for treating aggression in children with posttraumatic stress disorder?

   A. Lithium.
   B. Risperidone.
   C. Fluoxetine.
   D. Clonidine.
   E. Divalproex sodium.

Chapter 38

Genetics

Fundamentals Relevant to Child and Adolescent Psychiatry

Select the single best response for each question.

38.1 How frequently do DNA mutations occur in every replication cycle?

    A. 1 per each 100,000 base pairs (bp).
    B. 1 per each 10,000 bp.
    C. 1 per each 1,000 bp.
    D. 1 per each 500 bp.
    E. 1 per each 100 bp.

38.2 Nonharmful changes in DNA can be passed on to subsequent generations. Mutations may or may not have effects on functioning. Which of the following describes a mutation that occurs in more than 1% of the population?

    A. Genetic drift.
    B. Polymorphism.
    C. Hardy-Weinberg equilibrium.
    D. Single nucleotide polymorphisms (SNPs).
    E. None of the above.

38.3 Which of the following statements regarding chromosomes is *false?*

    A. They are in the nucleus.
    B. The human genome consists of 22 pairs of autosomal chromosomes and a pair of sex chromosomes—XY in males or XX in females.
    C. The autosomal chromosomes are numbered 1 through 22 in order of increasing size.
    D. The shorter arms are designated "p," whereas the longer arms are designated "q."
    E. An ordered list of loci within a particular genome provides a genetic map.

38.4 All of the following statements regarding the regulation of gene expression are correct *except*

    A. Each of an individual's nucleated cells (other than eggs or sperm) contains the same DNA and associated genes.
    B. Gene transcription can be induced or silenced by transcription factors.
    C. Genes can be induced by exposure to exogenous compounds.
    D. Histone acetylation can enhance DNA transcription.
    E. DNA methylation can promote DNA transcription.

38.5   According to up-to-date research, which of the following statements regarding the Mendelian patterns of inheritance of medical and psychiatric disorders is *false?*

    A. Most psychiatric disorders follow Mendelian patterns of inheritance.
    B. Huntington disease is inherited as an autosomal dominant disorder.
    C. Both dominant and recessive patterns of inheritance have been associated with Alzheimer's disease.
    D. X-linked dominant inheritance has been suggested in Rett syndrome.
    E. Recessive pattern of inheritance is associated with cystic fibrosis.

38.6   Linkage studies examine the relationship between a phenotype and a genetic locus. The degree of linkage is expressed by a lod score. Which of the following lod scores is considered evidence of linkage?

    A. >0.5.
    B. >1.
    C. >2.
    D. >3.
    E. >4.

Chapter 39

Psychiatric Emergencies

Select the single best response for each question.

39.1 All of the following statements regarding assessing suicidal youth in an emergency room are correct *except*

A. Parental consent should be obtained prior to assessment.
B. Safety is a primary concern.
C. Assessment includes a careful physical examination and mental status examination.
D. Lethality and intent are two important aspects for assessment.
E. Precipitants and predisposing factors need to be addressed.

39.2 Which of the following statements regarding youth evaluated in emergency settings for suicidal behavior is *false?*

A. About 14% of patients evaluated in the emergency room for suicidality never attend an outpatient mental health appointment.
B. Patients with higher levels of suicidal behavior and depression are more likely to attend outpatient appointments.
C. Patients who actively express suicidal ideation and intent should be hospitalized.
D. Patients who have low levels of suicidality and who agree to participate in outpatient sessions with family support may require outpatient treatment only.
E. A no-suicide contract is an important and valid indicator of future risk.

39.3 An intervention is defined as *seclusion* if the patient is placed alone in a room under which of the following circumstances?

A. The patient is behind a locked door.
B. The door is either held by staff or locked with a spring-loaded latch.
C. Free movement of the patient is inhibited.
D. The patient is actively separated and taken to a specific location away from the group.
E. All of the above.

39.4 All of the following statements regarding chemical restraints in an emergency department setting are correct *except*

A. *Chemical restraint* is defined as the use of medication for behavioral control.
B. To avoid chemical restraint, medications should be prescribed in a manner consistent with the diagnosis.
C. Pharmacological management of aggression is preferable to the use of restraints.
D. There is a clear consensus on the most appropriate medication strategy for the pediatric emergency psychiatry patient.
E. Some atypical antipsychotics are effective for the treatment of aggression and self-injurious behavior in children with pervasive developmental disorder (PDD).

39.5   Which of the following recommendations for restraint of children and adolescents is *correct?*

A. Makeshift restraints are preferable to those prescribed for adults.
B. In certain circumstances, it is appropriate to tie down only one limb.
C. There are no randomized trials on the most appropriate method or position for restraint.
D. The prone restraint position is better for the clinician but not for the patient.
E. Patients with medical conditions should never be restrained supine.

C h a p t e r 4 0

Family Transitions

Challenges and Resilience

Select the single best response for each question.

40.1   In which decade did a white, middle-class, intact nuclear household headed by a breadwinner father and a homemaker mother represent the model family?

    A. 1920s.
    B. 1930s.
    C. 1950s.
    D. 1980s.
    E. None of the above.

40.2   Which of the following statements regarding changing family structures and gender roles in the United States is *false?*

    A. More than 70% of all mothers were in the workforce by 2001.
    B. The assumption that mothers' work outside the home harms children has not been supported by research.
    C. Divorce rates continue to climb up, especially for first marriages.
    D. Research shows children raised by gay and lesbian couples fare as well as those who are raised by heterosexual ones.
    E. Most adoptions are now open.

40.3   Family systems–oriented practice is guided by a developmental, multisystemic perspective on human problems and processes of change. All of the following statements regarding family systems practice approaches are accurate *except*

    A. Tools such as the genogram and timeline are of only limited value in elucidating key elements of family systems.
    B. The family is viewed as a transactional system evolving over the life course and across the generations.
    C. Family processes can heighten risk or foster positive adaptation.
    D. Key members in the family system must be identified.
    E. It is important to identify processes that promote resilience.

40.4   Which of the following situations can increase the risk for child and family dysfunction?

    A. Sudden death.
    B. Lingering death.
    C. Ambiguous loss.
    D. Disenfranchised losses.
    E. All of the above.

40.5 Which of the following are tasks that may facilitate adaptation for children and strengthen the family as a functional unit, according to Walsh and McGoldrick (2004)?

    A. Share acknowledgment of reality of death.
    B. Share experiences of loss.
    C. Reorganize family system.
    D. Transform bonds with deceased.
    E. All of the above.

Chapter 41

Psychiatric Aspects of Chronic Physical Disorders

Select the single best response for each question.

41.1 All of the following statements regarding the psychological adjustment of children with chronic health problems are correct *except*

A. Suffering from chronic illnesses increases risks for emotional adjustment problems.
B. Patients with chronic illnesses are more likely to suffer from externalizing syndrome.
C. Disease-related factors are relatively less significant than family/child-related factors.
D. Disease involving the central nervous system (CNS) has a significant impact on adjustment.
E. Patients with multiple chronic physical conditions are at higher risk for psychiatric disorders.

41.2 Which of the following statements regarding models of adaptation to the effects of chronic illness is *true*?

A. Wright's model posited a central role for the effect of chronic illness.
B. According to Wright, an individual with chronic illness highly values a physical status "like everyone else."
C. More recent models that emphasize the interplay between child and parent have been developed.
D. The transactional model emphasizes the interplay between chronic illness and exposure to negative life events.
E. All of the above.

41.3 All of the following statements concerning the impact on families of a child's chronic illness are correct *except*

A. High levels of parental attention, reassurance, and empathy are essential for strengthening the child's ability to cope with his or her illness.
B. Most families with a medically ill child are well adjusted and productive.
C. Parents must deal with their feelings of loss of control over their child's life.
D. Overconcern with medical information can cause parents to neglect both their child's and their family's psychosocial needs.
E. Siblings may sometimes withdraw from engagement in activities with the affected child.

41.4 Which of the following statements regarding psychopharmacological management of youth with chronic physical disorders is *false*?

A. Medically ill children represent the exception to the axiom "start low, go slow" when initiating treatment with psychotropic medication.
B. Drug levels for psychotropic medications are not reliable indicators of efficacy or toxicity.
C. It is best to use one medication at a time and to choose a drug with a short half-life.
D. Most psychotropic drugs are highly protein bound.
E. Drug metabolism and drug-drug interactions may be altered in medically ill patients.

41.5   Which of the following is the most common cause of delirium in pediatric patients?

    A. Cancer.
    B. Trauma.
    C. Central nervous system (CNS) infections.
    D. Diabetes.
    E. All of the above.

C h a p t e r   4 2

Children of Parents With Psychiatric and Substance Abuse Disorders

Select the single best response for each question.

42.1 Which of the following interventions for families at high risk because of parental mental illness is supported by the Institute of Medicine Committee on Prevention?

    A. Indicated prevention programs.
    B. Selective prevention programs.
    C. Universal prevention programs.
    D. All of the above.
    E. None of the above.

42.2 There are several well-established risk factors for depression and other disorders. Some of them are specific for depression. All of the following are specific risks for depression *except*

    A. Social isolation.
    B. Extensive family history of depression.
    C. Prior history of depression.
    D. Depressogenic cognitive style.
    E. Bereavement.

42.3 Children growing up with parents with a psychiatric disorder are at significantly higher risk of developing a mental disorder during their life span. All of the following statements regarding risks and outcomes are correct *except*

    A. The risk increases significantly when both parents are ill.
    B. Parent-child interaction with parents with certain psychiatric disorders can be a risk factor for children.
    C. The relationship between risk factors and later outcome for children is deterministic.
    D. The risk and protective factors can be additive, interactive, and accumulative in nature.
    E. It is not the diagnosis of the parent but the chronicity, severity, and amount of impairment that is associated with effects on the child.

42.4 According to a study by Beardslee and Podorefsky (1988), which of the following characteristics do children with good functioning exhibit?

    A. They are active in pursuing and accomplishing age-appropriate developmental tasks.
    B. They are committed to relationships.
    C. They understand they are not to blame for their parent's illness.
    D. All of the above.
    E. None of the above.

42.5 Which of the following programs is *not* ordinarily used as a prevention program for children of parents with substance abuse disorders?

    A. FRIENDS.
    B. Nurse-Family Partnership.
    C. Strengthening Families Program (SFP).
    D. Family Check-up Preventive Intervention (FCU).
    E. All of the above.

Chapter 43

Legal and Ethical Issues

Select the single best response for each question.

43.1 Which of the following statements regarding the concept of *parens patriae* is *true*?

    A. It is related to child privacy.
    B. It is related to state taking over guardianship.
    C. It is related to involuntary hospitalization.
    D. It is related to children being charged as adults.
    E. It is related to mandatory warning process.

43.2 According to a consensus developed at a White House Conference on Children in 1970, which of the following rights is specific to a child's well-being?

    A. The right to grow in a society with respect.
    B. The right to grow up nurtured by affectionate parents.
    C. The right to be a child during childhood.
    D. The right to have social mechanisms to enforce the foregoing rights.
    E. All of the above.

43.3 Informed consent in treatment and research and maintaining appropriate professional boundaries and confidences are related to which of the following concepts?

    A. Confidentiality.
    B. Autonomy.
    C. Beneficence.
    D. Justice.
    E. None of the above.

43.4 According to American Academy of Child and Adolescent Psychiatry guidelines, important factors to consider in evaluating the need for involuntary hospitalization of young patients include all of the following *except*

    A. A qualified psychiatrist's evaluation.
    B. Diagnosis by DSM criteria.
    C. Severity of impairment in one area of daily functioning.
    D. Likelihood of benefit from the proposed treatment.
    E. Prior consideration of less restrictive treatment procedures.

43.5 All of the following elements must be presented by the plaintiff to the court during a professional negligence lawsuit against a child psychiatrist *except*

    A. Intentionality.
    B. Duty.
    C. Dereliction.
    D. Damage.
    E. Direct causation.

C h a p t e r   4 4

Telepsychiatry

Select the single best response for each question.

44.1 Which of the following terms is correctly described by the definition "use of interactive televideo communication (ITV) to deliver medical care that is usually delivered in person"?

    A. E-health.

    B. Telemedicine.

    C. Telepsychiatry.

    D. Bandwidth.

    E. Telecommunication connectivity.

44.2 Based on current data, child and adolescent telepsychiatry programs have been sited in all of the following settings *except*

    A. Inpatient psychiatric hospitals.

    B. Community medical and mental health centers.

    C. Urban daycare and rural schools.

    D. Corrections and residential settings.

    E. Private practice.

44.3 A growing literature has examined telepsychiatry with children and adolescents. Based on up-to-date research data on this issue, which of the following statements is *false?*

    A. Telepsychiatry with children and adolescents has shown to be feasible, acceptable, and sustainable in consultation to primary care clinicians.

    B. Studies measuring satisfaction showed that providers, families, and youth are very satisfied with their care.

    C. Scientific evidence of its efficacy has been well supported.

    D. Cost effectiveness remains to be demonstrated.

    E. All of the above.

44.4 All of the following statements regarding regulatory and ethical issues in telemedicine are correct *except*

    A. The Joint Commission for the Accreditation of Healthcare Organizations (JCAHO; now known as the Joint Commission) has regulations applicable to telemedicine at the national level.

    B. Most states require telepsychiatrists to be licensed only in the state in which they practice.

    C. Familiarity with laws regarding involuntary commitment and reporting child maltreatment across states is essential.

    D. Televideo transmission needs to be compliant with the Health Insurance Portability and Accountability Act (HIPAA).

    E. Until nationally accepted telepsychiatry care guidelines are available, telepsychiatrists should adhere to existing procedures for in-person care.

C h a p t e r   4 5

Principles of Psychopharmacology

Select the single best response for each question.

45.1 Which of the following goals needs to be reached during a psychiatric assessment of youth before considering psychopharmacological treatment?

    A. Psychiatric symptoms that reflect possible underlying psychiatric disorders must be identified.

    B. Determine which elements of the disorder need to be addressed by psychopharmacological treatments.

    C. Decide which elements of the disorder may need a combination of psychosocial intervention with medications.

    D. Determine which modalities might be most suitable for the particular patient.

    E. All of the above.

45.2 Which of the following medications is least likely to affect electrocardiogram (ECG) at therapeutic doses?

    A. Alpha-2-adrenergic agonists (clonidine or guanfacine).

    B. Thioridazine or pimozide.

    C. Escitalopram or citalopram.

    D. Clozapine or ziprasidone.

    E. Lithium or tricyclic antidepressants.

45.3 All of the following statements regarding the principles of diagnosing and treating youth with psychiatric disorders are correct *except*

    A. Primary psychiatric diagnosis and possible comorbid conditions need to be identified.

    B. Treatment planning should be based on a biopsychosocial formulation.

    C. Treating target symptoms is more important than treating the psychiatric disorders.

    D. In many treatment settings, an authoritative approach is advisable for clinicians.

    E. The efficacy and safety of a medication is only one of the factors to consider when selecting psychopharmacological agents.

45.4 Which of the following statements regarding the differences in pharmacokinetics between children and adults is *false*?

    A. Youths have proportionally more liver tissue than adults when adjusted for body weight.

    B. Children may have higher glomerular filtration rates than adults when adjusted for body weight.

    C. Children may have higher weight-based dosing for hydrophilic drugs.

    D. Children may have higher weight-based dosing for lipophilic drugs.

    E. There is greater variability of oral drug absorption in youth compared to adults.

45.5 Which of the following elements should be considered during the informed consent and assent processes?

A. The process needs to be completed prior to the initiation of the psychopharmacological treatment.
B. Parents or legal guardians should be competent and able to make decisions freely without coercion.
C. Parents or legal guardians should have an understanding of the nature of the patient's illness and the potential risks, benefits, and side effects of the proposed treatment.
D. The expected prognosis with and without the proposed treatment should be discussed.
E. All of the above.

Chapter 46

Medications Used for Attention-Deficit/Hyperactivity Disorder

Select the single best response for each question.

46.1 Emerging neuropsychological and neuroimaging literature suggests that the underlying neural substrate of attention-deficit/hyperactivity disorder (ADHD) is a dysfunction of which of the following?

   A. The parietal-temporal region.
   B. The limbic lobe.
   C. The frontostriatal region.
   D. The parietal lobe.
   E. The hippocampus.

46.2 The most commonly abused substance in adolescents and adults with attention-deficit/hyperactivity disorder (ADHD) is

   A. Alcohol.
   B. Marijuana.
   C. Stimulants.
   D. Benzodiazepines.
   E. Barbiturates.

46.3 Which of the following medications (brand names) is a long-acting preparation of amphetamine?

   A. Concerta.
   B. Metadate-CD.
   C. Focalin XR.
   D. Adderall XR.
   E. Daytrana.

46.4 Which of the following medications has *not* been shown to be effective in the treatment of attention-deficit/hyperactivity disorder (ADHD)?

   A. Desipramine.
   B. Nortriptyline.
   C. Bupropion.
   D. Modafinil.
   E. Venlafaxine.

Chapter 47

Antidepressants

Select the single best response for each question.

47.1 All of the following statements regarding antidepressant use in youth are correct *except*

    A. Half-lives of antidepressants are generally longer in children because of their lower weight.

    B. Randomized controlled trials (RCTs) are the gold standard for assessing both efficacy and safety of drugs.

    C. It is wrong to assume that antidepressants adverse effects are the same in children and in adults.

    D. The increased rates of suicidality in clinical trials using antidepressants occur not only in children but also in young adults.

    E. The difference in suicidality between active treatment and placebo is approximately 4% vs. 2%.

47.2 Which of the following antidepressants has not received any U.S. Food and Drug Administration (FDA)–approved pediatric indications?

    A. Citalopram (Celexa).

    B. Fluoxetine (Prozac).

    C. Fluvoxamine (Luvox).

    D. Sertraline (Zoloft).

    E. Imipramine.

47.3 Which of the following statements regarding fluoxetine is *false*?

    A. To date, there have been only two large randomized controlled trials (RCTs) in pediatric major depressive disorder (MDD) demonstrating superiority of fluoxetine over placebo.

    B. In contrast to other selective serotonin reuptake inhibitors (SSRIs), fluoxetine seems to be equally effective in children younger than 12 years.

    C. There are three positive RCTs in children and adolescents with obsessive-compulsive disorder (OCD).

    D. Fluoxetine is the only antidepressant to have more than one positive RCT for MDD, OCD, and anxiety disorders.

    E. Fluoxetine is the only antidepressant FDA-approved for treatment of pediatric MDD.

47.4 Which of the following atypical antidepressants is a norepinephrine and dopamine reuptake inhibitor?

    A. Duloxetine.

    B. Bupropion.

    C. Trazodone.

    D. Mirtazapine.

    E. Venlafaxine.

47.5 Which of the following antidepressants is currently a third-line treatment option for youth with treatment-resistant major depressive disorder (MDD) because of the increased risk of emergent suicidal thinking?

    A. Bupropion.
    B. Duloxetine.
    C. Mirtazapine.
    D. Venlafaxine.
    E. Trazodone.

Chapter 48

Mood Stabilizers

Select the single best response for each question.

48.1 You decide to start a 16-year-old girl on lithium for treatment of hypomania associated with her bipolar II disorder. Which of the following tests does *not* need to be ordered?

 A. Serum electrolytes.
 B. Lipid panel.
 C. Thyroid function tests.
 D. Complete blood count with differential.
 E. Electrocardiogram (ECG).

48.2 With the adolescent girl in the last question, you change the formulation of lithium from lithium carbonate to a slower-release preparation. For which of the following common side effects would this change have a beneficial effect?

 A. Acne.
 B. Weight gain.
 C. Hypothyroidism.
 D. Polyuria.
 E. Nausea and diarrhea.

48.3 Which of the following baseline studies should be ordered in children and adolescents for whom valproate is to be initiated?

 A. Complete blood count with differential.
 B. Serum electrolytes.
 C. Thyroid function tests.
 D. ECG.
 E. Urinalysis.

48.4 You start a 17-year-old girl on valproate. You order all the necessary baseline tests, which are within normal limits. Three months later, she develops irregular menstruation, weight gain, hirsutism, and acne. Which clinical condition should you be concerned about?

 A. Pregnancy.
 B. Hyperammonemia.
 C. Polycystic ovarian syndrome (PCOS).
 D. Pancreatitis.
 E. Liver failure.

48.5 You begin carbamazepine in a 15-year-old boy who is also on atypical antipsychotic medication. Which of the following potential drug-drug interactions should you be concerned about?

    A. A decrease in carbamazepine serum levels.

    B. An increase in carbamazepine serum levels.

    C. A decrease in serum levels of the atypical antipsychotic.

    D. An increase in serum levels of the atypical antipsychotic.

    E. None.

48.6 The U.S. Food and Drug Administration (FDA) has issued the following black box warning for lamotrigine: "Lamictal is not indicated for use in patients below the age of 16." Which of the following serious medical conditions was the FDA concerned about in this patient population?

    A. Leukopenia.

    B. Lupus.

    C. Agranulocytosis.

    D. Serious rash.

    E. Hepatic failure.

Chapter 49

Antipsychotic Medications

Select the single best response for each question.

49.1 Cytochrome P450 (CYP) enzymes metabolize antipsychotics. The CYP2C19 and 2C9 enzymes are relevant for which of the following antipsychotic medications?

    A. Aripiprazole.
    B. Clozapine.
    C. Molindone.
    D. Perphenazine.
    E. Risperidone.

49.2 Which of the following antipsychotic medications has the shortest half-life when administered orally?

    A. Aripiprazole.
    B. Olanzapine.
    C. Quetiapine.
    D. Risperidone.
    E. Ziprasidone.

49.3 The degree of receptor occupancy is one of the determinants of an antipsychotic's therapeutic and adverse effects. With a full antagonist, what percentage of dopamine receptor occupancy is needed for antipsychotic efficacy?

    A. 40%–50%.
    B. 50%–60%.
    C. 60%–70%.
    D. 70%–80%.
    E. 80%–90%.

49.4 All of the following statements regarding neuromotor adverse effects of antipsychotic medications in children and adolescents are accurate *except*

    A. Youth are more sensitive than adults to extrapyramidal side effects (EPS).
    B. In studies of youth with psychotic disorders, risperidone and olanzapine have been associated with substantial EPS.
    C. Withdrawal dyskinesias experienced by youth are usually irreversible.
    D. Meta-analytic studies have shown relatively low rates of tardive dyskinesia (TD) in youth.
    E. Even though neuroleptic malignant syndrome (NMS) appears to be rare in youth, vigilance is still needed.

49.5 Which of the following antipsychotics is *least* likely to cause prolactin-related side effects, such as hyperpro-lactinemia?

    A. Risperidone.
    B. Olanzapine.
    C. Ziprasidone.
    D. Quetiapine.
    E. Aripiprazole.

Chapter 50

Alpha-Adrenergics, Beta-Blockers, Benzodiazepines, Buspirone, and Desmopressin

Select the single best response for each question.

50.1 Research suggests that guanfacine may be useful for treatment of the hyperactivity, impulsiveness, and distractibility associated with which of the following disorders?

  A. Panic disorder.
  B. Pervasive developmental disorder (PDD).
  C. Impulse control disorder.
  D. Generalized anxiety disorder.
  E. None of the above.

50.2 Clonidine may be an effective treatment for which of the following disorders?

  A. Major depressive disorder.
  B. Bipolar disorder.
  C. Attention-deficit/hyperactivity disorder (ADHD).
  D. Social phobia.
  E. None of the above.

50.3 Prior to beginning an alpha-2 agonist and during treatment, which of the following clinical areas should be evaluated or tests obtained?

  A. Blood pressure.
  B. Kidney function.
  C. Liver function.
  D. Electrocardiogram (ECG).
  E. All of the above.

50.4 Beta-blockers have been reported to be effective, either alone or in combination with other medications, in treating which of the following disorders in children?

  A. Aggression.
  B. Panic disorder.
  C. Social phobia.
  D. Specific phobias.
  E. Posttraumatic stress disorder (PTSD).

50.5 There is considerable evidence to support the use of benzodiazepines to treat which of the following disorders in children?

    A. Panic disorder.
    B. Generalized anxiety disorder.
    C. Posttraumatic stress disorder (PTSD).
    D. Social phobia.
    E. None of the above.

Chapter 51

Medications Used for Sleep

Select the single best response for each question.

51.1 Which of the following neurotransmitters is responsible for the regulation of sleep?

   A. Gamma-aminobutyric acid (GABA).
   B. Melatonin.
   C. Histamine.
   D. Norepinephrine.
   E. All of the above.

51.2 Medications exert their sedative effect through different mechanisms, affecting different receptors. All of the following medications are correctly paired with their receptors/mechanisms *except*

   A. Benzodiazepines—benzodiazepine receptor.
   B. Trazodone—anticholinergic mechanism.
   C. Diphenhydramine—antihistamine mechanism.
   D. Mirtazapine—gamma-aminobutyric acid (GABA) receptor and chloride channels.
   E. Clonidine—alpha-adrenergic agonist.

51.3 Which of the following statements regarding melatonin is *false*?

   A. In the United States, melatonin is a widely sold licensed, over-the-counter drug.
   B. There are a number of placebo-controlled trials of melatonin in the treatment of pediatric insomnia.
   C. Melatonin has been used to treat insomnia in a number of pediatric populations.
   D. Melatonin has been used in the treatment of adolescents with delayed sleep phase syndrome.
   E. Melatonin is relatively short acting, with a short half-life that makes it more effective in treating initial insomnia.

51.4 Among the following sedative-hypnotic medications, which has the shortest half-life?

   A. Eszopiclone.
   B. Zaleplon.
   C. Zolpidem.
   D. Temazepam.
   E. Estazolam.

51.5 Which of the following medications has been reported to likely be associated with Stevens-Johnson syndrome?

   A. Mirtazapine.
   B. Chloral hydrate.
   C. Modafinil.
   D. Sodium oxybate.
   E. Pramipexole.

Chapter 52

Electroconvulsive Therapy, Transcranial Magnetic Stimulation, and Deep Brain Stimulation

Select the single best response for each question.

52.1 Rates of response to electroconvulsive therapy (ECT) in adolescents are similar to those reported in adults, with the exception of one disorder. For which disorder are ECT response rates in adolescents lower than those in adults?

    A. Bipolar mania.
    B. Bipolar depression.
    C. Schizophrenia.
    D. Major depressive disorder.
    E. Major depressive disorder with psychosis.

52.2 The American Academy of Child and Adolescent Psychiatry (AACAP) has established consensus eligibility criteria for electroconvulsive therapy (ECT) in adolescents. Which of the following are ECT indications?

    A. Adolescents unable to achieve a therapeutic medication dose because they are not able to tolerate an adequate psychopharmacological trial.
    B. Adolescents with treatment-resistant depression who have failed at least two adequate antidepressant drug trials of at least 8 weeks' duration at a therapeutic dose and serum level without even mild improvement.
    C. Adolescents with bipolar disorder who have failed at least one antipsychotic-mood stabilizer/antidepressant combination treatment trial of at least 6 weeks' duration without even mild improvement.
    D. Adolescents with schizophrenia with mood symptoms.
    E. All of the above.

52.3 In which of the following child or adolescent populations would use of electroconvulsive therapy (ECT) be contraindicated?

    A. Adolescents who are pregnant.
    B. Adolescents with mental retardation.
    C. Adolescents with a seizure disorder.
    D. Adolescents with a space-occupying central nervous system (CNS) lesion.
    E. Prepubertal children.

52.4 Prior to beginning electroconvulsive therapy (ECT) in an adolescent, which of the following clinical or medical assessments should be completed?

   A. Age-appropriate cognitive assessment.
   B. Consultation with a second child and adolescent psychiatrist who is knowledgeable about ECT but not involved in the current treatment of the patient.
   C. Complete physical examination.
   D. Laboratory evaluations of physiological parameters that may influence the administration of anesthesia.
   E. All of the above.

52.5 Modern electroconvulsive therapy (ECT) is generally well tolerated by patients, and side effects are usually mild and transient. In a study of more than 800 ECT treatments in patients younger than 19 years, the most frequently reported adverse event was

   A. Prolonged seizures.
   B. Nausea/vomiting.
   C. Subjective memory problems.
   D. Headaches.
   E. Tardive seizures.

52.6 Which type of transcranial magnetic stimulation (TMS) is used clinically to treat depression and other conditions?

   A. Single-pulse TMS.
   B. Paired-pulse TMS.
   C. Repetitive TMS.
   D. Nonrepetitive TMS.
   E. All of the above.

Chapter 53

Individual Psychotherapy

Select the single best response for each question.

53.1   Child psychiatry incorporates both uncovering and support in its general approach to psychotherapy. Which of the following techniques would a child therapist be less likely to employ in supportive therapy?

    A. Clarification.
    B. Education.
    C. Suggestion.
    D. Modeling.
    E. Reinforcement.

53.2   If a therapist treats a child through the parent (who takes the doctor's ideas home and tries them out on the young person), the therapy is called

    A. Uncovering psychotherapy.
    B. Supportive psychotherapy.
    C. Family therapy.
    D. Filial therapy.
    E. Collaborative therapy.

53.3   All of the following statements regarding individual psychotherapy are correct *except*

    A. Establishing a therapeutic alliance with the child is essential to performing effective therapy.
    B. The therapist should be calm, unhurried, willing to listen, and nonjudgmental.
    C. The child therapist should be a passive listener and occasional communicator to allow the child free expression.
    D. A thorough acquaintance with the concepts of transference and countertransference is important.
    E. Individual child psychotherapy requires a room where appropriate toys and games are available.

53.4   Which of the following concepts is relevant when a therapist makes interpretations during the individual therapy with a child?

    A. Ego ideal.
    B. Defense and coping.
    C. Secret unattainable desires.
    D. Transference.
    E. Countertransference.

Chapter 54

Parent Counseling, Psychoeducation, and Parent Support Groups

Select the single best response for each question.

54.1 Which of the following is a basic principle of parent counseling interventions?

    A. Education and therapy are provided directly to the child.

    B. Parents' expertise in caring for their children is not used, since parental shortcomings are frequently the source of their children's problems.

    C. It is assumed that parent-child conflicts are due to parental problems.

    D. Parents are helped to understand normal child development, their own child, and his or her needs and problems.

    E. None of the above.

54.2 What is an advantage of multifamily psychoeducation groups over individual family psychoeducation?

    A. Increased privacy.

    B. Flexibility to tailor to individual needs.

    C. Development of a support network.

    D. Ease of scheduling.

    E. All of the above.

54.3 Which of the following are age adjustments needed for psychoeducation with children and adolescents with mental illness?

    A. Less emphasis on social skills training.

    B. Less intensive treatment.

    C. Emphasis on the home environment.

    D. Shorter follow-up.

    E. Little attention given to environmental circumstances.

54.4 Family or parent psychoeducation interventions have been designed for all the following disorders *except*

    A. Attention-deficit/hyperactivity disorder (ADHD).

    B. Obsessive-compulsive disorder (OCD).

    C. Bipolar disorder.

    D. Eating disorder.

    E. Depressive disorders.

54.5 A variety of techniques are used in psychoeducation. The technique whereby a child develops a variety of pleasant or relaxing activities to use in affect regulation is called

    A. Toolkit.
    B. Thinking, feeling, doing.
    C. Naming the enemy.
    D. Mood chart.
    E. Daily routine tracking.

Chapter 55

Behavioral Parent Training

Select the single best response for each question.

55.1 Which of the following is *not* one of the four key concepts of contingency-based behavioral interventions?

    A. Shaping.
    B. Positive reinforcement.
    C. Negative reinforcement.
    D. Punishment.
    E. Extinction.

55.2 Which of the following is a key component of functional behavior analysis?

    A. Specifying behaviors (either positive or negative behaviors).
    B. Identifying each behavior's antecedents.
    C. Identifying each behavior's consequences.
    D. All of the above.
    E. None of the above.

55.3 Which of the following is considered a supplemental topic—rather than a core session topic—of parent training programs?

    A. Psychoeducation/background information.
    B. Praise and positive reinforcement.
    C. Parent stress/emotion management.
    D. Time-out.
    E. Home-school report card.

55.4 In regard to potential adverse effects resulting from behavioral parent training, those complications likely to be most serious relate to which of the following topics?

    A. Positive reinforcement.
    B. Attending.
    C. Token economy.
    D. Punishment.
    E. Developing a plan for homework.

55.5 Based on recent studies, all of the following statements regarding the outcomes of behavioral parent training (BPT) are accurate *except*

    A. Evidence shows that low socioeconomic status (SES) predicts higher dropout rates for behavioral parent training versus other psychosocial treatments.
    B. Having both parents attending the training may not affect posttreatment outcome.
    C. Severe marital discord can reduce efficacy of parent training.
    D. Children with conduct disorder, who are high on callous-unemotional traits, show poorer response.
    E. Therapist warmth, likeability, and communication skills are likely to contribute to more positive outcomes.

Chapter 56

Family Therapy

Select the single best response for each question.

56.1   Which form of family therapy uses the emotional reactions of family members to guide assessment and intervention?

    A. Structural family therapy.
    B. Experiential family therapy.
    C. Family systems therapy.
    D. Strategic family therapy.
    E. None of the above.

56.2   Who is viewed as the originator of structural family therapy?

    A. James Alexander.
    B. Carl Whitaker.
    C. Virginia Satir.
    D. Salvador Minuchin.
    E. D.W. Winnicott.

56.3   A number of frameworks and models have been developed for use in assessing and conceptualizing family issues and problems. Which of the following models asks the questions "Why can't people solve their own problems? What is constraining a person or family from overcoming the difficulty?"

    A. Linear causality.
    B. Emotion regulation.
    C. Clinical constraints.
    D. Developmental trajectories.
    E. Circular causality.

56.4   Which newer form of family therapy encourages therapists to observe how symptoms and behavior function and then seek to remedy the presenting problem?

    A. Functional family therapy.
    B. Solution-focused family therapy.
    C. Narrative family therapy.
    D. Emotionally focused therapy.
    E. Strategic family therapy.

56.5   D.W. Winnicott emphasized the significance of the social environment for normal human development and psychological growth. A critical component to this theory is

    A. The identified patient.
    B. Nuclear family emotional process.
    C. Multigeneration transmission process.
    D. Family projection process.
    E. The holding environment.

Chapter 57

Interpersonal Psychotherapy for Depressed Adolescents

Select the single best response for each question.

57.1 Which of the following statements regarding interpersonal psychotherapy for depressed adolescents (IPT-A) is *false?*

    A. IPT-A is a time-limited, manualized, psychotherapeutic intervention adapted from IPT for adults.

    B. It is based on the principle that depression occurs within an interpersonal context.

    C. Its goal is to decrease depressive symptoms.

    D. It can be used for the treatment of adolescents who have either psychotic or nonpsychotic depression.

    E. It is not recommended for adolescents who are mentally retarded, actively suicidal or homicidal, or have bipolar disorders.

57.2 Which of the following statements regarding the course of treatment using interpersonal psychotherapy for depressed adolescents (IPT-A) is *false?*

    A. IPT-A is usually delivered once a week for 12 weeks.

    B. IPT-A is an individual treatment that requires parental participation.

    C. There are three treatment phases: initial, middle, and termination.

    D. Each session begins with an assessment of the adolescent patient's mood using a 1–10 scale.

    E. The therapist and patient focus on tasks that are specific to the phase of treatment after reviewing of the symptoms.

57.3 Which of the following interpersonal problem areas may be identified during interpersonal psychotherapy for depressed adolescents (IPT-A)?

    A. Grief due to death.

    B. Interpersonal role disputes.

    C. Interpersonal role transitions.

    D. Interpersonal deficits.

    E. All of the above.

57.4 General techniques commonly used in interpersonal psychotherapy for depressed adolescents (IPT-A) include all of the following *except*

    A. Encouragement of affect and linkage with interpersonal events.

    B. Reinforcements of coping skills.

    C. Communication analysis.

    D. Decision analysis.

    E. Role-playing.

57.5 Interpersonal psychotherapy for depressed adolescents (IPT-A) has been examined in a number of randomized, controlled clinical trials. For which of the following target symptoms do the greatest amount of empirical data support the effectiveness of IPT-A?

    A. Anxiety symptoms.
    B. Symptoms related to abusing substances.
    C. Depressive symptoms.
    D. Obsessive-compulsive disorder (OCD)–like symptoms.
    E. Attention-deficit/hyperactivity disorder (ADHD) symptoms.

Chapter 58

Cognitive-Behavioral Treatment for Anxiety Disorders

Select the single best response for each question.

58.1   Cognitive-behavioral therapy (CBT) has been shown to be efficacious in treating which of the following childhood disorders?

    A. Social phobia/social anxiety disorder.

    B. Avoidant disorder.

    C. Generalized anxiety disorder.

    D. Overanxious disorder.

    E. All of the above.

58.2   There is widespread agreement that the key ingredient in cognitive-behavioral therapy (CBT) is the behavioral intervention known as

    A. Exposure.

    B. Cognitive restructuring.

    C. Extinction.

    D. Within-session habituation.

    E. None of the above.

58.3   A parent comes to you to express her concern about her 10-year-old daughter, Jackie, who is afraid of dogs and runs away whenever she sees one. You schedule a session with Jackie and her mother and arrange to have a well-behaved dog present. Although Jackie is highly fearful at first, you encourage her to remain in the office until her anxiety diminishes. You are employing a model of treatment based on

    A. Implosion therapy.

    B. Relaxation training.

    C. Extinction.

    D. Cognitive restructuring.

    E. None of the above.

58.4   Which of the following treatment approaches may not be effective in preadolescent children?

    A. Intensive exposure.

    B. Cognitive restructuring.

    C. Lack of parental involvement in homework assignments.

    D. All of the above.

    E. None of the above.

58.5 In controlled trials of cognitive-behavioral therapy (CBT) in children and adolescents, which of the following factors was associated with more positive outcomes?

    A. Higher levels of overall family dysfunction.
    B. Symptoms of depression, fear, and hostility in parents.
    C. Massed treatment sessions rather than once weekly.
    D. At least 6–8 weeks of treatment rather than 4 weeks.
    E. Comorbid symptoms of depression and trait anxiety in children.

Chapter 59

Cognitive-Behavioral Therapy for Depression

Select the single best response for each question.

59.1 Which of the following statements regarding cognitive-behavioral therapy (CBT) is *false?*

  A. CBT has been found to be efficacious in treating depressed youth.
  B. Early meta-analyses reported low mean effect sizes for CBT with depressed youth compared with more recent meta-analyses that found higher mean effect sizes.
  C. CBT delivered in clinical settings yields smaller effect sizes relative to CBT delivered in research settings.
  D. CBT can be effective in reducing suicidal ideation among depressed adolescents.
  E. None of the above.

59.2 Which of the following cognitive vulnerabilities observed in depressed children and adolescents can be targets of cognitive-behavioral therapy (CBT) interventions?

  A. Negative thoughts about self.
  B. Anticipation of rejection.
  C. Anticipation of failure.
  D. Perfectionistic standards.
  E. All of the above.

59.3 Which of the following statements regarding cognitive-behavioral therapy (CBT) is *false?*

  A. CBT is formulation based and prescriptive.
  B. CBT treatment is usually open ended.
  C. An agenda is set up and homework is usually assigned.
  D. Collaboration between the therapist and the patient is needed to work together toward specific goals.
  E. Negative thoughts are seen not as facts, but rather as hypotheses to be explored.

59.4 Which of the following is not a specific intervention commonly used in cognitive-behavioral therapy (CBT)?

  A. Rational problem-solving.
  B. Rationally disputing automatic thoughts.
  C. Affect regulation.
  D. Defense interpretation.
  E. Parent training.

59.5   In cognitive-behavioral therapy (CBT), patients are encouraged to test the validity and utility of their negative and upsetting thoughts by asking which of the following questions?

    A. What is the evidence that supports the thought?
    B. Is there any contradicting evidence?
    C. Is there another way to look at the situation?
    D. If the negative thought is true, is it really so big a deal?
    E. All of the above.

Chapter 60

Motivational Interviewing

Select the single best response for each question.

60.1 What is the major goal of motivational interviewing?

  A. Providing insight.
  B. Healing conflict.
  C. Resolving ambivalence.
  D. Improving relationships.
  E. Stabilizing affect.

60.2 Motivational interviewing uses a cluster of counseling skills referred to as OARS. Which of the following letter–skill pairings is correct?

  A. O = organization.
  B. A = affect resolution.
  C. R = resistance awareness.
  D. S = symptom relief.
  E. None of the above.

60.3 In the stages of change model, a patient who has some ambivalence and is willing to consider change, but who has not yet made a commitment, would be considered to be in what stage?

  A. Maintenance.
  B. Preparation.
  C. Precontemplation.
  D. Contemplation.
  E. Action.

60.4 Much of the research literature on the efficacy of motivational interviewing in adolescents has focused on which of the following disorders?

  A. Generalized anxiety disorder.
  B. Alcohol and substance use disorders.
  C. Social phobia.
  D. Panic disorder.
  E. Avoidant disorder.

60.5 Motivational interviewing is guided by which of the following principles?

  A. Express empathy.
  B. Develop discrepancy.
  C. Roll with resistance.
  D. Support self-efficacy.
  E. All of the above.

Chapter 6 1

Systems of Care, Wraparound Services, and Home-Based Services

Select the single best response for each question.

61.1 Which of the following statements regarding the historical roots of system of care (SOC) approaches and wraparound services is *false?*

    A. Congress funded the Child and Adolescent Service System Program (CASSP) in 1984.

    B. At the time CASSP was founded, a wide range of services were available to children with significant difficulties.

    C. The guiding principle of the CASSP was the SOC.

    D. The three core values of SOC are child and family centered, community based, and culturally competent.

    E. Wraparound services and intensive home-based services are common features of an SOC approach.

61.2 Which of the following is *not* a guiding principle of systems of care?

    A. Services should be individualized for the child and family.

    B. Services should be developmentally appropriate and least restrictive.

    C. Case management should be provided to coordinate care as needed.

    D. A smooth transition to adult services should be ensured.

    E. Caregivers need not be fully integrated in the treatment process.

61.3 Wraparound services are helpful when children and families have significant emotional and behavioral difficulties. Key elements of wraparound services include all of the following *except*

    A. The youth and family must be full and active partners at every level in every activity.

    B. The wraparound approach must be team driven.

    C. The services must encompass both community and inpatient settings.

    D. There must be an unconditional commitment to serve children and their families.

    E. The wraparound teams must have flexible approaches and adequate funding.

61.4 Home-based services serve children with mental health needs who are involved in the child welfare or juvenile justice systems. Which of the following programs is generally delivered in the office but has also been used as an in-home service?

    A. Brief Strategic Family Therapy.

    B. Multisystemic Therapy.

    C. Intensive In-Home Child and Adolescent Psychiatric Service.

    D. Massachusetts Mental Health Services Program for Youth (MHSPY).

    E. The Nurse-Family Partnership.

61.5   Which of the following interventions has been empirically validated for the treatment of substance abuse and conduct problems?

    A. Intensive In-Home Child and Adolescent Psychiatric Service.
    B. Functional Family Therapy.
    C. Multidimensional Treatment Foster Care.
    D. Brief Strategic Family Therapy.
    E. Nurse-Family Partnership.

Chapter 62

Milieu Treatment

Inpatient, Partial Hospitalization, and Residential Programs

Select the single best response for each question.

62.1 Which of the following statements regarding the historical perspective of milieu treatments is *false?*

    A. Therapeutic milieus began as orphanages and boarding schools for youth with mental handicaps and psychiatric illness.
    B. Later, they evolved into child care institutions and group foster homes.
    C. In the past 15 years there has been a marked proliferation of unregulated facilities.
    D. Managed care has lessened problems of access to hospital inpatient units (IUs).
    E. There was a decreased use of IUs in the 1990s.

62.2 Which of the following components is essential for providing effective milieu treatment?

    A. Estimation of ability to form therapeutic alliance.
    B. Determination of critical factors prior to admission.
    C. Consideration of multiple domains in the life of the mentally ill child and family.
    D. Availability of aftercare by other services in the continuum of care.
    E. All of the above.

62.3 In determining whether a patient warrants an inpatient admission for suicidality, which of the following factors is considered to be least risky?

    A. Dysfunctional family patterns.
    B. Clearly abnormal mental state in a suicide attempter.
    C. Stated persistent wish to die.
    D. Adequate supervision and support not possible outside therapeutic milieu.
    E. Unresolved biopsychosocial risk factors unlikely to change sufficiently to allow safe return home.

62.4 Some milieu treatment programs are more successful than others in providing effective care. Components of effective milieu treatment include all of the following *except*

    A. Optimization of safety for patient, peers, and staff.
    B. Limitation of dysfunctional family involvement.
    C. Presence of treatment plan addressing factors identified in case formulation.
    D. Availability of financial support for duration of required treatment.
    E. Discharge when lesser level of care will suffice and is appropriate.

62.5   According to Pottick et al. (2004), which of the following is the most frequent presenting problem in acute specialty mental health inpatient programs?

   A. Suicidality.
   B. Aggression.
   C. Depressed or anxious mood (including self-harm).
   D. Family problems.
   E. Alcohol or drug use.

62.6   In regard to future directions in the field of milieu treatment, critical issues to be addressed include which of the following?

   A. Overcoming barriers to translating evidence-based practice into milieu treatment settings.
   B. Improving aftercare services.
   C. Decreasing readmission rates.
   D. Expanding and evaluating use of standardized measures for milieu treatments.
   E. All of the above.

Chapter 6 3

School-Based Interventions

Select the single best response for each question.

63.1 Since the mid-twentieth century, mental health consultation and service to schools has undergone significant expansion, stimulated by a number of broad sociocultural movements coincident with that period. Which of the following is *not* one of the major sociocultural movements contributing to the expanded role of mental health in education?

A. The community mental health movement after the Vietnam War.
B. The civil rights movement of the 1960s.
C. The dramatic changes in social norms from the 1960s through the 1980s.
D. The growth of the school-based health clinic movement in the 1990s.
E. Recent trends toward greater academic accountability in school settings.

63.2 Which of the following statements regarding models of school consultation and clinical care is *false?*

A. In the case consultation model, the consultation may be direct or indirect.
B. In the systems consultation model, individual students' needs are specifically addressed.
C. In the school-based health center model, a broad range of mental health services are provided by mental health practitioners.
D. In the school-linked health center model, off-site hospitals or community clinics are contracted to provide mental health services to school students.
E. In the expanded school mental health programs model, schools partner with community organizations to coordinate and integrate the variety of existing programs into a coherent whole.

63.3 School climate greatly influences the desirability and effectiveness of mental health interventions. Key components of a positive school climate include all of the following *except*

A. A supportive, welcoming atmosphere.
B. A variety of learning experiences.
C. Low expectations for achievement and self-regulation.
D. Fair and effective discipline.
E. Opportunities for participation in extracurricular activities.

63.4 Classroom accommodations provided for students with attention-deficit/hyperactivity disorder (ADHD) include all of the following *except*

A. Provide verbal and visual cues to stay on task.
B. Use small-group instruction.
C. Simplify and repeat directions.
D. Provide duplicate materials.
E. Allow student to observe others before performing tasks.

63.5 A child with a suspected disability should undergo a special education evaluation to determine eligibility for special education services. All of the following statements concerning Individualized Education Programs (IEPs) are correct *except*

    A. IEPs can include specific accommodations.
    B. IEPs can include curriculum modification.
    C. IEPs are reviewed and revised annually.
    D. Every year a comprehensive reevaluation is conducted to determine continued eligibility for an IEP.
    E. Children in an IEP are afforded special disciplinary consideration.

Chapter 64

Collaborating With Primary Care

Select the single best response for each question.

64.1 Optimal mental health care requires collaboration between the primary care physician and mental health specialists. Collaborative mental health care can be considered along a spectrum encompassing all of the following levels *except*

    A. Primarily primary care.
    B. Primarily primary care with consultation.
    C. Shared care.
    D. Shared care and lower levels of care.
    E. Primarily mental health care.

64.2 For the physician treating a child with attention-deficit/hyperactivity disorder (ADHD) who has been unresponsive to ADHD medications or who experiences exacerbation of a previously controlled depression, which level of collaborative mental health care is warranted?

    A. Primarily primary care.
    B. Primarily primary care with consultation.
    C. Shared care.
    D. Shared care and higher levels of care.
    E. Primarily mental health care.

64.3 What kind of "primary" mental health care services can primary care physicians provide?

    A. Anticipatory guidance.
    B. Mental health screening.
    C. Earlier identification.
    D. Earlier intervention.
    E. All of the above.

64.4 The resources available to assist the primary care physician vary across communities. Which of the following resources is least required by pediatricians or family physicians who provide collaborative health care in the primary care clinic?

    A. Local or regional connections with mental health professionals.
    B. Clear and regular communication.
    C. A mental health professional in the clinic.
    D. Onsite structured interviews and psychological testing.
    E. Continuing education.

64.5   What information should be documented in the patient's chart by the primary care physician after consulting a child and adolescent psychiatrist?

    A. Name of the consultant.
    B. The reason for the consultation.
    C. Reference to the case being summarized.
    D. Discussion of the diagnosis and recommendations for treatment.
    E. All of the above.

Chapter 65

Juvenile Justice

Select the single best response for each question.

65.1 Which of the following Supreme Court rulings made the execution of juveniles illegal?

    A. *Kent v. United States* (1966).
    B. *Roper v. Simmons* (2005).
    C. *In re Gault* (1967).
    D. All of the above.
    E. None of the above.

65.2 According to a study by the Northwestern Juvenile Project (Teplin et al. 2002), which of the following are the most common psychiatric disorders/conditions among both male and female juvenile detainees?

    A. Substance abuse.
    B. Disruptive behaviors (oppositional defiant disorder and conduct disorder).
    C. Posttraumatic stress disorder (PTSD).
    D. Mood disorders.
    E. Other anxiety disorders.

65.3 Several medical conditions predispose children to violent and aggressive behavior. For example, youth in juvenile justice are more likely than members of the general population to have been exposed during the postnatal period to which of the following?

    A. Lead.
    B. Alcohol.
    C. Other illicit substances.
    D. Head trauma.
    E. Verbal abuse.

65.4 When did the zero-tolerance policy become mandated by the federal government?

    A. 1989.
    B. 1993.
    C. 1994.
    D. 2002.
    E. 2004.

65.5 Which of the following factors increases suicide risk among incarcerated youth?

    A. Depression.
    B. History of impulsivity and drug abuse.
    C. History of abuse.
    D. Separation from biological parents.
    E. All of the above.

Chapter 1

Assessing Infants and Toddlers

Select the single best response for each question.

1.1   Infant psychiatry focuses on which of the following age groups?

    A. From birth to first birthday.
    B. From birth through age 3 years.
    C. From birth to preschool years.
    D. From conception to age 3 years.
    E. From conception to preschool years.

The correct response is option C.

Infant psychiatry is a strength-based, prevention-focused subspecialty of child and adolescent psychiatry that has brought attention to the mental health needs of children from birth through the preschool years. Infant psychiatry focuses on early identification of risk contexts and mental health disorders in infants, young children, and their families and requires a different assessment approach than that used with older children and adolescents. **(p. 3)**

1.2   Which of the following is the strongest outcome predictor of early childhood development?

    A. Presence or absence of pregnancy complications.
    B. Birth weight.
    C. Child's temperament.
    D. Parental relationship.
    E. Primary caregiving relationship.

The correct response is option E.

The quality of the primary caregiving relationship is the strongest determinant of early childhood development.

In early childhood, assessment focuses primarily on the child-caregiver relationship rather than on the young child as an individual. When working with young children and their families, the primary focus of assessment shifts from the child to the young child's important caregiving relationships. A primary reason for this is that the individual characteristics of the infant or toddler have limited predictive value for the child's future development. The child's important caregiving relationships, on the other hand, are far more predictive of subsequent outcomes (Shonkoff and Phillips 2000; C.H. Zeanah and Zeanah, in press; P.D. Zeanah et al. 2005). **(pp. 3–4)**

Shonkoff JP, Phillips DA: From Neurons to Neighborhoods: The Science of Early Childhood Development Committee on Integrating the Science of Early Childhood Development. Washington, DC, National Academy Press, 2000

Zeanah CH, Zeanah PD: Infant mental health: the case for early experience, in Handbook of Infant Mental Health, 3rd Edition. Edited by Zeanah CH. New York, Guilford, in press

Zeanah PD, Stafford B, Nagle GN, et al: Addressing Social-Emotional Development and Infant Mental Health in the State Early Childhood Comprehensive Systems Initiative. Los Angeles, University of California Los Angeles, 2005

1.3   Which of the following assessment or diagnostic tools uses the DSM-IV multiaxial system?

    A. Diagnostic Criteria: Zero to Three, Revised (DC:0–3R).
    B. Child Behavior Checklist 1½–5.
    C. Infant-Toddler Social and Emotional Assessment (ITSEA).
    D. Ages and Stages Questionnaires: Social-Emotional.
    E. None of the above.

The correct response is option A.

DC:0–3R, which has incorporated some of the criteria from the Research Diagnostic Criteria: Preschool Age, provides descriptions of clinical presentations commonly seen in infants and young children. Its multiaxial system emphasizes the centrality of the parent-child relationship (Zero to Three Diagnostic Classification Task Force 2005). The use of the multiaxial system in infant psychiatry is as important as the consistent use of Axis I diagnosis. When applying the DSM-IV multiaxial system, developmental status (Axis II), medical or biological conditions (Axis III), environmental factors (Axis IV), and child's level of functioning or impairment (Axis V) contribute to the understanding of the child and family. The DC:0–3R system includes a relationship classification axis (Axis II) and a social-emotional functioning axis (Axis V).

Perhaps the best known adult-report measure about children's behavior is the Child Behavior Checklist (CBCL), for ages 1½–5 (Achenbach and Rescorla 2000). The CBCL has been used to track treatment outcomes as well as for assessment (e.g., Lieberman et al. 2005). It can be scored by hand or using a computer program, which also generates a profile with comparison norms.

ITSEA (Briggs-Gowan 1998) and its companion, the Brief Infant-Toddler Social and Emotional Assessment (BITSEA) (Briggs-Gowan and Carter 2002), assess problems and strengths in children 12–36 months, using a 3-point Likert scale. The ITSEA has strong evidence supporting its concurrent validity with well-accepted observational and parent report measures (Carter et al. 1999).

The Ages and Stages Questionnaires: Social-Emotional screening system includes a 6-month screen, which focuses primarily on infant cues and regulation patterns related to calming the infant, feeding, sleeping, and stooling (Squires et al. 2002). **(pp. 5, 10–12)**

Achenbach T, Rescorla L: Manual for the ASEBA Preschool Form. Burlington, University of Vermont, 2000

Briggs-Gowan M: Preliminary acceptability and psychometrics of the Infant-Toddler Social and Emotional Assessment (ITSEA): a new adult-report questionnaire. Infant Mental Health Journal 19:422–445, 1998

Briggs-Gowan M, Carter AS: Brief Infant Toddler Social Emotional Assessment (BITSEA) Manual, Version 2.0. New Haven, CT, Yale University, 2002

Carter AS, Little C, Briggs-Gowan MJ, et al: The Infant-Toddler Social and Emotional Assessment (ITSEA): comparing parent ratings to laboratory observations of task mastery, emotion regulation, coping behaviors, and attachment status. Infant Mental Health Journal 20:375–392, 1999

Lieberman AFP, Van Horn PJ, Ippen CGP: Toward evidence-based treatment: child-parent psychotherapy with preschoolers exposed to marital violence. J Am Acad Child Adolesc Psychiatry 44:1241–1248, 2005

Squires J, Bricker D, Twombly E: Ages and Stages Questionnaires: Social-Emotional. A Parent-Completed, Child-Monitoring System for Social-Emotional Behaviors. 6 Month ASQ:SE Questionnaire (for Infants Ages 3 Through 8 Months). Baltimore, MD, Paul H. Brookes, 2002. Available at: http://eip.uoregon.edu/pdf/6month_asqse.pdf. Accessed August 10, 2007.

Zero to Three Diagnostic Classification Task Force: Diagnostic Classification of Mental Health and Development Disorders of Infancy and Early Childhood: DC:0–3R. Washington, DC, Zero to Three Press, 2005

1.4   Which of the following is *not* considered a key element of the infant/toddler assessment?

    A. History of presenting problem.
    B. Medical history.
    C. Developmental history.
    D. IQ.
    E. Family history.

The correct response is option D.

IQ testing is not considered a key element of the infant/toddler assessment.

The comprehensive assessment of infants and toddlers should include multiple appointments, the use of multiple informants, and multiple modes of assessment, including formal and informal observations; structured assessment tools; and medical, developmental, family, and social history (in addition to history of presenting problems). **(p. 6; see also Table 1–1)**

1.5   Which of the following is the only diagnostic interview with published data to support its reliability for assessing infants and toddlers?

    A. Preschool Age Psychiatric Assessment (PAPA).
    B. Diagnostic Infant Preschool Structured Interview.
    C. Crowell procedure.
    D. Beck Depression Inventory.
    E. Parenting Stress Index.

The correct response is option A.

The PAPA is the only diagnostic interview for which reliability data have been published (Egger et al. 2006). The instrument is an interviewer-based psychiatric diagnostic interview focused on children 2–5 years old.

The Diagnostic Infant Preschool Structured Interview (Scheeringa M: "Diagnostic Infant Preschool Structured Interview," unpublished manual, 2005) is a respondent-based interview of parents of children, ages 18–60 months.

In the Crowell procedure (Crowell and Feldman 1988), the parent and child (of at least 6 months developmental age) are observed in a series of activities including free play, cleanup, a bubbles sequence, and four puzzle tasks as well as a separation and reunion.

Some clinical problems within the infant-parent relationship may stem from parent distress or psychopathology. The Beck Depression Inventory–II (Beck et al. 1996) and the Parenting Stress Index–Short Form (Haskett et al. 2006) may be helpful in assessing the need for further parental assessment. **(p. 10)**

    Beck A, Steer RA, Brown G: Beck Depression Inventory II. San Antonio, TX, Harcourt Assessment, 1996
    Crowell JA, Feldman SS: Mothers' internal models of relationships and children's behavioral and developmental status: a study of mother-child interaction. Child Dev 59:1273–1285, 1988
    Egger HL, Erkanli A, Keeler G, et al: Test-retest reliability of the Preschool Age Psychiatric Assessment (PAPA). J Am Acad Child Adolesc Psychiatry 45:538–549, 2006
    Haskett ME, Ahern LS, Ward CS, et al: Factor structure and validity of the Parenting Stress Index–Short Form. J Clin Child Psychol 35:302–312, 2006

Chapter 2

Assessing the Preschool-Age Child

Select the single best response for each question.

2.1   The significant developmental differences between preschool- and school-age children require a tailored approach to obtaining a history and mental status exam. Which of the following principles should be kept in mind when evaluating a preschool-age child?

A.   The most meaningful evaluation occurs when the child is evaluated without the primary caregiver.
B.   The mental status examination should be conducted in the context of play.
C.   The preschooler should be evaluated in one session to avoid conflicting results.
D.   It is desirable to include only the primary caregiver when evaluating the child.
E.   All of the above.

The correct response is option B.

The mental status exam of the preschooler must be conducted in the context of play. While this may seem an obvious component of any child assessment, it is essential to a valid preschool mental status exam. Both the availability of age-appropriate toys to facilitate representational play, if the child is capable, and the examiner's willingness and ability to engage the child in play are essential. Concretely, this means the examiner should not wear a white coat or carry a chart or examination tools. The examiner should be able to adopt a playful posture, which often involves sitting on the floor, following the child's play, and assuming a more imaginative and whimsical demeanor. Clinicians unwilling or unable to engage in elaborate play will not be well suited to work with preschoolers.

The preschool child does not function as a psychologically autonomous individual and remains inextricably tied to the primary caregiver for adaptive and emotional functioning. This idea was succinctly expressed by Winnicott (1965), whose famous phrase "There is no such thing as a baby" emphasized the importance of the dyad very early in life. This adage remains applicable during the preschool period, despite the important developmental transitions in the primary relationship. Therefore, because the caregiver-child dyad more accurately represents the psychological status and functioning of the preschooler, the dyad is the most meaningful unit of observation or assessment. This means that, whenever possible, the mental status exam of a preschool child should be conducted with the child and caregiver together rather than with the child individually. Although an individual play interview of the preschooler alone may be necessary in some circumstances (e.g., with preschoolers without the benefit of primary caregivers), observation of the child with the caregiver present is generally the most appropriate method.

Another key principle of preschool assessment is that due to significant state- and relationship-related variation in the mental status of the young child, it is necessary to observe a preschooler on more than one occasion and with more than one caregiver. For this reason, assessments are best done over a series of several sessions on different days and, whenever possible, with different caregivers. In general, this requires an extended evaluation conducted over several days or weeks. (pp. 15–16)

Winnicott DW: The Maturational Process and the Facilitating Environment: Studies in the Theory of Emotional Development. New York, International Universities Press, 1965

2.2   The Washington University School of Medicine Infant/Preschool Mental Health (WUSM IPMH) clinic uses a standardized format for evaluating preschool-age children. Which of the following statements correctly describes this evaluation?

    A. The assessment is conducted in one 3-hour session.
    B. Free play is observed with the primary caregiver.
    C. A semistructured observation with secondary caregivers is included.
    D. Emotional, psychological, family, and developmental history is obtained only from the mother.
    E. None of the above.

The correct response is option E.

None of the above statements is correct.

A standard format for a preschool mental health assessment has been established in the WUSM IPMH clinic. This format has been used successfully for nearly two decades; however, many variations on this format have been used in other clinics and may prove more feasible and equally useful.

The preschool assessment is conducted in four 50-minute sessions over 4 consecutive weeks. In the first session, all primary caregivers (both parents, or grandparent and parent, if available) are asked to come in without the child to obtain a comprehensive history.

During the first session, a complete emotional, psychological, family, and developmental history of the child is obtained from caregivers. In the second session, free play is observed with secondary caregivers. During the third session, a semistructured observation with the primary caregiver takes place. The child and caregiver share a snack, dyadic play, and then separation and reunion are observed. In the fourth and final session, observations and findings, biopsychosocial formulation, differential diagnosis, and treatment plan are reviewed. **(p. 16; see also Table 2–1)**

2.3   Which of the following actions should be taken by parents to prepare their preschooler for the play evaluation?

    A. Parents should provide honest information to the child about the purpose of the evaluation.
    B. Parents should not disclose to their child that they have already met with the examiner.
    C. Parents should avoid discussing with the child that the examination will involve play.
    D. It is best to inform the child about the examination over several days to a week so he/she may ask questions.
    E. Parents should not prepare their child for the examination.

The correct response is option A.

Once a comprehensive history has been obtained, play-assessment sessions are the next step. At the completion of the session in which the history was obtained, it is very important to instruct the parents on how to prepare the child for the play session. If the child comes to the session with a basic knowledge of the purpose of the encounter, it is likely to be far more fruitful and productive. To inform the child about the assessment and the reasons for it in a nonjudgmental way, using clear simple and understandable language is the most important first step in the assessment as well as the therapeutic process. The clinician should encourage the parents to be as honest as possible with the child about the nature of the concern. This may be the first time that caregivers engage in a direct and candid exchange with the child about the problem. It is, of course, also important to make sure the child understands that the assessment will involve play and not any frightening or painful medical examinations or procedures. To avoid unnecessary anticipatory anxiety, and in keeping with limitations in the young child's sense of time, informing the child about the evaluation on the day prior may be most sensible. Further, it is also useful for parents, as well as the examiner, to disclose to the child that they have already met with the clinician to tell them about the child, the family, and the nature of the problem. **(pp. 17–18)**

2.4   Which of the following statements regarding conduct of the free-play assessment with the preschooler is *true*?

    A. A brief separation between the parent and child midway through the free-play session is useful.

    B. The clinician should avoid disclosing to the child what was learned about his or her problems from the meeting with the parents.

    C. When the parent asks questions of the therapist during the play session, the therapist should freely answer the questions in order to reduce the parents' anxiety.

    D. The examiner should not respond to the child's bids to engage in play.

    E. All of the above.

The correct response is option A.

It may be useful to enact a brief separation between parent and child midway through the free-play session. This allows observation of how the parent separates from the child, how the child responds to that separation, and how the parent and child reunite.

At the onset of the session, it is important for the clinician to communicate two basic principles: first, to explain to the child the purpose of the session and to disclose what the therapist knows from meeting with the parent about the nature of the child's problems, and second, to state that the child may play with the toys however he or she would like.

It is often necessary to redirect parents' natural attempts to engage in conversational exchanges with the therapist. This will derail the dyadic interaction, which is the central purpose of this session. Advise parents that there will be another time to ask questions and relay further details of history.

The role of the examiner in this dyadic free-play observation is to serve as a "participant-observer" in the play. That is, the examiner should be prepared to respond to any bids from the child to engage in play. The examiner, though, should follow and never lead the child's play. **(p. 18)**

2.5   Several standardized semistructured interviews may be useful in the dyadic assessment of parent and child. Which of the following are characteristics of the Parent-Child Early Relational Assessment (PCERA)?

    A. The parent blows bubbles to elicit affect from the child.

    B. Tasks of escalating difficulty are performed by the child and parent and videotaped for further review.

    C. The parent and child perform a structured task in which block designs are made from sample cards.

    D. None of the above.

    E. All of the above.

The correct response is option C.

Several standardized semistructured interviews, originally developed for research, are now available and may be useful in the clinical setting. In one such interview, the PCERA (Clark 1985), the clinician observes, through a one-way mirror, the dyad performing several tasks. The primary caregiver and child share a snack and then perform a structured task in which block designs are made from sample cards. Next, they engage in free play, and, lastly, a brief separation and reunion is enacted. This interview provides an interesting and varied format in which the quality of parent-child relationship, parenting, and child's behaviors toward the caregiver, are observed.

The Crowell procedure (Crowell and Fleischmann 1993) is a similar interview that adds blowing bubbles to specifically elicit affect in the child.

Other similar useful dyadic observational assessments include "The Teaching Task" (Egeland et al. 1995), in which tasks of escalating difficulty are performed by the dyad while parent-child interactions are observed and videotaped for later review. **(pp. 18–19)**

Clark R: The Parent-Child Early Relational Assessment, Manual and Instrument. Madison, University of Wisconsin Department of Psychiatry, 1985

Crowell J, Fleischmann MA: Use of structured research procedure in clinical assessments of infants, in Handbook of Infant Mental Health, 2nd Edition. Edited by Zeanah CH. New York, Guilford, 1993, pp 210–221

Egeland B, Weinfeld N, Hiester M, et al: Teaching Tasks Administration and Scoring Manual. Minneapolis, University of Minnesota Institute of Child Development, 1995

Chapter 3

Assessing the Elementary School–Age Child

Select the single best response for each question.

3.1   The key developmental milestones for the school-age child are related to

   A. Separation and individuation.
   B. Initiation and rapprochement.
   C. Object constancy and individual consolidation.
   D. Peer identity and social identity formation.
   E. Intimacy and generativity.

The correct response is option D.

The key developmental milestones for this age group are focused on the tasks of identity formation that are related to autonomy, peer identity, and social identity (Gemelli 1996). **(p. 27)**

   Gemelli R: Normal Child and Adolescent Development. Washington, DC, American Psychiatric Press, 1996

3.2   Which of the following is key to a successful evaluation?

   A. Seeing the child first.
   B. Seeing the parent(s) first.
   C. Seeing the child and parent(s) together.
   D. Seeing the referral professional first.
   E. Establishing a collaborative relationship between the clinician and the child and his or her family.

The correct response is option E.

Key to the evaluation process is the establishment of a collaborative relationship between the clinician and the child and his or her family.

   In middle childhood, the specific roles of the parent and child in the evaluation process may vary with different clinical situations. It is therefore helpful to discuss the clinician's interview plan with the presenting family members and to ask for input from the parents. It is appropriate to ask them whether they would prefer to begin the substantive discussions in the presence of their child or separately. It is also helpful to ask the parents for input about what will make their child feel more comfortable: sitting in the room, remaining in the waiting room, or sitting nearby, outside of the office.

   Studies have shown that obtaining factual information from a child is an important part of the clinical assessment (Herjanic and Reich 1982). It is now standard practice to obtain information from multiple informants regarding a child's functioning and symptoms and to realize that the information from these informants may not agree. Low correlation does not necessarily refute the validity of any of the reports; rather, the reports are combined to best understand the child's symptoms and the impact of those symptoms on the child's functioning (Graham and Rutter 1968; Rutter and Graham 1968). **(pp. 28, 31)**

Graham P, Rutter M: The reliability and validity of the psychiatric assessment of the child, II: interview with the parent. Br J Psychiatry 114:581–592, 1968

Herjanic B, Reich W: Development of a structural psychiatric interview for children: agreement between child and parent on individual symptoms. J Abnorm Child Psychol 10:307–324, 1982

Rutter M, Graham P: The reliability and validity of the psychiatric assessment of the child, I: interview with the child. Br J Psychol 114:563–579, 1968

3.3   Key procedural information that should be covered in the first evaluation session includes all of the following *except*

    A. Office/departmental procedures.
    B. Plan/process of the evaluation.
    C. Communication with school.
    D. Confidentiality.
    E. Safety plans.

The correct response is option C.

Key procedural information to cover in the first evaluation session includes the explanation of office/departmental procedures, ways of reaching the clinician, the process of the evaluation, the confidentiality of the information disclosed, the review of safety plans, and the opportunity to ask questions about the process. **(pp. 28–29 [Table 3–1])**

3.4   For the clinician, appropriate steps in the evaluation of a child whose parents are divorced include all of the following *except*

    A. Attempt to include both parents in gathering information.
    B. Agree to complete a custody evaluation.
    C. Clarify which parent has primary custody and request a copy of the custody agreement.
    D. Clarify health insurance responsibility.
    E. Clarify the role of the clinician.

The correct response is option B.

Custody evaluations are a highly specialized and contentious type of evaluation. Specialized training and procedures are standard practice for these evaluations (American Academy of Child and Adolescent Psychiatry 1997). Clinicians need to be clear with parents about the limits if custody issues are involved and that the evaluation is not a formal custody evaluation. Referrals to court mediators and custody evaluators are appropriate for these requests.

Many children presenting for evaluation will have experienced parental marital conflict, separation, and/or divorce. In separation or divorce cases, it is particularly critical that at the initial appointment the clinician discuss and establish plans and goals for completing the evaluation. Whether one or both parents accompany the child, it is critical to inquire about custody arrangements, including which parent has primary custody and health insurance responsibility and what are the guardianship visitation and custody sharing arrangements. Requesting a copy of the custody agreement is advised. These discussions are critical for both establishing the fundamental collaborative relationship and clarifying the role of the clinician. It is important to address issues related to access to medical records, court involvement, and limitations related to roles.

Even if the role of the clinician is not to conduct a custody evaluation, if custody disputes are ongoing, clinical records may be subpoenaed by the court. Although one parent may claim that the noncustodial parent has very little interest in or involvement with the child you are evaluating, it is good practice to attempt to include both parents in your information-gathering process. A direct request from a clinician regarding observations and concerns about the child may result in a very different response than was predicted by the other parent. In most cases, both parents do have some role with the child. Including both parents in the diagnostic process therefore underscores for the child and parents that both relationships are important and impacting the child. In addition, it sets the stage for future therapeutic interventions that may necessitate coparenting despite the end of the marital relationship. **(pp. 33–34)**

> American Academy of Child and Adolescent Psychiatry: Practice parameters for child custody evaluation. J Am Acad Child Adolesc Psychiatry 36 (10 suppl):57S–68S, 1997

3.5   Common presenting problems in school-age children include all of the following *except*

   A. Sexualized behavior.
   B. Academic difficulties.
   C. Peer difficulties.
   D. School refusal.
   E. Social anxiety.

The correct response is option A.

A less common presenting problem in school-age children is related to sexualized behavior between peers or siblings. In these situations, typically a parent or other adult has learned about these behaviors either by interrupting them or via a disclosure from an involved child.

School-age children generally present with refusal of school, social/separation anxiety, poor academic performance or lack of academic motivation, and peer difficulties such as aggression and bullying toward peers or being the recipient of peer victimization and teasing, with subsequent social withdrawal or aggression. **(pp. 32–33)**

Chapter 4

Assessing Adolescents

Select the single best response for each question.

4.1   Which of the following statements concerning the assessment of adolescents is *true?*

    A. Because mothers and fathers may have divergent views about the adolescent's problems, only one parent should be interviewed.

    B. Involve as few informants as possible in collecting information to minimize conflicting opinions.

    C. Understanding how the adolescent was referred for treatment is not important.

    D. Prior medical records from primary care physicians should be obtained as part of the assessment.

    E. Data from rating scales or psychological testing are rarely helpful in establishing the correct diagnosis.

The correct response is option D.

Prior records from the primary care physician, prior mental health treatment records, school records, and records from other involved agencies should be obtained as part of a comprehensive assessment. Data from rating scales, standardized diagnostic interviews, or psychological testing can also be helpful in establishing the correct diagnosis and an accurate problem list, leading to a plan of treatment. Finally, understanding how the adolescent has been referred for treatment is an important piece of information to have prior to beginning the assessment. Did the parents self-refer? Was the school involved, or the juvenile court? Do the parents or the adolescent believe there is a problem, or are they only following through on a forced assessment?

Involving as many informants as possible provides the broadest data set from which to base the diagnostic assessment and proposed treatment plan. Mothers and fathers frequently have divergent views about the adolescent's problems and their underlying causes (Chess et al. 1966; Youngstrom et al. 2000). Whenever possible, both parents should be involved. They can be interviewed with the child, as a couple, or separately. Many times a combination of formats is best. Other primary caregivers can be included with the permission of the legal guardian. **(p. 48)**

> Chess S, Thomas A, Birch HD: Distortions in developmental reporting made by parents of behaviorally disturbed children. J Am Acad Child Adolesc Psychiatry 5:226–234, 1966
>
> Youngstrom E, Loeber R, Stouthamer-Loeber M: Patterns and correlates of agreement between parent, teacher, and male adolescent ratings of externalizing and internalizing problems. J Consult Clin Psychol 68:1038–1050, 2000

4.2   In the initial assessment of an adolescent, which of the following strategies is usually most productive?

    A. Interview one parent, then the adolescent, then the other parent.

    B. Interview the adolescent alone first, then the parent or parents.

    C. Interview both parents, then the adolescent.

    D. Interview the parents together with the adolescent.

    E. None of the above.

The correct response is option D.

In most cases, starting the initial assessment with parent(s) and adolescent together can be productive. How long to continue this interview is a decision based on the interaction of the parties. At a minimum, this allows the clinician to assess the relationship between the adolescent and the parent(s). An introduction to the problems causing the referral gives the clinician information on which to base the interview with the adolescent alone. The level of resistance and oppositional behavior can be seen. In order to minimize the perception of the clinician as solely a parental agent, this interview may be short and quickly transition to the adolescent alone. **(p. 49)**

4.3   What information obtained from adolescents should be shared with the parents?

    A. All details obtained from the adolescent should be shared with the parents.
    B. No information obtained from the adolescent should be shared with the parents.
    C. Safety issues involving the adolescent, such as suicidal behavior, should be shared with the parents.
    D. None of the above.
    E. All of the above.

The correct response is option C.

Parents should be told that the clinician will give them the overview of problems and diagnoses, without specific details of statements and behaviors reported by the adolescent, *unless the adolescent would be at risk of harm if the parents were not informed.* In cases of suicidal behaviors, dangerous sexual behaviors (multiple partners and/ or unprotected sex), dangerous driving behaviors, and the like, the safety of the adolescent takes precedence over confidentiality.

In the beginning of the assessment process it is vital that both parent and adolescent understand the structure and process of the evaluation. Confidentiality issues must be explained to both the parent and adolescent. In order for adolescents to feel comfortable providing details about their life, symptoms, actions, and feelings, they need to know how much of what they disclose will be communicated to a parent. If adolescents assume that everything they say will be communicated directly to the parent, this places a huge roadblock on the flow of information. However, some will assume everything will be kept confidential, causing difficulties when significant issues need to be disclosed to parents. Conversely, parents often think it is their right to know every detail divulged by the adolescent in the interview. After all, they are bringing their underage child for assessment, and they are paying for it too! Coming to an understanding of just how confidentiality is handled will avoid some uncomfortable situations and allows for a much easier first interview with the adolescent. What is the proper balance between confidentiality for the adolescent and sufficient communication with the parent? In order to facilitate communication by the adolescent, he or she should feel that the clinician is, at least in part, his or her advocate. **(p. 49)**

4.4   An evidence-based approach that has been successfully used for interviewing adolescents is

    A. Psychodynamic interviewing.
    B. Dialectical behavioral interviewing.
    C. Cognitive-behavioral interviewing.
    D. Interpersonal interviewing.
    E. Motivational interviewing.

The correct response is option E.

An evidence-based approach that has been successfully used in adolescents, particularly substance-abusing teens, is called *motivational interviewing*, or *motivational enhancement therapy*. Motivational interviewing uses Carl Rogers' client-centered approach, focusing on the person's current interests or concerns, thus likely providing the adolescent with a more positive experience. This enhances the interviewer's role as advocate for the adolescent rather than agent of the parent. However, as opposed to a true Rogerian therapy, motivational interviewing is directive. The approach specifically focuses on the resolution of ambivalence, guiding the person toward positive change. The interviewer elicits from the adolescent thoughts about change, reinforces them, and deals with resistance in ways intended to reduce it. The goal is to resolve ambivalence so that a person moves toward change. **(p. 50)**

4.5 Goals for the initial parent interview include all of the following *except*

    A. Data collection.
    B. Sharing differential diagnostic possibilities.
    C. Understanding the parent's point of view.
    D. Establishing a relationship with the parents.
    E. None of the above.

The correct response is option B.

Sharing of differential diagnostic possibilities is not a goal of the initial parent interview.

The clinician should have multiple goals for the initial parent interview. First and foremost, it provides an opportunity for the clinician to establish a relationship with the parent(s) that sets the stage for the ongoing treatment of the adolescent, and possibly for the success or failure of that treatment. Absent a positive, collaborative relationship with an adolescent's parents, treatment is arduous at best.

A second goal of the interview is to understand the presenting problems from the parent's point of view. This is best done without the presence of the adolescent. The adolescent has likely heard about his or her problems many times in the past. Hearing the recitation of problems in front of a stranger often creates a hostile, antagonistic, and resistive response from the adolescent. Conversely, many parents will not discuss their concerns about the adolescent frankly in the presence of their child. Therefore, an interview with the parent alone is crucial.

Data collection is a third primary aim of the parent interview. The present illness should be thoroughly explored from the parent's perspective. Similar to the adolescent interview, a screen for other psychiatric disorders should be completed with the parents. **(p. 52)**

4.6 A respondent-based interview that is highly structured and designed to be administered by trained lay interviewers is

    A. Diagnostic Interview Schedule for Children, Version IV (DISC-IV).
    B. Schedule for Affective Disorders and Schizophrenia for School-Age Children (K-SADS).
    C. Child Adolescent Psychiatric Assessment (CAPA).
    D. Child Behavior Checklist (CBCL).
    E. Behavior Assessment System for Children (BASC).

The correct response is option A.

Diagnostic interviews allow a comprehensive assessment of psychiatric diagnoses and are of two primary types: interviewer-based and respondent-based interviews. Respondent-based interviews such as the National Institute of Mental Health DISC-IV (Shaffer et al. 2000) are highly structured and use trained lay interviewers. The interviewer follows a predetermined script and is not allowed to deviate from the script or interpret the subject's response.

The K-SADS (Ambrosini 2000; Chambers et al. 1985) and the CAPA (Angold and Costello 2000) are examples of interviewer-based diagnostic interviews. These are semistructured interviews that allow the interviewer to make judgments during the interview. They require a clinician or highly trained interviewer and thus are more expensive to administer.

Rating scales screen for problem symptoms or behaviors using parent, adolescent, or teacher reports. They should be used to help focus the clinician on problem areas to explore. These instruments generally compare responses for the individual being assessed to standardized population norms. Rating scales may be broad-band scales assessing problems across broad dimensions of behavior, such as the CBCL (Achenbach and Rescorla 2001) and the BASC (Kamphaus et al. 2007). **(p. 54)**

Achenbach TM, Rescorla LA: Manual for ASEBA School-Age Forms and Profiles. Burlington, University of Vermont, Research Center for Children, Youth, and Families, 2001

Ambrosini PJ: Historical development and present status of the Schedule for Affective Disorders and Schizophrenia for School-Age Children (K-SADS). J Am Acad Child Adolesc Psychiatry 39:49–58, 2000

Angold A, Costello E: The Child and Adolescent Psychiatric Assessment (CAPA). J Am Acad Child Adolesc Psychiatry 39:39–48, 2000

Chambers WJ, Puig-Antich J, Hirsch M, et al: The assessment of affective disorders in children and adolescents by semi-structured interview: test-retest reliability of the Schedule for Affective Disorders and Schizophrenia for School-Age Children. Arch Gen Psychiatry 42:696–792, 1985

Kamphaus RW, VanDeventer MC, Brueggemann A, et al: Behavior Assessment System for Children, in The Clinical Assessment of Children and Adolescents: A Practitioner's Handbook. Edited by Smith SR, Handler L. Mahwah, NJ, Lawrence Erlbaum, 2007, pp 311–326

Shaffer D, Fisher P, Lucas CP, et al: NIMH Diagnostic Interview Schedule for Children, Version IV (NIMH DISC-IV): description, differences from previous versions, and reliability of some common diagnoses. J Am Acad Child Adolesc Psychiatry 39:28–38, 2000

Chapter 5

Classification of Psychiatric Disorders

Select the single best response for each question.

5.1   DSM-I (American Psychiatric Association 1952) categories relating specifically to childhood or adolescence included all of the following *except*

   A. Chronic brain syndrome associated with birth trauma.
   B. Schizophrenia reaction, childhood type.
   C. Special symptom reactions such as learning disturbance, enuresis, and somnambulism.
   D. Adjustment reactions.
   E. Hyperkinetic reaction of childhood.

The correct response is option E.

Hyperkinetic reaction of childhood was not included in DSM-I, but rather was added in DSM-II (American Psychiatric Association 1968).

   The developers of the first edition of DSM (DSM-I) did not include child and adolescent psychiatrists. There were only four categories relating specifically to childhood or adolescence: 1) chronic brain syndrome associated with birth trauma; 2) schizophrenic reaction, childhood type; 3) special symptom reactions such as learning disturbance, enuresis, and somnambulism; and 4) the adjustment reactions (habit disturbance, conduct disturbance, neurotic traits) of infancy, childhood, and adolescence. **(p. 62)**

   American Psychiatric Association: Diagnostic and Statistical Manual: Mental Disorders. Washington, DC, American Psychiatric Association, 1952
   American Psychiatric Association: Diagnostic and Statistical Manual of Mental Disorders, 2nd Edition. Washington, DC, American Psychiatric Association, 1968

5.2   All of the following statements regarding DSM-II (American Psychiatric Association 1968) are correct *except*

   A. It was intended to coincide with the *International Classification of Diseases*, 8th Revision (ICD-8).
   B. The developers tried to avoid terms that implied either the nature of a disorder or its cause.
   C. It reflected the growing importance of biological theories and research findings.
   D. It emphasized psychoanalytic theory.
   E. Descriptive phenomenology assumed a larger role.

The correct response is option D.

DSM-II deemphasized psychoanalytic theory.

   DSM-II (American Psychiatric Association 1968) was intended to coincide with ICD-8 (World Health Organization 1969) in the context of ongoing dialogue and constructive tension between the United States and international approaches to diagnostic classification in psychiatry. The developers of DSM-II tried to avoid terms that implied either the nature of a disorder or its causes and to be "explicit about causal assumptions when they are integral to a diagnostic concept" (p. viii). DSM-II reflected the growing importance of biological theories and research findings in understanding mental disorders. Descriptive phenomenology assumed a larger role than it had previously. **(p. 62)**

American Psychiatric Association: Diagnostic and Statistical Manual of Mental Disorders, 2nd Edition. Washington, DC, American Psychiatric Association, 1968

World Health Organization: International Classification of Diseases, 8th Revision. Geneva, Switzerland, World Health Organization, 1969

5.3   All of the following statements regarding DSM-III (American Psychiatric Association 1980) are correct *except*

A. It was highly controversial when introduced.

B. Assumed etiology was included for most disorders.

C. It was modeled on the Feighner criteria.

D. It provided specific phenomenological diagnostic criteria for each disorder, in contrast to the global clinical impression of DSM-IV (American Psychiatric Association 1994).

E. Each diagnosis had inclusion and exclusion criteria, and a five-part multiaxial system was introduced.

The correct response is option B.

Except when etiology was clearly known, as in organic mental disorders, no assumptions about etiology were included.

DSM-III (American Psychiatric Association 1980) was highly controversial when it was introduced. DSM-III was modeled on the Feighner criteria, and the subsequent related Research Diagnostic Criteria. DSM-III provided specific phenomenological diagnostic criteria for each disorder. Some observers called this the "Chinese menu" approach, in contrast to the global clinical impressions of DSM-II (American Psychiatric Association 1968). Each diagnosis had inclusion criteria. Exclusion criteria were also added. DSM-III introduced a five-part multiaxial system that allowed for the coding of most psychiatric disorders on Axis I, personality and specific developmental disorders on Axis II, medical conditions on Axis III, and psychosocial stressors and the highest level of adaptive functioning in the past year on Axes IV and V, respectively. **(pp. 62–63)**

American Psychiatric Association: Diagnostic and Statistical Manual of Mental Disorders, 2nd Edition. Washington, DC, American Psychiatric Association, 1968

American Psychiatric Association: Diagnostic and Statistical Manual of Mental Disorders, 3rd Edition. Washington, DC, American Psychiatric Association, 1980

American Psychiatric Association: Diagnostic and Statistical Manual of Mental Disorders, 4th Edition. Washington, DC, American Psychiatric Association, 1994

5.4   All of the following statements about DSM-IV (American Psychiatric Association 1994) are correct *except*

A. It was a reconceptualization of its predecessor.

B. There was greater coordination and agreement with the ICD development process.

C. For most DSM-IV disorders, a single criteria set was provided that applies to children, adolescents, and adults.

D. A number of disorders were moved from Axis II to Axis I, and only personality disorders and mental retardation remained on Axis II.

E. The category "attention-deficit and disruptive behavior disorders" replaced the DSM-III-R (American Psychiatric Association 1987) category of disruptive behavior disorders.

The correct response is option A.

DSM-IV was a modification and refinement of its predecessor rather than a reconceptualization.

There was even greater coordination with the ICD development process, and DSM-IV and ICD-10 (World Health Organization 1992) agree more closely than their predecessors did. "For most (but not all) DSM-IV disorders, a single criteria set is provided that applies to children, adolescents, and adults" (American Psychiatric Association 1994, p. 37). The overarching category of developmental disorders that was previously coded on Axis II was dropped. Pervasive developmental disorders and learning disorders (formerly academic skills disorders), motor skills disorder, and communication disorders (formerly language and speech disorders) were moved to Axis I from Axis II. Only personality disorders (rarely, if ever, used in children and adolescents), and mental retardation remain on Axis II. The category "attention-deficit and disruptive behavior disorders" replaced the DSM-III-R category of disruptive behavior disorders. **(pp. 63–64)**

American Psychiatric Association: Diagnostic and Statistical Manual of Mental Disorders, 3rd Edition, Revised. Washington, DC, American Psychiatric Association, 1987

American Psychiatric Association: Diagnostic and Statistical Manual of Mental Disorders, 4th Edition. Washington, DC, American Psychiatric Association, 1994

World Health Organization: International Statistical Classification of Diseases and Related Health Problems, 10th Revision. Geneva, Switzerland, World Health Organization, 1992

5.5 Other diagnostic systems have been developed for populations of patients or professionals who have not been well served by either the DSM or ICD models. All of the following statements are correct *except*

    A. The *Diagnostic and Statistical Manual for Primary Care* (DSM-PC) was developed collaboratively by the American Academy of Pediatrics and the American Psychiatric Association.

    B. DSM-PC was designed to be used by pediatricians and faculty physicians to classify emotional and behavioral problems.

    C. DSM-PC includes a simplified single cluster approach.

    D. The Diagnostic Classification on Infancy and Early Childhood (DC:0–3) was revised in 2005.

    E. The goals of DC:0–3 were to increase the recognition of mental health and developmental challenges in young children.

The correct response is option C.

The DSM-PC includes a system for coding "situations" that might be producing a child's symptoms and three clusters of "child manifestations": developmental variations, problems requiring intervention, and disorders (for those children who meet DSM-IV [American Psychiatric Association 1994] criteria for a disorder).

A collaboration between the American Academy of Pediatrics and the American Psychiatric Association (including representatives of the American Academy of Child and Adolescent Psychiatry) produced the DSM-PC, Child and Adolescent Version (American Academy of Pediatrics 1996). This was designed to be used by pediatricians and family physicians to classify emotional and behavioral problems seen in office primary care practice.

The DSM system has very limited utility for infants and toddlers. To address the need for diagnoses and criteria tailored for very young children, the Zero to Three/National Center for Clinical Infant Programs Diagnostic Classification Task Force (1994) developed a diagnostic classification system. This was recently revised (Zero to Three 2005) based on clinical experience using the 1994 system as well as empirical research. The goals of this system are to increase the recognition of mental health and developmental challenges in young children and to use diagnostic criteria effectively. **(p. 66)**

American Academy of Pediatrics: The Classification of Child and Adolescent Mental Diagnoses in Primary Care: Diagnostic and Statistical Manual for Primary Care (DSM-PC), Child and Adolescent Version. Chicago, IL, American Academy of Pediatrics, 1996

American Psychiatric Association: Diagnostic and Statistical Manual of Mental Disorders, 4th Edition. Washington, DC, American Psychiatric Association, 1994

Zero to Three/National Center for Clinical Infant Programs Diagnostic Classification Task Force: Diagnostic Classification of Mental Health and Developmental Disorders of Infancy and Early Childhood. Arlington, VA, The Zero to Three/National Center for Clinical Infant Programs, 1994

Zero to Three: Diagnostic Classification of Mental Health and Developmental Disorders of Infancy and Early Childhood, Revised (DC:0–3R). Arlington, VA, The Zero to Three/National Center for Clinical Infant Programs, 2005

Chapter 6

The Process of Assessment and Diagnosis

Select the single best response for each question.

6.1 Child assessment differs from adult assessment in a number of ways. Which of the following describes aspects of the child assessment that are different from the adult assessment?

    A. Multiple sources constitute the field for data collection with children.

    B. Child assessments frequently require information from the school.

    C. For younger children, verbal communication is much less important than play.

    D. Children rarely seek out an evaluation.

    E. All of the above.

The correct response is option E.

All of the above are differences in the child and adult assessment.

    The prime source of information in the evaluation of an adult is the person himself. Multiple sources, especially the parents, constitute the field for data collection with children. The overwhelming majority of child assessments need information from the school regarding not only academic status but also social relatedness to peers and adults. It would be quite unusual for a psychiatrist to request information from the employer of an adult patient.

    The interchange between psychiatrist and adult patient is generally verbal, with some data gathered from nonverbal communication. Although this is true for most adolescents, the younger the child, the more central the role of play in the evaluation process. How a child plays and what he plays is a window to the child and his world. In assessing the infant or preschool child, there is less emphasis on verbal production, and the clinician needs to be well versed in the popular toys, video games, and so forth, that form an important part of a child's life.

    The issue of volitional participation is another area of difference. Children are brought to the evaluation; they rarely seek it out. Infants and children are brought because, in general, their behavior is bothersome to others, not necessarily to themselves. **(p. 70)**

6.2 In conducting the parent interview, clinicians should *not*

    A. Request information about the child's interests, activities, or strengths.

    B. Ask what preparation the parents have given the child for the evaluation.

    C. Ask parents for their understanding of the problem.

    D. Explain that the evaluation will invariably lead to treatment by the clinician.

    E. Discuss confidentiality of sessions between the child and the clinician.

The correct response is option D.

It is important to make it clear to the parents that an evaluation is not treatment and that it may or may not lead to intervention. The clinician needs to focus on getting the data, formulating the data, arriving at a diagnosis, and establishing a treatment plan (which may or may not involve the evaluating clinician).

The parental interview serves to gather information that may help the clinician in approaching the child, such as favorite activities, interests, and strengths. The parent interview gives the clinician an opportunity to determine what preparation, if any, the parents have given to the child for the evaluation and, if necessary, to recommend other approaches that may facilitate the child's participation. The clinician aims to assess parental understanding of the problem and expectations of the assessment as well as parenting strengths and weaknesses.

The confidentiality of the sessions between the child and the clinician needs to be discussed upfront with the parents and child. Parents are reminded that unless there is an overriding reason (such as a danger to self or others) the specifics of the interactions between the clinician and child are confidential. **(pp. 72–73)**

6.3   Which of the following is the most important source of an outside report the clinicians should obtain (with permission) when assessing a child?

   A. Friends.
   B. Teachers.
   C. Siblings.
   D. Noncaregiving relatives.
   E. Group activities.

The correct response is option B.

The clinician should obtain (with permission) information from others in the child's community. This information gives other viewpoints about the child. Bringing this information back to the interview with parents, child, or family may stimulate further disclosure and discussion essential to diagnosis and treatment. The most important of these "outside" reports is the school report. Teachers spend long periods of time with the child, and they observe the child's response to work demands and learning. They are able to compare the child with same-age peers. The school is also the natural setting for interactions with other children. At school the child's behavior and symptoms can be different from anywhere else. The behavior in school must be compared with the behavior at home and in the office (on a one-to-one basis). **(p. 73)**

6.4   In constructing a case formulation, Ebert et al. (2000) suggested that the clinician examine child and family factors along a time axis and categorize them as predisposing, precipitating, perpetuating, or prognostic. According to this approach, parents going through a divorce would be considered what type of factor?

   A. Predisposing.
   B. Precipitating.
   C. Perpetuating.
   D. Prognostic.
   E. None of the above.

The correct response is option B.

One of the most crucial phases of the evaluation process is the formulation, which is too often misunderstood or neglected. In organizing the formulation, Ebert et al. (2000) suggested looking at factors along a time axis grouped as predisposing, precipitating, perpetuating, and prognostic. *Predisposing factors* are genetic heritability, intrauterine or perinatal insults, neglect, and so on. *Precipitating factors* are defined as stressors that test the coping mechanisms and cause signs and symptoms to occur, such as physical illness, loss, or divorce. *Perpetuating factors* are those that reinforce symptomatology, such as continuous trauma or parental style. *Prognostic factors* are those that influence a child's symptom future, duration of illness, severity of illness, time of onset of illness, and so on. **(p. 74)**

Ebert MH, Loosen PT, Nurcombe B: Current Diagnosis and Treatment in Psychiatry. New York, McGraw-Hill, 2000

6.5   The major purpose of the parental feedback interview is

      A. To develop a concrete treatment plan to help their child.
      B. To gather additional information about the relationship between the child and parents.
      C. To test hypotheses concerning the case formulation.
      D. To inform the parents and child what has been found and what the clinician would recommend to address the issues that led to the assessment.
      E. To provide referral sources to the parents for either further assessment or treatment of their child.

The correct response is option D.

The purpose of the interpretative or feedback interview is to inform the parents and child of what has been found and what the clinician, with their help, would recommend to address the issues for which they came. This often is more complicated than in adult psychiatry, in which one generally has one patient. In the evaluation of a child, both parents and child need to hear and understand what the clinician says, and their participation in the process needs to be encouraged and enlisted. Also, the issues for which they came may be the tip of the iceberg and may lead to discovery of other problems that were not initially apparent. **(pp. 75–76)**

Chapter 7

Diagnostic Interviews

Select the single best response for each question.

7.1 The process of making a psychiatric diagnosis is fraught with numerous potential biases. Which of the following clinician practices is *least* likely to result in a biased diagnosis?

   A. Making diagnoses before all relevant information is collected.
   B. Collecting information selectively.
   C. Neglecting to be systematic in collecting and/or organizing information.
   D. Preventing the clinician's particular expertise from influencing diagnosis assignment.
   E. Assuming correlation between symptoms and illness.

The correct response is option D.

The subjective and variable nature of the symptom reports used to generate psychiatric diagnoses remains a limitation. Information derived from patients, their families, and other observers (e.g., teachers) is subtle, complex, and often conflicting (Achenbach 1987). Clinicians' diagnoses are potentially fraught with numerous biases (Angold 1999), including 1) making diagnoses before all relevant information is collected; 2) collecting information selectively when confirming and/or ruling out a diagnosis; 3) neglecting to be systematic in collecting and organizing information; 4) allowing the clinician's particular expertise to influence diagnosis assignment (e.g., a physician in a mood disorders clinic diagnosing most patients' disorders as depression, regardless of each patient's clinical presentation); and 5) assuming correlations between symptoms and illnesses that in reality are spurious or nonexistent (e.g., equating all irritability with mania). **(pp. 79–80)**

> Achenbach TE: Child/adolescent behavioral and emotional problems: implications of cross-informant correlations for situational specificity. Psychol Bull 101:213–232, 1987
> Angold AF: Interviewer-based interviews, in Diagnostic Assessment in Child and Adolescent Psychopathology. Edited by Shaffer D, Lucas CP, Richters JE. New York, Guilford, 1999, pp 34–64

7.2 Various diagnostic tools have been developed to enhance the reliability of the information gathered and the diagnosis assignment. Which of the following statements is *false*?

   A. Clinicians and researchers commonly use diagnostic interviews and questionnaires.
   B. Patients, parents, and teachers usually complete questionnaires.
   C. Structured diagnostic interviews are primarily used by clinicians in daily clinical practice.
   D. The instruments vary as to whether they are administered by clinicians or trained nonclinical interviewers.
   E. Structured interviews specific for children and adolescents have been developed.

The correct response is option C.

Structured diagnostic interviews are designed to elicit information from children and/or their parents about various aspects of functioning and mental health, including specific inquiries about symptom criteria for psychiatric disorders. They are primarily used for psychiatric research, both in epidemiological surveys and in clinical studies. Structured interviews were first developed to examine mental health problems in adults; interviews for use with children and adolescents and their families were subsequently developed.

The creation of diagnostic criteria helped structure the diagnostic process. However, even when the same diagnostic criteria are used, disagreements may still arise because of differences in wording of the questions or variable interpretations of either the question or the response.

The two types of diagnostic tools commonly used by clinicians and researchers are diagnostic interviews and questionnaires. Questionnaires are usually completed by patients, parents, or other significant individuals (e.g., teachers) and generally focus on broader domains of psychopathology but may focus more narrowly on specific illness states or symptoms.

The instruments vary as to whether they are administered by clinicians or trained interviewers, although some researchers have research assistants administer measures originally designed for use by clinicians. **(p. 80)**

7.3   The term *face validity* refers to

    A. How well a category as defined appears to describe a recognized illness.
    B. How well the category predicts a pertinent aspect of care, such as treatment needs or prognosis.
    C. Whether the category has meaning in terms of what it is designed to describe.
    D. How often different interviews assign the same diagnosis.
    E. How consistently respondents report the same symptoms over time.

The correct response is option A.

Validity reflects the degree to which a measure or classification system accurately characterizes the entity it is examining. Types of validity include *face validity*, or how well a category as defined appears to describe a recognized illness, *predictive validity*, or how well the category predicts a pertinent aspect of care, such as treatment needs or prognosis, and *construct validity*, or whether the category has meaning in terms of what it is designed to describe.

Reliability reflects agreement, including how often different interviewers assign the same diagnosis *(inter-rater reliability)*, how consistently respondents report the same symptoms or diagnoses over time *(test-retest reliability)*, and how internally consistent the measure is (i.e., the degree to which different sections of the measure give similar information). **(pp. 80, 81)**

7.4   "The percentage of individuals in a sample who do not have the disorder and are accurately identified by the interview as not having the disorder" defines which of the following terms?

    A. Sensitivity.
    B. Specificity.
    C. Predictive value positive.
    D. Predictive value negative.
    E. None of the above.

The correct response is option B.

In assessing a diagnostic instrument's utility at identifying cases, the following concepts are important:

- *Sensitivity:*   the percentage of individuals in a sample who have the disorder and are accurately identified by the interview.
- *Specificity:*   the percentage of individuals in a sample who do not have the disorder and are accurately identified by the interview as not having the disorder.
- *Predictive value positive:*   the percentage of individuals in the defined sample positively identified by the interview who actually have the disorder.
- *Predictive value negative:*   the percentage of individuals in the defined sample identified by the interview as not having the disorder who, in fact, do not have the disorder.

(p. 82)

7.5   Interviews are usually described as either structured or semistructured, depending on how much freedom the interviewer has to ask questions and interpret the responses. *Semistructured* interviews are designed for clinical research and allow the interviewer some leeway in wording questions and interpreting responses. All of the following instruments are semistructured *except*

    A. Schedule for Affective Disorders and Schizophrenia for School-Aged Children—Present and Lifetime (K-SADS-PL).
    B. Washington University Schedule for Affective Disorders and Schizophrenia for School-Aged Children (WASH-U-KSADS).
    C. Schedule for Affective Disorders and Schizophrenia for School-Aged Children—Epidemiological (K-SADS-E).
    D. Anxiety Disorders Interview Schedule for DSM-IV: Child and Parent Version (ADIS-CP).
    E. National Institute of Mental Health Diagnostic Interview Schedule for Children Version IV (NIMH DISC-IV).

The correct response is option E.

Structured interviews are designed for epidemiological research and typically follow a set script, allowing them to be administered by trained nonclinical interviewers. The NIMH DISC-IV is a *structured* interview.

Semistructured interviews are designed for clinical research and usually allow the interviewer some leeway in wording questions and interpreting responses. These instruments are generally preferred by clinicians. **(pp. 82–83; see also Table 7–1)**

Chapter 8

Rating Scales

Select the single best response for each question.

8.1   Which of the following terms is used to describe whether a scale is stable over time?

    A. Internal reliability.
    B. Interrater reliability.
    C. Test-retest reliability.
    D. Reliability.
    E. Psychometric properties.

The correct response is option C.

Test-retest reliability, or stability, assesses whether a scale is stable over time.

    Internal reliability, or internal consistency, represents the degree to which individual items are consistent with each other. Items that are not internally consistent detract from the scale.

    Interrater reliability represents the agreement, or concordance, between different informants.

    Reliability refers to the consistency with which a scale's items measure the same construct, the same way, every time. Lack of reliability is termed *random error*.

    Psychometric properties estimate the measurement error to determine whether a scale is appropriate for an application. **(p. 90)**

8.2   Which of the following types of concurrent validity is defined as the extent of correlation of related variables?

    A. Content validity.
    B. Face validity.
    C. Criterion validity.
    D. Discriminative validity.
    E. Convergent validity.

The correct response is option E.

There are two types of concurrent validity: *discriminative validity* compares scores for groups that do and do not have a characteristic; *convergent validity* is the extent of correlation of related variables.

    Validity indicates whether a scale accurately assesses what it was designed to assess. *Content validity* assesses whether the scale's items represent the construct being measured. *Face validity* is a type of content validity that is determined by subjectively judging whether items measure the content area. *Criterion validity* is assessed in relation to other scales with established validity in measuring the same construct. There are two subtypes: *predictive validity* asks whether the scale correlates with an event that will occur in the future; *concurrent validity* refers to a scale's correlation with an event assessed at the same time the scale is administered. **(p. 90)**

8.3   A "broad-band" rating scale that includes multiple versions for different reporters and age groups and that can be scored using factors that approximate DSM-IV-TR (American Psychiatric Association 2000) diagnostic criteria is

A. The Behavior Assessment System for Children, 2nd Edition (BASC-2).
B. The Child Behavior Checklist (CBCL).
C. The Child Symptom Inventories (CSI).
D. The Eyberg Child Behavior Inventory (ECBI).
E. The Sutter-Eyberg Student Behavior Inventory-Revised (SESBI-R).

The correct response is option B.

The CBCL (Achenbach and Rescorla 2000, 2001) has been the gold standard for research and clinical work among broad-band behavior rating scales since its development in the 1960s. The CBCL has multiple versions for different reporters and age groups, including the parent-report (CBCL) and Teacher Report Form (TRF) for youths 6–18 years old, the CBCL for preschoolers (CBCL/1½–5), the Caregiver-Teacher Report Form for pre-schoolers (C-TRF), and the Youth Self-Report (YSR) for youths over 11 years old. These scales were updated in 2001 with new normative data and several modifications to item content and subscale structure. In addition to the problem behavior domains familiar to users of earlier versions of the CBCL (e.g., anxious/depressed, so-matic complaints, aggressive behavior), all of the newer scales can also be scored using factors that approximate the diagnostic criteria of DSM-IV-TR (American Psychiatric Association 2000).

The BASC-2 (Reynolds and Kamphaus 2004) is an updated version of the BASC, a widely used broad-band measure of behavior problems. The BASC-2 includes a Parent Rating Scale (PRS) and a Teacher Rating Scale (TRS). In addition to individual clinical scales, the TRS and PRS provide composite scores for internalizing, ex-ternalizing, adaptive skills, and behavioral symptom index, an overall measure of problem behaviors.

The CSI (Gadow and Sprafkin 1997, 1998, 2002) are a series of scales based on DSM-IV (American Psy-chiatric Association 1994) diagnostic criteria for multiple disorders. The disorders covered vary by age group but include the most common disorders of childhood and adolescence as well as less common disorders such as schizophrenia, reactive attachment disorder, and somatization disorder.

The non-broad-band ECBI and SESBI-R (Eyberg and Pincus 1999) are well-established scales for assessing externalizing behaviors corresponding to diagnoses of attention-deficit/hyperactivity disorder (ADHD), oppo-sitional defiant disorder (ODD), and conduct disorder. The ECBI is completed by parents and the SESBI-R by teachers. These scales use the same format with item overlap. Respondents rate each item on two dimensions: an Intensity Scale (I) assesses behavior frequency, and a Problem Scale (P) assesses reporters' perception of whether the behavior is problematic. **(pp. 91–94)**

Achenbach TM, Rescorla LA: Manual for the ASEBA School-age Forms and Profiles. Burlington, VT, University of Vermont Research Center for Children, Youth, and Families, 2000

Achenbach TM, Rescorla LA: Manual for the ASEBA Preschool Forms and Profiles. Burlington, VT, University of Vermont Research Center for Children, Youth, and Families, 2001

American Psychiatric Association: Diagnostic and Statistical Manual of Mental Disorders, 4th Edition. Washing-ton, DC, American Psychiatric Association, 1994

American Psychiatric Association: Diagnostic and Statistical Manual of Mental Disorders, 4th Edition, Text Re-vision. Washington, DC, American Psychiatric Association, 2000

Eyberg S, Pincus D: Eyberg Child Behavior Inventory and Sutter-Eyberg Student Behavior Inventory-Revised Professional Manual. Odessa, FL, Psychological Assessment Resources, 1999

Gadow KD, Sprafkin J: Early Childhood Inventory, 4: Norms Manual. Stony Brook, NY, Checkmate Plus, 1997

Gadow KD, Sprafkin J: Adolescent Symptom Inventory, 4: Norms Manual. Stony Brook, NY, Checkmate Plus, 1998

Gadow KD, Sprafkin J: Childhood Symptom Inventory-4 Screening and Norms Manual. Stony Brook, NY, Checkmate Plus, 2002

Reynolds CR, Kamphaus RW: Behavior Assessment System for Children, 2nd Edition Manual. Circle Pines, MN, American Guidance Service Publishing, 2004

8.4 Of the following rating scales, which assesses the same aspects of depression with adolescents that it assesses with adults and additionally discriminates depressed teens from those with anxiety and conduct disorders?

    A. Children's Depression Inventory (CDI).
    B. Children's Depression Rating Scale-Revised (CDRS-R).
    C. Reynolds Adolescent Depression Scale (RADS).
    D. Beck Depression Inventory-II (BDI-II).
    E. Reynolds Child Depression Scale (RCDS).

The correct response is option D.

The BDI-II (Beck 1996) is the most popular depression-rating scale for adolescents. It assesses the same aspects of depression with adolescents that it assesses with adults: cognitive, behavioral, affective, and somatic. Most impressively, the BDI-II discriminates outpatient depressed teens from those with anxiety and conduct disorders. The BDI-II is likely most effective at assessing depression in adolescents.

The CDI (Kovacs 1992) is a downward extension of the BDI to preadolescents, although it is also used with teens. It is the most studied and utilized scale of juvenile depression.

The CDRS-R (Poznanski and Mokros 1999) is a clinician-rated scale patterned on the Hamilton Depression Rating Scale but developed specifically for children and widely used with teens. It has three unique features: it integrates information from both child and parent, includes behaviors observed during the interview, and contains several items that are not specific to depression.

The RADS (Reynolds 1987) and the RCDS (Reynolds 1989) are two related scales based on DSM-III (American Psychiatric Association 1980) criteria for depression. They have parent versions. These scales have shown very good reliability and convergent validity with multiple samples. They function well with diverse samples of ethnically heterogeneous community and clinical samples, although their main use has been in the schools. They offer the opportunity to assess children and adolescents with similar but developmentally suitable scales, making them useful for longitudinal applications. **(pp. 98–102)**

American Psychiatric Association: Diagnostic and Statistical Manual of Mental Disorders, 3rd Edition. Washington, DC, American Psychiatric Association, 1980

Beck AT: Beck Depression Inventory (BDI-II) Manual, 2nd Edition. San Antonio, TX, The Psychological Corporation, 1996

Kovacs M: Children's Depression Inventory Manual. North Tonawanda, NY, Multi-Health Systems, 1992

Poznanski EO, Mokros HB: Children's Depression Rating Scale-Revised (CDRS-R). Los Angeles, CA, Western Psychological Services, 1999

Reynolds WM: Reynolds Adolescent Depression Scale: Professional Manual. Odessa, FL, Psychological Assessment Resources, 1987

Reynolds WM: Reynolds Child Depression Scale: Professional Manual. Odessa, FL, Psychological Assessment Resources, 1989

8.5 A friend contacts you and expresses concern that her 8-year-old son may have attention-deficit/hyperactivity disorder (ADHD). She asks if there is a good rating scale available at no cost that a parent can use. You tell her to search online for the following:

    A. Vanderbilt ADHD Parent Rating Scale (VADPRS).
    B. Conners' Rating Scale–Revised (CRS-R).
    C. ADHD Rating Scale–IV (ADHD-RS-IV).
    D. Social Communication Questionnaire (SCQ).
    E. Vineland Adaptive Behavior Scales, 2nd Edition (VABS-II).

The correct response is option A.

The VADPRS (Wolraich 2003a) and the Vanderbilt ADHD Teacher Rating Scale (VADTRS) (Wolraich 2003b) are DSM-IV (American Psychiatric Association)–based scales that are free online (www.nichq.org). Similar to the Conners scales, both parent-report (Wolraich et al. 2003) and teacher-report (Wolraich et al. 1998) forms are available.

The CRS-R (Conners 2002) covers core ADHD subscales as well as comorbid problems, such as oppositional defiant disorder (ODD) and conduct disorder. There are both regular and abbreviated versions for the parent, teacher, and youth self-report forms. The multiple indices of problem areas along with a normative base, strong psychometrics, and multiple uses make the CRS-R excellent for comprehensive assessment.

The ADHD-RS-IV (DuPaul et al. 1998) is a brief scale that is directly derived from DSM-IV criteria for ADHD with the expected ADHD subscales. It does not address comorbid disorders. It can be completed by parents (home form) and teachers (school form). Cutoff scores are provided for multiple percentiles to allow variable guidelines for interpretation. The ADHD-RS-IV is important in several regards. This is one of the most extensively studied ADHD scales, with strong psychometric properties including being one of few ADHD scales to have established test-retest reliability, considerable evidence of discriminative validity, sensitivity to medication effects, and cross-cultural validity (Dopfner et al. 2006; Swanson et al. 2006).

The SCQ (Rutter et al. 2003), previously known as the Autism Screening Questionnaire, is a parent-report measure used specifically to screen children for deficits in social skills or communication. It is based on the Autism Diagnostic Interview, and items correspond to DSM-IV criteria for the diagnosis of autism.

VABS-II (Sparrow et al. 2005) comprises the prototypical measure of functioning. The original version of the VABS has been used extensively, particularly with youth diagnosed with developmental impairments. The VABS-II has recently been released and includes a number of improvements, including current norms and a wider age range. It is completed as a semistructured interview with caregivers of individuals from birth through adulthood. **(pp. 94–97)**

American Psychiatric Association: Diagnostic and Statistical Manual of Mental Disorders, 4th Edition. Washington, DC, American Psychiatric Association, 1994

Conners CK: Conners Rating Scales–Revised. North Tonawanda, NY, Multi-Health Systems, 2002

Dopfner M, Steinhausen HC, Coghill D, et al: Cross-cultural reliability and validity of ADHD assessed by the ADHD Rating Scale in a pan-European study. European Child and Adolescent Psychiatry 15:46–55, 2006

DuPaul GJ, Power TJ, Anastopoulos AD, et al: ADHD Rating Scale-IV: Checklist, Norms, and Clinical Interpretation. New York, Guilford, 1998

Rutter M, Bailey A, Lord C, et al: Social Communication Questionnaire. Los Angeles, CA, Western Psychological Services, 2003

Sparrow SS, Balla DA, Cicchetti DV: Interview Edition Survey Form Manual: Vineland Adaptive Behavior Scales. Minneapolis, MN, NCS Pearson Assessments, 2005

Swanson JM, Greenhill LL, Lopez FA, et al: Modafinil film coated tablets in children and adolescents with attention-deficit/hyperactivity disorder: results of a randomized, double-blind, placebo-controlled, fixed dose study followed by abrupt discontinuation. J Clin Psychiatry 67:137–147, 2006

Wolraich ML: Vanderbilt ADHD Parent Rating Scale (VADPRS). Cambridge, MA, American Academy of Pediatrics and The National Initiative for Children's Healthcare Quality, 2003a

Wolraich ML: Vanderbilt ADHD Teacher Rating Scale (VADTRS). Cambridge, MA, American Academy of Pediatrics and The National Initiative for Children's Healthcare Quality, 2003b

Wolraich ML, Feurer ID, Hannah JN, et al: Obtaining systematic teacher reports of disruptive behavior disorders utilizing DSM-IV. J Abnorm Child Psychol 26:141–152, 1998

Wolraich ML, Lambert W, Doffing MA, et al: Psychometric properties of the Vanderbilt ADHD diagnostic parent rating scale in a referred population. J Pediatr Psychol 28:559–567, 2003

Chapter 9

Pediatric Evaluation and Laboratory Testing

Select the single best response for each question.

9.1 A comprehensive medical history, the use of collateral informants, and close collaboration with the pediatric provider are essential in the evaluation of children and adolescents who present with psychiatric and behavioral symptoms. All of the following statements are correct *except*

    A. The presence of regular pediatric visits, well-child visits, and immunizations as scheduled should be established.

    B. History gathering begins with the child's delivery.

    C. A history of labor and delivery, including gestational age, Apgar scores, nature of delivery, and complications, should be reviewed.

    D. History gathering should include the family pedigree and family medical and psychiatric history.

    E. Family history of sudden cardiac death and hypercholesterolemia may need to be elicited.

The correct response is option B.

History gathering begins with the child's conception, gestation, and delivery. Questions about the circumstances of conception, prenatal care, ease of pregnancy or complications, and their treatments should be asked. A history of in utero exposure to medications, substances, and environmental toxins should be obtained, as well as any history of travel that may have taken place outside of the country and associated immunizations that occurred during the pregnancy. A history of labor and delivery should be reviewed and should include gestational age, Apgar scores, nature of delivery, and complications such as hyperbilirubinemia, respiratory distress, infections, or congenital abnormalities (Thomas et al. 1997).

    A comprehensive medical history, the use of collateral informants, and close collaboration with the pediatric provider is essential in the evaluation of children and adolescents who present with psychiatric and behavioral symptoms. The history gathering should include the family pedigree and review of the family medical and psychiatric history from both parents, with emphasis on diseases or disorders that may present initially in very young children. Specific inquiries about a family history of sudden cardiac death and hypercholesterolemia are relevant in children who may be treated with psychotropic medications. **(pp. 111–112)**

> Thomas JM, Benham AL, Gean M, et al: Practice parameters for the psychiatric assessment of infants and toddlers (0–36 months). J Am Acad Child Adolesc Psychiatry 36 (suppl):21S–36S, 1997

9.2 Assessing a child's development is an integral component of the overall medical evaluation. All of the following statements are accurate *except*

    A. The Denver Development Screening Tool (DDST) is used for children up to 6 years of age.

    B. The medical history for the 6- to 11-year-old child focuses on growth, development, and skills acquisition.

    C. During the period between 6 and 11 years of age, the head grows rapidly.

    D. Adolescent physical development is characterized by physical growth and sexual development.

    E. The peak of growth in male adolescents comes 2–3 years later than that in females.

The correct response is option C.

Middle childhood (ages 6–11 years) is characterized by physical growth, with episodic growth spurts lasting approximately 8 weeks and final growth at an average rate of 3–3.5 kg and 6–7 cm per year. Head growth slows during this phase of development, reflecting a slowing of brain growth, with head circumference increasing only about 2–3 centimeters from 6 to 11 years of age.

A detailed investigation of the child's development is an integral component of a psychiatric assessment (American Academy of Pediatrics Committee on Children with Disabilities 2001, 2006). One of the scales most commonly used by pediatricians is the DDST to screen for developmental problems in children up to 6 years of age (Frankenburg et al. 1975). The screen assesses gross and fine motor, personal/social, and language development. Corrections and allowance are made for prematurity until 2 years of age.

The medical history for the 6- to 11-year-old child (middle childhood) focuses on growth, development, and skills acquisition.

Adolescent physical development is characterized by physical growth and sexual development. Between 10 and 20 years of age, youths undergo rapid changes in body structure as well as changes in psychological and social development. Hormonal interactions result in a complex and predictable pattern of sexual and physical development starting at approximately 10 years of age in girls and approximately 13 years of age in boys. Growth acceleration for both sexes also occurs at this time, with increased growth velocity beginning in early adolescence and peaking at sexual maturity, with boys typically peaking 2–3 years after girls have stopped growing. **(p. 112)**

American Academy of Pediatrics Committee on Children with Disabilities: Developmental surveillance and screening of infants and young children. Pediatrics 108:192–196, 2001

American Academy of Pediatrics Committee on Children with Disabilities: Identifying infants and young children with developmental disorders in the medical home: an algorithm for developmental surveillance and screening. Pediatrics 118:405–420, 2006

Frankenburg WK, Dodds J, Fandal A: Denver Developmental Screening Test. Denver, CO, LADOCA, 1975

9.3   Which of the following syndromes has a recognizable behavioral phenotype?

    A. Fragile X syndrome.
    B. Prader-Willi syndrome.
    C. Angelman's syndrome.
    D. Turner syndrome.
    E. All of the above.

The correct response is option E.

Preschool- and school-age children who have genetic syndromes that were not discovered pre- or postnatally may present for an initial assessment with social-emotional or behavioral concerns as their chief complaint. Some of these genetic disorders have recognizable behavioral phenotypes (King et al. 2005) (Table 9–1). **(pp. 112–113, 114 [Table 9–1])**

King BH, Hodapp RM, Dykins EM: Mental retardation. Kaplan and Sadock's Comprehensive Textbook of Psychiatry, 8th Edition. Edited by Kaplan HI, Sadock BJ. Baltimore, MD, Lippincott Williams & Wilkins, 2005, pp 3076–3106

Benarroch F, Hirsch HJ, Gentsil L, et al: Prader-Willi syndrome: medical prevention and behavioral challenges. Child Adolesc Psychiatr Clin North Am 16:695–708, 2007

Buntinx IM, Hennekam RC, Brouwer OF, et al: Clinical profile of Angelman syndrome at different ages. Am J Med Genet 56:176–183, 1995

Collacott RA, Cooper SA, Branford D, et al: Behavior phenotype for Down's syndrome. Br J Psychiatry 172:85–89, 1998

Table 9–1.   Selected genetic syndromes with behavioral phenotypes

Syndrome	Behavioral phenotype
Angelman's syndrome	Developmental delay, hyperactivity diminishing with age, short attention span (Buntinx et al. 1995)
Cornelia de Lange's (Brachmann de Lange) syndrome	Developmental delay, hyperactivity, self-injury, aggression, sleep disturbance, diminished social relatedness, repetitive and stereotyped behaviors, "autistic-like" behaviors (Hyman et al. 2002)
Down syndrome	Developmental delay, stubbornness, inattention, opposition, depression and dementia (adults) (Collacott et al. 1998)
Fetal alcohol syndrome	Cognitive deficits, hyperactivity, short attention span, distractibility, impaired concentration, withdrawal (Kelly et al. 2000)
Fragile X syndrome	Cognitive deficits, inattention, hyperactivity, distractibility, disturbance in language/communication, social anxiety, social deficits, poor eye contact, cognitive abnormalities (Reiss and Hall 2007)
Lesch-Nyhan syndrome	Self-injurious behavior, self-biting, compulsive behaviors, coprolalia, copropraxia (Jinnah and Friedman 2000)
Neurofibromatosis I	Attentional problems, social withdrawal, hyperactivity, cognitive deficits (Lewis et al. 2004)
Noonan syndrome	Cognitive deficits, social problems, attention deficits, anxiety (Verhoeven et al. 2008).
Prader-Willi syndrome	Developmental delay, excessive food-seeking behaviors, oppositional behaviors, interpersonal problems, repetitive behaviors, affective dysregulation, and increased risk of ADHD, obsessive-compulsive disorder, and mood and psychotic symptoms (Benarroch et al. 2007)
Rett syndrome	Autistic symptoms, including loss of language and repetitive stereotypic behaviors (Ben Zeev Ghidoni 2007).
Rubenstein-Taybi syndrome	Developmental delay, short attention span, impulsivity, moodiness, hyperacusis, autistic behaviors (Stevens et al. 1999)
Smith-Lemli-Opitz syndrome	Self-stimulation, self-destructive behaviors, autism spectrum disorders (Sikora et al. 2006)
Smith-Magenis syndrome	Affective lability, temper tantrums, impulsivity, anxiety, physical aggression, destruction, argumentativeness, sleep difficulties (Shelley and Robertson 2005)
Sotos syndrome	Cognitive deficits, social deficits, peer difficulties (De Boer et al. 2006)
Tuberous sclerosis complex	Attention deficits, hyperactivity, impulsivity, learning disability, cognitive deficits (Lewis et al. 2004)
Turner syndrome	Uneven cognitive profile, increased risks of anxiety, low self-esteem, depression related to physical appearance (Kesler 2007)
Velocardiofacial syndrome (22q11 deletion)	Cognitive deficits; repetitive, stereotyped behaviors; higher rates of ADHD, anxiety disorders, affective disorders, and psychotic disorders; autistic spectrum disorders (Gothelf 2007)
Williams syndrome	Cognitive unevenness, hypersociability, social anxiety, fears, inattention, hyperactivity, hyperacusis (Feinstein and Singh 2007)

Note.   ADHD = attention-deficit/hyperactivity disorder.

De Boer L, Roder I, Wit JM: Psychosocial, cognitive, and motor functioning in patients with suspected Sotos syndrome: a comparison between patients with and without NSD1 gene alterations. Dev Med Child Neurol 48:582–588, 2006

Feinstein C, Singh S: Social phenotypes in neurogenetic syndromes. Child Adolesc Psychiatr Clin North Am 16:631–647, 2007

Ben Zeev Ghidoni B: Rett syndrome. Child Adolesc Psychiatr Clin N Am 16:723–743, 2007

Gothelf D: Velocardiofacial syndrome. Child Adolesc Psychiatr Clin North Am 16:677–693, 2007

Hyman P, Oliver C, Hall S: Self injurious behavior, self restraint and compulsive behaviors in Cornelia de Lange syndrome. Am J Ment Retard 107:146–154, 2002

Jinnah GA, Friedman T: Lesch-Nyhan disease and its variants, in The Molecular and Metabolic Basis of Inherited Disease, 6th Edition. Edited by Scriver CR, Sly WS, Childs B, et al. New York, McGraw-Hill, 2000, pp 2537–2570

Kelly SJ, Day N, Streissguth AP: Effects of prenatal alcohol exposure on social behavior in humans and other species. Neurotoxicol Teratol 22:143–149, 2000

Kesler SR: Turner syndrome. Child Adolesc Psychiatr Clin North Am 16:709–722, 2007

Lewis JC, Thomas HV, Murphy KC, et al: Genotype and psychological phenotype in tuberous sclerosis. J Med Genet 41:203–207, 2004

Reiss AL, Hall SS: Fragile X syndrome: assessment and treatment implications. Child Adolesc Psychiatr Clin N Am 16:663–675, 2007

Shelley BP, Robertson MM: The neuropsychiatry and multisystem features of the Smith-Magenis syndrome: a review. J Neuropsychiatry Clin Neurosci 17:91–97, 2005

Sikora DM, Pettit-Kekel K, Penfield J, et al: Smith-Lemli Opitz (SLOS). Am J Med Genet A 140:1511–1518, 2006

Stevens CA, Schmitt C, Sperger S: Behavior in Rubenstein-Taybi syndrome. Proc Genet Ctr 18:144–145, 1999

Verhoeven W, Wingbermuhle E, Egger J, et al: Noonan syndrome: psychological and psychiatric aspects. Am J Med Genet A 146A:191–196, 2008

9.4   All of the following baseline laboratory assessments should be obtained when children and adolescents present with behavioral symptoms whose history or physical findings suggest an organic etiology *except*

   A.   Complete blood count.
   B.   Renal function tests.
   C.   Hepatic function tests.
   D.   Thyroid function tests.
   E.   Lipid profile.

The correct response is option E.

A lipid profile is not necessary in children and adolescents with behavioral symptoms whose history or physical findings suggest an organic etiology. Baseline tests should include complete blood count; serum electrolytes; blood glucose; renal, hepatic, and thyroid function tests, urinalysis, and drug screening, both urine and serum. **(p. 119; see also Table 9–3)**

9.5   Which of the following statements regarding cardiac risk and assessment of children and adolescents is *false?*

   A.   Cardiac evaluation and testing are suggested if positive for a family or medical history of sudden cardiac death, symptoms of palpitation, fainting, chest pain, exercise intolerance, arrhythmia, syncope, and hypertension.
   B.   Electrocardiograms (ECGs) are often used in psychiatric practice for monitoring the effects of drugs known to adversely affect cardiac function.
   C.   An ECG should be obtained prior to initiation of certain psychotropic medications.
   D.   Lithium can potentially cause benign reversible T-wave changes and impair SA nodal function.
   E.   Current recommendations advocate routine ECGs before initiating stimulant treatment.

The correct response is option E.

The current policy recommendation is that healthy children do not need an ECG before initiating stimulant treatment (Perrin et al. 2008).

Current recommendations for the assessment of children and adolescents in psychiatric practice do not include routine ECGs for screening. A family or medical history of sudden cardiac death, symptoms of palpitations, fainting, exercise intolerance, chest pain, arrhythmias, syncope, and hypertension would suggest further cardiac evaluation and testing (Vetter et al. 2008). ECGs are most commonly used in psychiatric practice for monitoring the effects of medications known to adversely affect cardiac function or in those individuals with psychiatric disorders known to occur with cardiac symptoms, such as individuals with eating disorders who purge (hypokalemia).

Medications used in psychiatric practice that have cardiac effects include the tricyclic antidepressants (TCAs), the antipsychotic medications ziprasidone and thioridazine, and lithium. Clinicians using these medications should obtain an ECG prior to initiation and perform regular ECG monitoring, especially when used in high doses or when combined with other QTc-prolonging agents. Lithium therapy can cause benign reversible T-wave changes and impair SA nodal function, suggesting that an ECG should be obtained prior to initiation. **(pp. 119–120)**

Perrin JM, Friedman RA, Knilans TK: Cardiovascular monitoring and stimulant drugs for attention-deficit/hyperactivity disorder. Pediatrics 122:451–453, 2008

Vetter VL, Elia J, Erickson C, et al: Cardiovascular monitoring of children and adolescents with heart disease receiving medications for attention-deficit/hyperactivity disorder: a scientific statement from the American Heart Association Council on Cardiovascular Disease in the Young, Congenital Cardiac Defects Committee, and the Council on Cardiovascular Nursing. Circulation 117:2407–2426, 2008

C h a p t e r   1 0

Neurological Examination, Electroencephalography, and Neuroimaging

Select the single best response for each question.

10.1 Which of the following are characteristic of upper motor neuron lesions?

    A. Bilateral distribution.
    B. Flaccid paralysis.
    C. Hypotonia.
    D. Decreased or absent deep tendon reflexes.
    E. Babinski reflex positive.

The correct response is option E.

Characteristics of upper motor neuron lesions include a positive Babinski reflex; spastic paralysis with hypertonia; accompanying encephalopathy, developmental delay, mental retardation, and seizures; asymmetric distribution of cortical lesions; and increased deep tendon reflexes.

    Flaccid paralysis with hypotonia, generally preserved mental status, bilateral distribution of lesions, decreased or absent deep tendon reflexes, absent Babinski reflex, and fasciculations and fibrillations are characteristics of lower motor neuron lesions. **(p. 125 [Table 10–2])**

10.2 Which part of the neurological examination is the least objective in the nonverbal and/or young patient?

    A. Motor examination.
    B. Sensory examination.
    C. Coordination assessment.
    D. Gait examination.
    E. Cranial nerve assessment.

The correct response is option B.

The sensory examination can be challenging and is the least objective part of the examination in the nonverbal and/or young patient.

    The motor examination typically consists of assessment of muscle tone and strength. However, children younger than 4 years typically cannot understand directions adequately for a full muscular strength assessment. In such patients, having the patient perform different tasks will give at minimum an idea of how the muscles oppose gravity and whether they can withstand the resistance of their own body (e.g., getting up from the prone position without using furniture).

    Coordination assessment may be accomplished by holding toys so the patient has to reach across the midline to reach them—any tremors, dysmetria, or dyscoordination may be noted.

Gait should be assessed in all patients, as observation of the trunk and limbs is important. If the patient wears any splints or uses any assistive devices, he or she should ideally be observed with and without them.

Cranial nerve assessment is easily observed during the interview. Any asymmetry should be further evaluated during the extremity motor examination to elucidate whether this represents only facial involvement or the whole body and whether this would localize to the peripheral nerve, brainstem, or contralateral motor cortex. **(pp. 124–125)**

10.3   Which part of the neurological examination may be accomplished by holding toys so that the patient has to reach across the midline to reach them?

    A. Motor examination.
    B. Sensory examination.
    C. Coordination assessment.
    D. Gait assessment.
    E. Cranial nerve assessment.

The correct response is option C.

Coordination assessment may be accomplished by holding toys so the patient has to reach across the midline to reach them—any tremors, dysmetria, or dyscoordination may be noted. **(p. 125)**

10.4   Which of the following EEG rhythms are the predominant pattern when children are awake with their eyes closed?

    A. Delta.
    B. Theta.
    C. Alpha.
    D. Beta.
    E. None of the above.

The correct response is option C.

EEG waves are highly influenced by the patient's state (i.e., whether the patient is alert and awake, drowsy, or asleep) and age, as well as by the presence of medications, structural lesions, and disease states. Typical rhythms are classified according to their frequency as delta (1–3/sec), theta (4–7/sec), alpha (8–12/sec), and beta (13–20/sec). Delta can be seen in deeper stages of sleep and also in pathological states, such as encephalopathy. Alpha is the predominant pattern while awake with the eyes closed, best seen in the posterior head leads. Beta can be seen during sleep states, particularly in infants and children, and can also be seen in patients who have received medications such as benzodiazepines. Theta waves can be seen during awake states in children, although more commonly in drowsy states. **(pp. 126–127)**

10.5   Which of the following EEG findings commonly reflect primary generalized epilepsy and may be elicited by hyperventilation or photic stimulation?

    A. Spike and slow-wave discharges.
    B. Sharp and slow-wave complex discharges.
    C. Focal epileptiform discharges.
    D. Periodic lateralized epileptiform discharges.
    E. Rhythmic slowing.

The correct response is option A.

Spike and slow-wave discharges are reflective of primary generalized epilepsy.

Sharp and slow-wave complex discharges may be seen in patients with tonic seizures, who may have accompanying developmental delay or mental retardation (i.e., Lennox-Gastaut syndrome). Focal epileptiform discharges may be seen in patients with partial-onset seizures. Periodic lateralized epileptiform discharges reflect acute or subacute infection, vascular insult, or trauma. Rhythmic slowing may be related to structural lesions, a recent seizure, encephalopathy, or migraine. **(p. 128 [Table 10–3])**

Chapter 11

Psychological and Neuropsychological Testing

Select the single best response for each question.

11.1 According to the American Education Research Association, clinically relevant requirements for the ethical administration and interpretation of tests include all of the following *except*

   A. Test publishers have a number of responsibilities.
   B. Test users must be qualified in the area in which they are conducting an assessment.
   C. Testing must be guided by the best interests of the patient.
   D. Decisions must be based on test data that are current.
   E. Tests must be ready for readministration within 1 year.

The correct response is option E.

A given instrument typically is not readministered within 1 year because of "practice effects," which may artificially raise scores (Hausknecht et al. 2007).

Widely accepted standards for psychological and educational testing, published in 1985 and revised in 1999, outline requirements for the ethical administration and interpretation of tests (American Educational Research Association et al. 1999). Clinically relevant highlights include the following:

* *Test publishers have a number of responsibilities.* Test manuals must describe the test's construction, reliability and validity studies, and normative data. Tests must be marketed responsibly, including information regarding any potential for misuse and other limitations, such as the degree of appropriateness for nonnative English speakers, people from countries other than the United States, and people with various types of motor or sensory impairments.
* *Test users must be qualified* in the areas in which they are conducting an assessment. Typically, those qualified to perform testing are licensed, doctoral-level psychologists and their trainees and employees who have been appropriately trained and are working under their supervision.
* *Testing must be guided by the best interests of the patient.*
* *Decisions must be based on test data that are current.* As a general rule, tests conducted within the past year are considered current.

(p. 136)

American Educational Research Association, American Psychological Association, National Council on Measurement in Education: Standards for Educational and Psychological Testing, 3rd Edition. Washington, DC, American Educational Research Association, 1999

Hausknecht JP, Halpert JA, Di Paolo NT, et al: Retesting in selection: a meta-analysis of coaching and practice effects for tests of cognitive ability. J Appl Psychol 92:373–385, 2007

11.2 A psychological test must be appropriately constructed and standardized. Interpretation is based on some type of standardized score, which in turn is based on the standard deviation (SD), or dispersion, of test scores for the sample. Correct statements regarding the SD include all of the following *except*

    A. About 68% of scores fall within one standard deviation of the mean.
    B. 80% of scores fall within two standard deviations.
    C. For most tests, the mean of standardized scores is low.
    D. Some tests are constructed with a mean of 50.
    E. Some tests are constructed with a mean of 0.

The correct response is option B.

Just over 95% of scores fall within two standard deviations of the mean.

About 68% of scores fall within one standard deviation of the mean. For many psychological tests, the standardized scores are constructed so that the mean is 100 and the standard deviation is 15 points. However, some tests are constructed with a mean of 50 and a standard deviation of 10 points (referred to as *t* scores), and some are constructed with a mean of 0 and a standard deviation of 1 (referred to as *z* scores). **(pp. 136–137)**

11.3 Which of the following is the correct definition of reliability?

    A. The degree to which the test measures what it claims to measure.
    B. The degree to which the questions and tasks are representative of the universe of behavior the test was designed to sample.
    C. A test that, if repeated or if administered by another examiner, would yield approximately the same score.
    D. The extent to which a test estimates a person's performance on some outcome measure or criterion.
    E. A theoretical, intangible quality or trait in which individuals differ.

The correct response is option C.

A test must have adequate *reliability*. This means that a test, if repeated or if administered by another examiner, would yield approximately the same score within acceptable measurement error.

A test also must have adequate *validity*. The generally accepted definition of validity is the degree to which the test measures what it claims to measure (Gregory 2007, p. 121).

Content validity is determined by "the degree to which the questions, tasks, or items on a test are representative of the universe of behavior the test was designed to sample" (Gregory 2007).

Criterion-related validity refers to the extent to which a test estimates a person's performance on some outcome measure, or criterion.

Construct validity is the most complex type of validity. A construct is some theoretical, intangible quality or trait in which individuals differ (Messick 1995). Tests are designed to tap underlying constructs. **(p. 137)**

Gregory RJ: Psychological Testing: History, Principles, and Applications, 5th Edition. Boston, MA, Allyn & Bacon, 2007
Messick S: Validity of psychological assessment: validation of inferences from persons' responses and performances as scientific inquiry into score meaning. Am Psychol 50:741–749, 1995

11.4 All of the following are IQ tests *except*

    A. Stanford-Binet.
    B. Wechsler Intelligence Scale for Children.
    C. Differential Ability Scales.
    D. Bayley-III.
    E. Kaufman.

The correct response is option D.

The instruments sometimes referred to as "IQ tests" are individually administered tests designed to provide an overall appraisal of an individual's intellectual ability as well as variability (strengths and weaknesses) in particular areas. The Bayley Scales of Infant and Toddler Development, Third Edition (Bayley-III; Bayley 2005) (for ages 1–42 months) is not considered an IQ test.

Commonly used tests of intellectual ability include the Stanford-Binet Intelligence Scales, 5th Edition (Roid 2003); Wechsler Intelligence Scale for Children, 4th Edition (Wechsler 2003); Differential Ability Scales, 2nd Edition (Elliott 2007); Kaufman Assessment Battery for Children, 2nd Edition (Kaufman and Kaufman 2004); and Woodcock-Johnson Tests of Cognitive Abilities and Achievement, 3rd Edition (Woodcock et al. 2001). **(pp. 138, 143)**

Bayley N: Bayley Scales of Infant and Toddler Development, 3rd Edition. San Antonio, TX, Harcourt Assessment, 2005

Elliott CD: Differential Ability Scales, 2nd Edition. San Antonio, TX, Psychological Corporation, 2007

Kaufman AS, Kaufman NL: Kaufman Assessment Battery for Children, 2nd Edition. Circle Pines, MN, American Guidance Service, 2004

Roid GH: Stanford-Binet Intelligence Scales, 5th Edition. Itasca, IL, Riverside Publishing, 2003

Wechsler D: Wechsler Intelligence Scale for Children, 4th Edition. San Antonio, TX, Harcourt Assessment, 2003

Woodcock WR, McGrew KS, Mather N, et al: Woodcock-Johnson Tests of Cognitive Abilities and Achievement, 3rd Edition. Itasca, IL, Riverside Publishing, 2001

11.5   Assessment of intellectual deficiency (mental retardation) must include which of the following measures?

    A. The Iowa Tests of Basic Achievement.
    B. Standard Achievement Test.
    C. Woodcock-Johnson Tests of Achievement.
    D. Halstead-Reitan Test Battery.
    E. Test of adaptive functioning.

The correct response is option E.

Assessment of intellectual deficiency must include an assessment of *adaptive functioning* (i.e., personal and social skills used for everyday living) in addition to cognitive skills.

The interchangeable terms *intellectual deficiency* and *mental retardation* generally refer to intelligence test results two standard deviations below the mean, which would be a score of 70 on a test with a mean of 100 and a standard deviation of 15. When a youngster's subtest scores are widely distributed (this large amount of spread is referred to as *scatter*), the overall IQ score may not be a good representation of his or her ability. In fact, there often is no single score that can adequately describe that person's overall intellectual ability. However, when the majority of subtest scores, as well as the full-scale IQ (when interpretable), are within the deficient range, a diagnosis of intellectual deficiency can be considered. **(p. 142)**

Chapter 12

Intellectual Disability (Mental Retardation)

Select the single best response for each question.

12.1 In 1992, the American Association on Mental Retardation (AAMR), now the American Association on Intellectual Disability and Developmental Disabilities (AAIDD), proposed a new classification system for intellectual disability based on intensity of supports needed as opposed to the traditional system of classification by IQ score. For the new proposed classification, where would someone be classified if he or she requires additional support to navigate through everyday situations?

    A. Intermittent support.
    B. Limited support.
    C. Extensive support.
    D. Pervasive support.
    E. None of the above.

The correct response is option B.

The AAMR/AAIDD has been responsible for defining intellectual disability and providing diagnostic criteria since 1921. The most recent definition (American Association on Mental Retardation 2002) describes key assumptions essential to the application of the definition, including consideration of the individual's environment, diverse factors that affect valid assessment of strengths and challenges, the coexistence of strengths, and identification of needed supports to improve life functioning. The following is the proposed classification system for individuals with intellectual disabilities:

- *Intermittent support:* Higher-functioning individuals, who require little intervention in order to function, except during times of uncertainty or stress (mild intellectual disability under the old system of classification).
- *Limited support:* Individuals who may require additional support to navigate through everyday situations (moderate disability).
- *Extensive support:* Individuals who rely on around-the-clock daily support to function (severe disability).
- *Pervasive support:* Requiring daily interventions and lifelong support necessary to help the individual function in every aspect of daily routines (profound disability).

(p. 153)

American Association on Mental Retardation: Mental Retardation: Definition, Classification and Systems of Supports, 10th Edition. Washington, DC, American Association on Mental Retardation, 2002

12.2   Which of the following predisposing factors is associated with the highest percentage of cases of intellectual disability?

    A. Environmental influences.
    B. Pregnancy and perinatal complications.
    C. Acquired medical conditions.
    D. Heredity.
    E. Chromosomal changes and exposure to toxins during prenatal development.

The correct response is option E.

Predisposing factors include chromosomal changes and exposure to toxins during prenatal development (e.g., Down syndrome, fetal alcohol spectrum disorder), which affect 30% of cases; heredity, which affects approximately 5% of cases and includes single-gene abnormalities (e.g., tuberous sclerosis complex), chromosomal defects (e.g., fragile X syndrome), and inborn errors of metabolism inherited through autosomal-recessive mechanisms (e.g., Tay-Sachs disease); pregnancy and perinatal complications (e.g., trauma, prematurity, hypoxia) affecting 10% of cases; acquired medical conditions (e.g., lead poisoning) affecting 5% of cases; and environmental influences (severe deprivation) and other predisposing disorders such as autism (15%–20% of cases) (American Psychiatric Association 2000). **(p. 155)**

> American Psychiatric Association: Diagnostic and Statistical Manual of Mental Disorders, 4th Edition, Text Revision. Washington, DC, American Psychiatric Association, 2000

12.3   Which of the following risk factors for intellectual disability of unknown etiology is the strongest predictor of disability?

    A. Lower level of maternal education.
    B. Children born to older women.
    C. Low birth weight.
    D. Males.
    E. Multiple births.

The correct response is option C.

Risk factors for intellectual disability of unknown etiology continue to be studied. Croen et al. (2001) examined infant and maternal characteristics of over 11,000 children born between 1987 and 1994 in California with intellectual disability of unknown cause. The sample was further stratified into groups of children with mild, severe, and unspecified levels of disability. Findings showed that low birth weight was the strongest predictor of disability, both mild and severe. Similar findings have been reported elsewhere (Trevathan et al. 1997). Males and children born to black women and older women were also at increased risk for both mild and severe intellectual disability. Lower level of maternal education was also associated with increased risk, independent of race, for severe disability in this sample. A lower level of maternal education is correlated with lower socioeconomic status, which has been shown to be a strong and consistent predictor of mild but not severe forms of intellectual disability (Durkin et al. 1998). Additional risk factors for mild disability included multiple births and second or later born children; for severe disability, children born to Asian and Hispanic mothers. **(p. 155–156)**

> Croen LA, Grether JK, Selvin S: The epidemiology of mental retardation of unknown cause. Pediatrics 107:1410–1414, 2001
>
> Durkin MS, Schupf N, Stein Z, et al: Mental retardation, in Public Health and Preventive Medicine. Edited by Wallace R. Stamford, CT, Appleton & Lange, 1998, pp 1049–1058
>
> Trevathan E, Murphy CC, Yeargin-Allsopp M: Prevalence and descriptive epidemiology of Lennox-Gastaut syndrome among Atlanta children. Epilepsia 38:1283–1288, 1997

12.4   Which of the following genetic causes of intellectual disability is associated with a deletion at 22q11.2?

      A. Angelman syndrome.

      B. Williams syndrome.

      C. Prader-Willi syndrome.

      D. Velocardiofacial syndrome (VCFS).

      E. Rett syndrome.

The correct response is option D.

VCFS, as its name implies, is a disorder that typically involves abnormalities in the palate, heart, and face. The most common features are cleft palate; heart defects; characteristic facial features; and learning, speech, and feeding difficulties. VCFS is also known as Shprintzen syndrome, DiGeorge syndrome, or craniofacial syndrome. Myriad physical anomalies can be associated with a deletion at 22q11.2 (more than 35 genes are present in the region most commonly affected), and increasingly these disorders are being grouped as 22q11 deletion syndromes. Speech difficulty, with defects in phonation, language acquisition, and comprehension, is a significant concern for children with chromosome 22q11.2 deletion syndrome. Expressive language skills are below that expected for cognitive development and generally are more delayed than receptive skills. Social language skills are even more problematic.

Angelman syndrome is a neurogenetic disorder that occurs at a rate of about 1 per 10,000 to 1 per 20,000 worldwide (Williams 2005). Prevalence in populations with severe intellectual disability is 1.4% (King et al. 2005). The clinical presentation is varied, with some features present in virtually all individuals with Angelman syndrome (severe developmental delays with severe speech impairment, ataxia of gait and/or tremulous movement of the limbs, frequent laughter/happy demeanor, excitable personality, often with hand flapping, and short attention span). Other signs and symptoms present in 20%–80% of individuals include delayed head growth resulting in microcephaly by age 2 years, seizures, abnormal electroencephalogram with large amplitude slow-spike waves, protruding tongue, feeding problems, drooling, sleep disturbance, hypopigmented skin, strabismus, and prognathia (Williams 2005).

Williams syndrome is caused by a microdeletion on chromosome 7q11.23, has a prevalence of 1/7,500, and is associated with a specific pattern of facial features, personality (excessively friendly, anxious), connective tissue abnormalities, heart disease, failure to thrive, and growth deficiency (Morris 2006). Individuals with Williams syndrome most often have mild to moderate intellectual and learning disabilities, although in some cases low-average to average intelligence has been reported (Mervis and Becerra 2007).

Prader-Willi syndrome can be caused by either paternal deletion (about 70% of cases) or maternal uniparental disomy (about 29% of cases) on chromosome 15q11.13, the same region implicated in Angelman syndrome. Prader-Willi syndrome is found in 1 per 29,500 births and is characterized by hypotonia, intellectual disability, failure to thrive giving way to hyperphagia, early obesity, hypogonadism, short stature with small hands and feet, sleep apnea, and behavioral problems (Horsthemke and Buiting 2006). Compulsive food-seeking and -hoarding behaviors are seen as early as 2 years of age and are lifelong challenges. Other compulsive behaviors are commonly observed, leading to an increased risk of developing obsessive-compulsive disorder. Impulse-control disorders and affective disorders that interfere with adaptive functioning are also often found (King et al. 2005).

Rett syndrome affects primarily females (with reports of rare cases involving males; Zeev et al. 2002) and is one of the most common causes of severe intellectual disability in females, with an incidence of 1/10,000 by the age of 12 years (Leonard et al. 1997). Females with Rett syndrome have a period of ostensibly normal development for the first 6–18 months of life (although more recent studies suggest the existence of subtle behavioral abnormalities in the first 6 months [Burford et al. 2003]), followed by a regression or loss of intellectual functioning and fine and gross motor skills, social withdrawal, the development of stereotypic hand-wringing movements, and a reduced life span. **(pp. 157–159)**

Burford B, Kerr AM, Macleod HA: Nurse recognition of early deviation in development in home videos of infants with Rett disorder. J Intellect Disabil Res 47:588–596, 2003

Horsthemke B, Buiting K: Imprinting defects on human chromosome 15. Cytogenet Genome Res 113:292–299, 2006

King BH, Hodapp RM, Dykens EM: Mental retardation, in Kaplan and Sadock's Comprehensive Textbook of Psychiatry, 8th Edition, Vol 2. Edited by Kaplan HI, Sadock BJ. Baltimore, MD, Lippincott Williams & Wilkins, 2005, pp 3076–3106

Leonard H, Bower C, English D: The prevalence and incidence of Rett syndrome in Australia. Eur Child Adolesc Psychiatry 6 (suppl):8–10, 1997

Mervis CB, Becerra AM: Language and communicative development in Williams syndrome. Ment Retard Dev Disabil Res Rev 13:3–15, 2007

Morris CA: The dysmorphology, genetics, and natural history of Williams-Beuren syndrome, in Williams-Beuren Syndrome: Research, Evaluation, and Treatment. Edited by Morris CA, Lenhoff HM, Wang PP. Baltimore, MD, Johns Hopkins University Press, 2006, pp 3–17

Williams CA: Neurological aspects of the Angelman syndrome. Brain Dev 27:88–94, 2005

Zeev BB, Yaron Y, Schanen NC, et al: Rett syndrome: clinical manifestations in males with MECP2 mutations. J Child Neurol 17:20–24, 2002

12.5   Which of the following atypical antipsychotic medications has the most scientific evidence to support its use in treating children with extreme irritability, aggression, or self-injury in the setting of intellectual disability?

    A. Aripiprazole.
    B. Olanzapine.
    C. Quetiapine.
    D. Risperidone.
    E. Ziprasidone.

The correct response is option D.

Bramble (2007) recently surveyed child and adolescent psychiatrists specializing in intellectual disability in the United Kingdom. These clinicians ranked risperidone as their most commonly prescribed antipsychotic drug. The evidence supporting expanded indications for risperidone, including behavioral disturbances in persons with intellectual disability, is now greater than that which exists for any other psychotropic drug. Thus, the presence of a pervasive developmental disorder and/or disruptive behavior is most predictive of antipsychotic drug use in children (de Bildt et al. 2006). In a randomized, placebo-controlled crossover trial of risperidone for disruptive behavior in 20 individuals with developmental disabilities of mixed etiology, with a response definition of a 50% reduction in mean Aberrant Behavior Checklist total scores, half of the subjects responded to active treatment (Zarcone et al. 2001). **(p. 164)**

Bramble D: Psychotropic drug prescribing in child and adolescent learning disability psychiatry. J Psychopharmacol 21:486–491, 2007

de Bildt A, Mulder EJ, Scheers T, et al: Pervasive developmental disorder, behavior problems, and psychotropic drug use in children and adolescents with mental retardation. Pediatrics 118:e1860–e1866, 2006

Zarcone JR, Hellings JA, Crandall K, et al: Effects of risperidone on aberrant behavior of persons with developmental disabilities, I: a double-blind crossover study using multiple measures. Am J Ment Retard 106:525–538, 2001

Chapter 13

Autism Spectrum Disorders

Select the single best response for each question.

13.1   In which of the following DSM editions did autism become an official and codified diagnosis?

   A. DSM-I.
   B. DSM-II.
   C. DSM-III.
   D. DSM-III-R.
   E. DSM-IV.

The correct response is option C.

It was not until DSM-III (American Psychiatric Association 1980) was published that autism became an official and codified diagnosis.

In 1943, Leo Kanner, author of the first U.S. textbook on child psychiatry, published a paper in which he described 11 children "whose condition differs so markedly and uniquely from anything reported so far, that each case merits—and, I hope will eventually receive—a detailed review of its fascinating peculiarities" (Kanner 1943, p. 217). The following year, Hans Asperger described in a German publication a similar disorder (Asperger 1944/1991). Both reports had the word *autistic* in their title. Kanner's report was initially much better known in the West. **(p. 173)**

> American Psychiatric Association: Diagnostic and Statistical Manual of Mental Disorders, 3rd Edition. Washington, DC, American Psychiatric Association, 1980
> Asperger H: "Autistic psychopathology" in childhood (1944), in Autism and Asperger Syndrome. Edited by Frith U. Cambridge, UK, Cambridge University Press, 1991, pp 37–92
> Kanner L: Autistic disturbances of affective contact. Nerv Child 2:217–250, 1943

13.2   A DSM-IV-TR (American Psychiatric Association 2000) diagnosis of autism requires all of the following *except*

   A. Qualitative impairments in social interaction.
   B. Qualitative impairments in communication.
   C. Restricted repetitive and stereotyped patterns of behavior, interests, and activities.
   D. Delays or abnormal functioning in at least one of above areas prior to age 3 years.
   E. Low IQ.

The correct response is option E.

Approximately 50% of persons with autism may have normal verbal expressions and IQ scores, despite having moderate to severe social skills deficits.

In DSM-IV-TR (American Psychiatric Association 2000), *autism* is defined by the presence of severe and pervasive impairments in reciprocal social interaction and in verbal and nonverbal communication skills. There must also be symptoms of restrictive and repetitive behaviors, and/or stereotyped patterns of interest that are abnormal in their intensity or focus. **(p. 174)**

> American Psychiatric Association: Diagnostic and Statistical Manual of Mental Disorders, 4th Edition, Text Revision. Washington, DC, American Psychiatric Association, 2000

13.3   Evaluation instruments designed for autism include all of the following *except*

A. Checklist for Autism in Toddlers (CHAT).
B. Autism Diagnostic Interview—Revised (ADI-R).
C. Autism Diagnostic Observation Schedule—Generic (ADOS-G).
D. Childhood Autism Rating Scale (CARS).
E. Vineland Adaptive Behavior Scales (VABS).

The correct response is option E.

Although not a diagnostic interview for autism per se, the VABS have been used to evaluate the social skills of children who may have autism (Volkmar et al. 1993). The development of supplementary norms designed to enhance the use of the VABS in persons with autism (Carter et al. 1998) should add to its usefulness in evaluating individuals with social communication disorder.

CHAT was developed for use by pediatricians and nurses with children who are 18–24 months of age (Baron-Cohen et al. 1992). It takes less than 10 minutes to administer and uses information from the parent as well as observation of the child.

For children 3 years of age and older, the ADI-R (Lord et al. 1994) and the ADOS-G (Lord et al. 2000) are universally recognized as the most comprehensive and valid diagnostic instruments available. The ADI-R is a semistructured interview of the child's primary caretaker that includes many items pertaining to social communication. The diagnosis is reached using an algorithm based on scores on clusters of items that correspond to social relationships; verbal and nonverbal communication; and restrictive, repetitive, and stereotyped patterns of behavior. The ADOS-G, designed to be used for both children and adults, consists of a number of age-appropriate social "presses" in which the examiner uses his or her behavior to elicit social responses from the child. The interview is scored using a template designed to measure the same domains as does the ADI-R. Interviewers must be trained, but the interview usually takes 1 hour or less to administer. The ADI-R and the ADOS-G yield independent and additive diagnostic information (Risi et al. 2006), and both should be used in making a diagnosis.

Two instruments, the CARS (Schopler et al. 1988) and the Autism Behavior Checklist (Krug et al. 1980), were developed prior to our current understanding of social communication, but they are still popular. **(pp. 176–177)**

Baron-Cohen S, Allen J, Gillberg C: Can autism be detected at 18 months? The needle, the haystack, and the CHAT. Br J Psychiatry 161:839–843, 1992

Carter AS, Volkmar FR, Sparrow SS, et al: The Vineland Adaptive Behavior Scales: supplementary norms for individuals with autism. J Autism Dev Disord 28:287–302, 1998

Krug DA, Arick JR, Almond PG: Behavior checklist for identifying severely handicapped individuals with high levels of autistic behavior. J Child Psychol Psychiatry 21:221–229, 1980

Lord C, Rutter M, Le Couteur A: Autism Diagnostic Interview—Revised: a revised version of a diagnostic interview for caregivers of individuals with possible pervasive developmental disorders. J Autism Dev Disord 24:659–685, 1994

Lord C, Risi S, Lambrecht L, et al: The Autism Diagnostic Observation Schedule—Generic: a standard measure of social and communication deficits associated with the spectrum of autism. J Autism Dev Disord 30:205–223, 2000

Risi S, Lord C, Gotham K, et al: Combining information from multiple sources in the diagnosis of autism spectrum disorders. J Am Acad Child Adolesc Psychiatry 45:1094–1103, 2006

Schopler E, Reichler R, Renner BR: The Childhood Autism Rating Scale (CARS). Los Angeles, CA, Western Psychological Services, 1988

Volkmar FR, Carter A, Sparrow SS, et al: Quantifying social development in autism. J Am Acad Child Adolesc Psychiatry 32:627–632, 1993

13.4 DSM-IV-TR (American Psychiatric Association 2000) pervasive development disorders (PDDs) include all of the following *except*

    A. Asperger's disorder.
    B. PDD not otherwise specified (NOS).
    C. Rett's disorder.
    D. Childhood disintegrative disorder (CDD).
    E. Fragile X syndrome.

The correct response is option E.

Fragile X is not categorized as a PDD. The cause of fragile X is a mutation in *FMR1* (including the occurrence of a greatly expanded trinucleotide repeat) at Xq27.3. Studies of persons who have fragile X syndrome have revealed social and communicative handicaps that resemble the symptoms of autism (Loesch et al. 2007; Rogers et al. 2001). *FMR1* is known to play a role in many neurodevelopmental processes, and some of these may involve systems that are defective in autism (Feinstein and Reiss 1998).

The criteria for Asperger's disorder are identical to those for autistic disorder (including the requirement that the symptoms be severe and pervasive) with the exception that there is no clinically significant delay in cognitive development or in the development of age-appropriate self-help skills, and no significant delay in language development.

DSM-IV-TR (American Psychiatric Association 2000) states that the diagnosis of PDD NOS should be used when there is a severe and pervasive impairment in the development of reciprocal social interaction or verbal and nonverbal communication, or when stereotyped behavior, interests, and activities are present, but the criteria for any of the more specific PDD diagnoses are not met.

Rett's disorder is caused by mutations in X-linked *MECP2*, encoding methyl-CpG-binding protein 2. It is almost exclusively found in females, although rare cases of Rett's disorder have been reported in males who have a concomitant XXY abnormality.

As currently described, the regression in childhood disintegrative disorder begins no earlier than 2 years and no later than 10 years of age. The clinical features of CDD can be quite similar to autistic disorder, distinguished only by the age at onset. Seizures are common in CDD (Hendry 2000). The most typical onset is between 2 and 4 years of age (Volkmar and Cohen 1989). **(pp. 177–178)**

American Psychiatric Association: Diagnostic and Statistical Manual of Mental Disorders, 4th Edition, Text Revision. Washington, DC, American Psychiatric Association, 2000

Feinstein C, Reiss AL: Autism: the point of view from fragile X studies. J Autism Dev Disord 28:393–405, 1998

Hendry CN: Childhood disintegrative disorder: should it be considered a distinct diagnosis? Clin Psychol Rev 20:77–90, 2000

Loesch DZ, Bui QM, Dissanayake C: Molecular and cognitive predictors of the continuum of autistic behaviours in fragile X. Neurosci Biobehav Rev 31:315–326, 2007

Rogers SJ, Wehner DE, Hagerman R: The behavioral phenotype in fragile X: symptom of autism in very young children with fragile X syndrome, idiopathic autism, and other developmental disorders. J Dev Behav Pediatr 22:409–417, 2001

Volkmar FR, Cohen DJ: Disintegrative disorder or "late onset" autism. J Child Psychol Psychiatry 30:717–724, 1989

13.5 Based on a 2001 study funded by the National Academy of Sciences, recommended targets for educational intervention in children with autism spectrum disorders include all of the following *except*

    A. Functional spontaneous communication.
    B. Social skills.
    C. Play skills.
    D. Cognitive development.
    E. Self-care skills.

The correct response is option E.

The National Academy of Sciences in 2001 funded a project of the National Research Council to study the educational services that should begin as soon as a child is suspected of having an autism spectrum disorder. The committee members recommended that interventions should focus on education in six areas: 1) functional spontaneous communication, 2) social skills, 3) play skills, 4) cognitive development taught in natural setting to facilitate generalization, 5) reduction of problem behaviors, and 6) functional academic skills. **(p. 183)**

National Academy of Sciences: Educating Children With Autism. Washington, DC, National Academy Press, 2001

Chapter 14

Developmental Disorders of Learning, Communication, and Motor Skills

Select the single best response for each question.

14.1   Which of the following is the most common learning disorder?

   A. Expressive language disorder.
   B. Receptive language disorder.
   C. Disorder of written expression.
   D. Reading disorder.
   E. Mathematics disorder.

The correct response is option D.

The DSM-IV (American Psychiatric Association 1994) definition of *reading disorder* uses a broader classification system for the complicated process often called "dyslexia." Dyslexia is the most common learning disorder and the most common diagnosis of children receiving special education services. The prevalence of dyslexia has been estimated to be as high as 17.4% in the school-age population (Shaywitz 2003).With more sophisticated testing, there is no longer a greater prevalence of dyslexia in boys (Rutter et al. 2004). The proportions of sex differences in developmental reading disability are estimated to be at about 1.5–2.1 in favor of males. **(p. 194)**

> American Psychiatric Association: Diagnostic and Statistical Manual of Mental Disorders, 4th Edition. Washington, DC, American Psychiatric Association, 1994
> Rutter M, Caspi A, Fergusson D, et al: Sex differences in developmental reading disability: new findings from four epidemiological studies. JAMA 291:2007–2012, 2004
> Shaywitz SE: Overcoming Dyslexia. New York, Knopf, 2003

14.2   "The ability to use working memory to retain sounds and then words" defines which of the following basic building blocks of reading?

   A. Phonological awareness.
   B. Rapid naming.
   C. Phonological memory.
   D. Word recognition.
   E. Spelling.

The correct response is option C.

Phonological memory is the ability to use working memory to retain sounds and then words. The relationship to poor reading is still not conclusive.

Phonological awareness is the metacognitive ability to understand the words we hear and read that have basic structure related to sound. Speech sounds, or phonemes, are patterns that make up words. Spoken language is done rapidly, without the listener deciphering each sound.

Rapid naming is the rapid automatized naming of letters and digits. This usually predicts reading skills over time (Schatschneider et al. 2004). Although some authors disagree, most would say the ability to name quickly enhances reading fluency.

Word recognition is the ability to recognize individual written words correctly. Word-level reading disability, or "dyslexia," is characterized by difficulty in single-word decoding. Without the ability to read a word, fluency and understanding are limited. This is the area where most research has been done. The inability to decode interferes with reading comprehension, word recognition, and reading fluency.

Spelling is the ability to encode words either in isolation or in context. Some children can spell but not decode. Spelling is a multidimensional skill that is related to both phonological processing and memory. **(pp. 194–195)**

Schatschneider C, Fletcher JM, Francis DJ, et al: Kindergarten prediction of reading skills: a longitudinal comparative analysis. Journal of Educational Psychology 96:265–282, 2004

14.3   Which of the following core cognitive processes is required for adequate reading comprehension?

   A. Language skills.
   B. Listening comprehension.
   C. Working memory.
   D. Inference.
   E. All of the above.

The correct response is option E.

Reading comprehension refers to the ability to understand information in written form. Core cognitive processes for comprehension include language skills, listening comprehension, working memory, and the higher-order processing of inference, prior knowledge, comprehension monitoring, and structure sensitivity. A deficit here affects all academic subject areas in which reading is required. **(pp. 195–196)**

14.4   Which of the following terms is used to describe problems that ensue when the brain fails to recognize and interpret a sound?

   A. Phonological disorder.
   B. Auditory processing disorder (APD).
   C. Fluency disorder.
   D. Expressive language disorder.
   E. Oral expression disorder.

The correct response is option B.

Auditory processing is a term used to describe what happens when a brain recognizes and interprets the sound (American Speech-Language-Hearing Association 1993). Children with APD often do not recognize subtle differences between sounds in words, even though the sounds themselves are loud and clear. It is not a sensory or hearing impairment. *Auditory processing disorder* is an umbrella term that describes a variety of problems with the brain that can interfere with processing auditory information.

Phonological disorder is the inability to use expected speech sounds appropriate for the child's age and dialect. Voice pitch, loudness, quality, nasal resonance, and vocal hygiene are important to assess.

Fluency disorder (stuttering) is the unexpected disturbance in the normal patterns and flow of speech. The nature and severity of dysfluency may vary at different levels of pragmatic complexity. More typical fluency disorders are hesitations, interjections, phrase revisions, unfinished words, and word repetitions. Less typical fluency problems such as syllable repetitions, sound repetition, prolongations, or blocks usually involve visible or audible tension with dysfluency.

Oral expression is the ability to convey information and ideas through speech. DSM-IV (American Psychiatric Association 1994) categorizes deficits in oral expression as *expressive language disorder*. Children usually understand language better than they can communicate. This deficit affects written language later in life. **(pp. 197–198)**

American Psychiatric Association: Diagnostic and Statistical Manual of Mental Disorders, 4th Edition. Washington, DC, American Psychiatric Association, 1994

American Speech-Language-Hearing Association: Definition of communication disorders. ASHA 35 (suppl):40–41, 1993

14.5   Which of the following statements concerning mathematics disability is *true?*

　　A. Research in dyslexia lags behind dyscalculia.
　　B. Several core deficits have been identified in the mathematics arena.
　　C. The prevalence of a math disability is estimated to be 10%–12%.
　　D. There is no evidence to support the heritability of math difficulties.
　　E. Federal guidelines break down mathematics disorder into the ability to perform calculations and problem solving.

The correct response is option E.

DSM-IV (American Psychiatric Association 1994) does not break down mathematics disability into the ability to do calculations and the ability of problem solving, as do the federal guidelines. The difficulty with defining a math disability is that *mathematics* is a broad term without consistent standards (Mazzocco and Myers 2003). Research in dyscalculia lags behind that of dyslexia. No core deficits or processes have been identified in the mathematics arena. The prevalence of a math disability is estimated to be 5%–6% (Shalev et al. 2005). There is strong evidence for the heritability of math difficulties. **(p. 196)**

American Psychiatric Association: Diagnostic and Statistical Manual of Mental Disorders, 4th Edition. Washington, DC, American Psychiatric Association, 1994

Mazzocco MMM, Myers GF: Complexities in identifying and defining mathematics learning disability in the primary school age years. Annals of Dyslexia 53:218–253, 2003

Shalev RS, Manor O, Gross-Tsur V: Developmental dyscalculia: a prospective six-year follow-up. Dev Med Child Neurol 47:121–125, 2005

Chapter 15

Attention-Deficit/ Hyperactivity Disorder

Select the single best response for each question.

15.1   All of the following are accurate statements regarding comorbidity with attention-deficit/hyperactivity disorder (ADHD) *except*

    A. Both oppositional defiant disorder (ODD) and conduct disorder are comorbidly present in at least 25% of children with ADHD.

    B. Learning and language disorders are comorbidly present in up to 25% of children with ADHD.

    C. Many children with ADHD have two or more comorbid disorders.

    D. Family studies suggest that ADHD with ODD/conduct disorder and ADHD alone are separate genetic subtypes.

    E. Compared with those with ADHD alone, those with comorbid anxiety are less likely to respond to psychosocial interventions.

The correct response is option E.

As in other psychiatric disorders, comorbidity is common in ADHD. Compared with those with ADHD alone, those with comorbid anxiety (without ODD/conduct disorder) show lower levels of impulsivity on laboratory measures of attention and a greater tendency to respond to psychosocial interventions (Jensen et al. 2001; March et al. 2000; Newcorn et al. 2001).

Both ODD/conduct disorder and anxiety disorders are present in 25%–33% of children with ADHD, whereas learning and language disorders afflict another quarter. Many children with ADHD will have two or more comorbid disorders.

Family studies suggest that ADHD with ODD/conduct disorder is a separate genetic subtype from ADHD alone (Biederman et al. 1992). **(p. 207)**

> Biederman J, Faraone SV, Keenan K, et al: Further evidence for family genetic risk factors in attention deficit hyperactivity disorder: patterns of comorbidity in probands and relatives psychiatrically and pediatrically referred samples. Arch Gen Psychiatry 49:728–738, 1992
>
> Jensen PS, Hinshaw SP, Kraemer HC, et al: ADHD comorbidity findings from the MTA study: comparing comorbid subgroups. J Am Acad Child Adolesc Psychiatry 40:147–158, 2001
>
> March JS, Swanson JM, Arnold LE, et al: Anxiety as a predictor and outcome variable in the multimodal treatment study of children with ADHD (MTA). J Abnorm Child Psychol 28:527–541, 2000
>
> Newcorn JH, Halperin JM, Jensen PS, et al: Symptom profiles in children with ADHD: effects of comorbidity and gender. J Am Acad Child Adolesc Psychiatry 40:137–146, 2001

15.2   All of the following statements concerning the etiology and risk factors of attention-deficit/hyperactivity disorder (ADHD) are correct *except*

    A. If a child has ADHD, there is a 10%–35% chance of first-degree relatives having the disorder.

    B. If a parent has ADHD, there is a 57% chance the child will develop ADHD.

    C. The rate of ADHD in biological relatives is 18% compared with 6% in the adopted relatives.

D. About 50% of the variance in ADHD traits is found to be attributable to genetics.

E. Nongenetic risk factors include perinatal stress, low birth weight, traumatic brain injury, and maternal smoking during pregnancy.

The correct response is option D.

Twin studies compare concordance rates for ADHD in monozygotic and dizygotic twins to determine the relative influence of genes and environment on the variance in symptoms of ADHD. About 75% of the variance in ADHD traits is found to be attributable to genetics (Faraone et al. 2005).

Family studies have consistently shown that if a child has ADHD, 10%–35% of first-degree relatives are likely to have the disorder as well (Biederman et al. 1992). If a parent has ADHD, the risk to the child of developing ADHD is as high as 57% (Biederman et al. 1995). Sprich et al. (2000) examined the rates of ADHD in the relatives of both adopted (i.e., nonbiological) and nonadopted children with ADHD. The rate of ADHD in biological relatives of children with ADHD was 18% compared with only 6% in the adopted relatives, suggesting a strong genetic effect.

A number of nongenetic risk factors for ADHD have been established (Nigg 2006). These include perinatal stress and low birth weight (Mick et al. 2002b), traumatic brain injury (Max et al. 1998), maternal smoking during pregnancy (Mick et al. 2002a) and very severe early deprivation (Kreppner et al. 2001). **(pp. 208–210; see also Table 15–2)**

Biederman J, Faraone SV, Keenan K, et al: Further evidence for family genetic risk factors in attention deficit hyperactivity disorder: patterns of comorbidity in probands and relatives psychiatrically and pediatrically referred samples. Arch Gen Psychiatry 49:728–738, 1992

Biederman J, Faraone SV, Mick E, et al: High risk for attention deficit hyperactivity disorder among children of parents with childhood onset of the disorder: a pilot study. Am J Psychiatry 152:431–435, 1995

Faraone SV, Perlis RH, Doyle AE, et al: Molecular genetics of attention-deficit/hyperactivity disorder. Biol Psychiatry 57:1313–1323, 2005

Kreppner JM, O'Connor TG, Rutter M: Can inattention/overactivity be an institutional deprivation syndrome? J Abnorm Child Psychol 29:513–528, 2001

Max JE, Arndt S, Castillo CS, et al: Attention-deficit hyperactivity symptomatology after traumatic brain injury: a prospective study. J Am Acad Child Adolesc Psychiatry 37:841–847, 1998

Mick E, Biederman J, Faraone SV, et al: Case-control study of attention-deficit hyperactivity disorder and maternal smoking, alcohol use, and drug use during pregnancy. J Am Acad Child Adolesc Psychiatry 41:378–385, 2002a

Mick E, Biederman J, Prince J, et al: Impact of low birth weight on attention-deficit hyperactivity disorder. J Dev Behav Pediatr 23:16–22, 2002b

Nigg JT: What Causes ADHD? New York, Guilford, 2006

Sprich S, Biederman J, Crawford MH, et al: Adoptive and biological families of children and adolescents with ADHD. J Am Acad Child Adolesc Psychiatry 39:1432–1437, 2000

15.3 All of the following statements regarding the pathophysiology of attention-deficit/hyperactivity disorder (ADHD) are correct *except*

A. Hippocampal volume is increased bilaterally in a large sample of children with ADHD relative to control subjects.

B. Children with ADHD show larger volumes of the dorsolateral prefrontal cortex (DLPFC), anterior cingulate, and caudate regions compared with control subjects.

C. Compared with children with ADHD, control subjects have increased activation in the prefrontal cortex (PFC) bilaterally when performing response inhibition tasks.

D. The parents of ADHD children (who had ADHD themselves) show decreased activity in the frontostriatal areas and anterior cingulate cortex (ACC).

E. ADHD may be seen as a disorder of both frontostriatal and frontocerebellar circuitry.

The correct response is option B.

Several studies have reported that ADHD subjects show smaller volumes than control subjects in the DLPFC, anterior cingulate, and caudate (Casey et al. 2007; Makris et al. 2007; Pliszka et al. 2006; Seidman et al. 2006; van't Ent et al. 2007).

The limbic areas have not been a major focus of study in ADHD, although recently hippocampal volume was found to be increased bilaterally in a large sample of children with ADHD relative to control subjects (Plessen et al. 2006).

A recent activation likelihood estimation meta-analysis of 16 neuroimaging studies contrasting subjects with ADHD and control subjects has been performed (Dickstein et al. 2006). In studies using response inhibition tasks, an increased likelihood of activation was seen for control subjects in the PFC bilaterally, ACC, left parietal lobe, and right caudate.

The parents of ADHD children (who had ADHD themselves) also showed decreased activity in the frontostriatal areas and ACC, but adults with ADHD had greater activation of the precuneus and inferior parietal lobule than control subjects.

In studies by Durston et al. (2007) and Mulder et al. (2008), children with ADHD and their unaffected siblings showed decreased activation of the cerebellum during the timing manipulation and decreased activation of the ACC during the expected presentation trials. Thus, ADHD may be seen as a disorder of both frontostriatal and frontocerebellar circuitry. **(pp. 209–211)**

Casey BJ, Epstein JN, Buhle J, et al: Frontostriatal connectivity and its role in cognitive control in parent-child dyads with ADHD. Am J Psychiatry 164:1729–1736, 2007

Dickstein SG, Bannon K, Xavier CF, et al: The neural correlates of attention deficit hyperactivity disorder: an ALE meta-analysis. J Child Psychol Psychiatry 47:1051–1062, 2006

Durston S, Davidson MC, Mulder MJ, et al: Neural and behavioral correlates of expectancy violations in attention-deficit hyperactivity disorder. J Child Psychol Psychiatry 48:881–889, 2007

Makris N, Biederman J, Valera EM, et al: Cortical thinning of the attention and executive function networks in adults with attention-deficit/hyperactivity disorder. Cereb Cortex 17:1364–1375, 2007

Mulder MJ, Baeyens D, Davidson MC, et al: Familial vulnerability to ADHD affects activity in the cerebellum in addition to the prefrontal systems. J Am Acad Child Adolesc Psychiatry 47:68–75, 2008

Plessen KJ, Bansal R, Zhu H, et al: Hippocampus and amygdala morphology in attention-deficit/hyperactivity disorder. Arch Gen Psychiatry 63:795–807, 2006

Pliszka SR, Lancaster J, Liotti M, et al: Volumetric MRI differences in treatment-naive vs chronically treated children with ADHD. Neurology 67:1023–1027, 2006

Seidman LJ, Valera EM, Makris N, et al: Dorsolateral prefrontal and anterior cingulate cortex volumetric abnormalities in adults with attention-deficit/hyperactivity disorder identified by magnetic resonance imaging. Biol Psychiatry 60:1071–1080, 2006

van't Ent D, Lehn H, Derks EM, et al: A structural MRI study in monozygotic twins concordant or discordant for attention/hyperactivity problems: evidence for genetic and environmental heterogeneity in the developing brain. Neuroimage 35:1004–1020, 2007

15.4 Research findings concerning the course and prognosis of attention-deficit/hyperactivity disorder (ADHD) include all of the following *except*

A. More than 60% of children with ADHD continue to suffer from the disorder during teenage years.

B. At a 3-year follow-up, the NIMH Multimodal Treatment Study of ADHD (MTA) found that 20% of the sample no longer met criteria for ADHD.

C. Follow-up studies in the adult population showed variable rates of ADHD depending on informants and presence or absence of comorbidity.

D. Adults with a childhood history of ADHD show higher rates of antisocial behavior, injuries and accidents, and employment and marital difficulties.

E. Adults with a childhood history of ADHD have higher rates of substance use disorders.

The correct response is option B.

At a 3-year follow-up, the NIMH MTA study found that 40% of the sample no longer met criteria for ADHD.

Very significant numbers (60%–85%) of children with ADHD continue to meet criteria for the disorder during the teenage years (Barkley et al. 1990; Biederman et al. 1996; Claude and Firestone 1995).

Four studies have followed fairly large samples of children with hyperactivity or ADHD into adulthood: the Montreal study (Weiss and Hechtman 2003), the New York study (Mannuzza et al. 1998), the Milwaukee study (Barkley et al. 2006), and, most recently, the Massachusetts General study (Biederman et al. 2006). These studies vary in the rates of ADHD found in adulthood as well as comorbidity of adult disorders. In general, studies tracking children with ADHD only (and no oppositional defiant disorder/conduct disorder) or that use patient self-report find that under 10% of children with ADHD still have it as adults (the New York study), whereas those including ADHD children with comorbidity and that use parent informants find rates of 49%–67% of ADHD at follow-up.

Adults with a childhood history of ADHD have higher than expected rates of antisocial behavior (Barkley et al. 2004), injuries and accidents (Barkley 2004), employment and marital difficulties, health problems, teen pregnancies (Barkley et al. 2006), and children out of wedlock (Johnston 2002). Biederman et al. (2006) found that adults with a childhood history of ADHD had higher rates of major psychopathology and substance use disorders than did control subjects. **(p. 211)**

Barkley RA: Driving impairments in teens and adults with attention-deficit/hyperactivity disorder. Psychiatr Clin North Am 27:233–260, 2004

Barkley RA, Fischer M, Edelbrock CS, et al: The adolescent outcome of hyperactive children diagnosed by research criteria, I: an 8-year prospective follow-up study. J Am Acad Child Adolesc Psychiatry 29:546–557, 1990

Barkley RA, Fischer M, Smallish L, et al: Young adult follow-up of hyperactive children: antisocial activities and drug use. J Child Psychol Psychiatry 45:195–211, 2004

Barkley RA, Fischer M, Smallish L, et al: Young adult outcome of hyperactive children: adaptive functioning in major life activities. J Am Acad Child Adolesc Psychiatry 45:192–202, 2006

Biederman J, Faraone S, Milberger S, et al: A prospective 4-year follow-up study of attention-deficit hyperactivity and related disorders. Arch Gen Psychiatry 53:437–446, 1996

Biederman J, Monuteaux MC, Mick E, et al: Young adult outcome of attention deficit hyperactivity disorder: a controlled 10-year follow-up study. Psychol Med 36:167–179, 2006

Claude D, Firestone P: The development of ADHD boys: a 12 year follow up. Canadian Journal of Behavioural Science 27:226–249, 1995

Johnston C: The impact of attention deficit hyperactivity disorder on social and vocational functioning in adults, in Attention Deficit Hyperactivity Disorder: State of the Science, Best Practices. Edited by Jensen PS, Cooper JR. Kingston, NJ, Civic Research Institute, 2002, pp 6-2–6-21

Mannuzza S, Klein RG, Bessler A, et al: Adult psychiatric status of hyperactive boys grown up. Am J Psychiatry 155:493–498, 1998

Weiss G, Hechtman L: Hyperactive Children Grown Up. New York, Guilford, 2003

15.5   All of the following statements regarding attention-deficit/hyperactivity disorder (ADHD) treatment are correct *except*

A. Pharmacological treatment of ADHD is the best-studied intervention in child and adolescent psychiatry.

B. Pharmacological intervention for ADHD is more effective than behavioral treatment alone.

C. Comorbid anxiety has been found to predict a poorer response to behavioral treatment.

D. According to recent American Academy of Child and Adolescent Psychiatry and Texas Children's Medication Algorithm Project (CMAP) guidelines, U.S. Food and Drug Administration (FDA)–approved agents should be the initial choice of medications.

E. The long-acting agents have similar safety and efficacy profiles compared with the immediate-release forms.

The correct response is option C.

In the Multimodality Treatment of ADHD (MTA) study, comorbid anxiety (as reported by the child's parent) predicted a better response to behavioral treatment relative to those without comorbidity (March et al. 2000), particularly when the ADHD patient had both an anxiety and a disruptive behavior disorder (oppositional defiant disorder or conduct disorder) (Jensen et al. 2001).

Pharmacological treatment of ADHD is the best-studied intervention in child and adolescent psychiatry. Both the American Academy of Child and Adolescent Psychiatry (Pliszka et al. 2007) and the Texas CMAP (Pliszka et al. 2006) have issued guidelines on the selection of appropriate agents for the pharmacological treatment of ADHD.

FDA-approved agents (stimulant or atomoxetine) should be the initial choice; the CMAP algorithm recommends a stimulant treatment as the first stage. Long-acting formulas of stimulants have been studied extensively, and they have been found to be similar in efficacy and safety to the immediate-release forms. **(pp. 213–216)**

Jensen PS, Hinshaw SP, Swanson JM, et al: Findings from the NIMH Multimodal Treatment Study of ADHD (MTA): implications and applications for primary care providers. J Dev Behav Pediatr 22:60–73, 2001

March JS, Swanson JM, Arnold LE, et al: Anxiety as a predictor and outcome variable in the multimodal treatment study of children with ADHD (MTA). J Abnorm Child Psychol 28:527–541, 2000

Pliszka SR, Crismon ML, Hughes CW, et al: The Texas Children's Medication Algorithm Project: revision of the algorithm for pharmacotherapy of attention-deficit/hyperactivity disorder. J Am Acad Child Adolesc Psychiatry 45:642–657, 2006

Pliszka S, AACAP Work Group on Quality Issues: Practice parameter for the assessment and treatment of children and adolescents with attention-deficit/hyperactivity disorder. J Am Acad Child Adolesc Psychiatry 46:894–921, 2007

Chapter 16

Oppositional Defiant Disorder and Conduct Disorder

Select the single best response for each question.

16.1   The most common comorbid disorder found with oppositional defiant disorder (ODD) is

    A. Separation anxiety disorder.
    B. Obsessive-compulsive disorder (OCD).
    C. Attention-deficit/hyperactivity disorder (ADHD).
    D. Major depressive disorder.
    E. Dysthymic disorder.

The correct response is option C.

ADHD is the most common comorbid condition found with ODD (Speltz et al. 1999), and conversely many children diagnosed with ADHD also have ODD (Lahey et al. 1999). It can be difficult at times to distinguish the behaviors between these two disorders and determine the root cause. Children with ADHD may be described as disobedient when actually their poor compliance is a result of inattention and forgetfulness rather than willful defiance.

Another important consideration is the possible presence of an anxiety disorder. Separation anxiety disorder and OCD initially may present with complaints of severe tantrums. Children with ODD appear to be at higher risk for developing an anxiety disorder (Lavigne et al. 2001). Similar consideration should be given for the mood disorders because antagonistic and disobedient behaviors are often associated features for children with mood disorders, and studies indicate children with ODD are at similar increased risk for a comorbid mood disorder (Lavigne et al. 2001). **(p. 224)**

> Lahey BB, Miller TL, Gordon RA, et al: Developmental epidemiology of the disruptive behavior disorders, in Handbook of the Disruptive Behavior Disorders. Edited by Quay HC, Hogan A. New York, Plenum, 1999, pp 23–48
> Lavigne JV, Cicchetti C, Gibbons RD, et al: Oppositional defiant disorder with onset in preschool years: longitudinal stability and pathways to other disorders. J Am Acad Child Adolesc Psychiatry 40:1393–1400, 2001
> Speltz ML, McClellan J, Deklyen M, et al: Preschool boys with oppositional defiant disorder: clinical presentation and diagnostic change. J Am Acad Child Adolesc Psychiatry 38:838–845, 1999

16.2   Which of the following family attributes are correlated with higher rates of oppositional behaviors?

    A. Parental discord.
    B. Domestic violence.
    C. Low family cohesion.
    D. Child abuse.
    E. All of the above.

The correct response is option E.

Various environmental factors are correlated with increased risk for oppositional defiant disorder (ODD). Lower socioeconomic status is associated with risk, but this is probably mediated by family stresses and resulting dysfunction. Many other family attributes are correlated with higher rates of oppositional behaviors, including poor parenting practices, parental discord, domestic violence, low family cohesion, child abuse, and parental mental disorder, especially substance abuse and antisocial personality disorder (Greene et al. 2002). Mothers of children at increased risk for oppositional and disruptive behaviors report feeling less competent as parents, have fewer solutions for child behavior problems, and are less assertive in management of child misbehavior (Cunningham and Boyle 2002). **(p. 226)**

Cunningham CE, Boyle MH: Preschoolers at risk for attention-deficit hyperactivity disorder and oppositional defiant disorder: family, parenting, and behavioral correlates. J Abnorm Child Psychol 30:555–569, 2002

Greene RW, Biederman J, Zerwas S, et al: Psychiatric comorbidity, family dysfunction, and social impairment in referred youth with oppositional defiant disorder. Am J Psychiatry 159:1214–1224, 2002

16.3   Oppositional defiant disorder (ODD) is most predictive of the later occurrence of which of the following disorders?

    A. Antisocial personality disorder.
    B. Conduct disorder.
    C. Obsessive-compulsive disorder.
    D. Substance use disorder.
    E. Mood disorder.

The correct response is option B.

The typical age at onset of ODD appears to be around 6 years old, when most children have outgrown earlier, normative oppositional behaviors. ODD demonstrates high stability over time, and stability correlates with severity of the symptoms (Loeber et al. 2000). Longitudinal studies have shown that children diagnosed with the disorder are at significant risk for continued disruptive behavior symptoms. While most children with ODD will not go on to develop conduct disorder, they are at greater risk for later development of it. Among boys with ODD, those who developed conduct disorder had higher numbers of ODD symptoms than those who did not, and the symptoms of ODD typically persisted after the onset of conduct disorder (Loeber et al. 1993). In boys with ODD, atypical family structure appears to increase the risk of progression to conduct disorder (Rowe et al. 2002). Just as conduct disorder is an associated and predictive condition for the later development of antisocial personality disorder, so too does ODD appear to be associated and predictive of conduct disorder. **(pp. 226–227)**

Loeber R, Keenan K, Lahey BB, et al: Evidence for developmentally based diagnoses of oppositional defiant disorder and conduct disorder. J Abnorm Child Psychol 21:377–410, 1993

Loeber R, Burke JD, Lahey BB, et al: Oppositional defiant and conduct disorder: a review of the past 10 years, part I. J Am Acad Child Adolesc Psychiatry 39:1468–1484, 2000

Rowe R, Maughan B, Pickles A, et al: The relationship between DSM-IV oppositional defiant disorder and conduct disorder: findings from the Great Smoky Mountains Study. J Child Psychol Psychiatry 43:365–373, 2002

16.4   Which of the following psychotherapeutic interventions have been shown to have the greatest efficacy in treating oppositional defiant disorder (ODD)?

    A. Cognitive-behavioral therapy.
    B. Family therapy.
    C. Parent management training.
    D. Psychodynamic psychotherapy.
    E. None of the above.

The correct response is option C.

Numerous interventions have been developed and tried, usually based on associated parental risk factors and individual social skills deficits that contribute to oppositional and defiant behavior. Reviews and meta-analytic studies have identified promising evidence-based treatment approaches. Of these, parent management training and child problem-solving skills training have demonstrated the greatest efficacy with ODD. Parent management training indirectly affects child behavior by improving parent skills in dealing with negative acts and promoting desired behaviors (Kazdin 2005). Child problem-solving skills training derives from cognitive-behavioral therapy techniques in correcting dysfunctional social interactions and focuses on delaying impulsive responses, increasing reflection on alternative solutions, anticipating consequences, and practicing self-assessment of behaviors (Kazdin 2000). Parent management and child problem-solving skills training can be combined, and reports indicate significant additional improvements when used together as opposed to using just one approach (Kazdin et al. 1992). As with most conditions, early intervention appears to increase the chances for improvement. **(p. 228)**

> Kazdin AE: Treatments for aggressive and antisocial children. Child Adolesc Psychiatr Clin N Am 9:841–858, 2000
> Kazdin AE: Parent Management Training: Treatment for Oppositional, Aggressive, and Antisocial Behavior in Children and Adolescents. New York, Oxford University Press, 2005
> Kazdin AE, Bass D, Siegel T: Cognitive problem-solving skills training and parent management training in the treatment of antisocial behavior in children. J Consult Clin Psychol 60:733–747, 1992

16.5 Conduct disorder is more prevalent in which of the following populations?

   A. Boys.
   B. Rural communities.
   C. Higher socioeconomic status families.
   D. Suburbs.
   E. Neighborhoods with low rates of crime.

The correct response is option A.

A striking and consistent finding is that conduct disorder is more prevalent among boys than girls, with rates three to four times higher (Loeber et al. 2000). This feature has prompted discussion that the diagnostic criteria be modified for girls because their antisocial behaviors tend to be less aggressive than boys. Conduct disorder is also more common among children and adolescents from low-socioeconomic-status families and from neighborhoods with high rates of crime and social disorganization (Burke et al. 2002). Although conduct disorder typically is perceived as a problem of inner-city youth, studies comparing prevalence between urban and rural populations have found conflicting results. **(p. 230)**

> Burke JD, Loeber R, Birmaher B: Oppositional defiant disorder and conduct disorder: a review of the past 10 years, part II. J Am Acad Child Adolesc Psychiatry 41:1275–1293, 2002
> Loeber R, Burke JD, Lahey BB, et al: Oppositional defiant and conduct disorder: a review of the past 10 years, part I. J Am Acad Child Adolesc Psychiatry 39:1468–1484, 2000

Chapter 1 7

Substance Abuse and Addictions

Select the single best response for each question.

17.1 All of the following statements regarding the definition and diagnosis of substance abuse or dependence are correct *except*

    A. Substance use per se is sufficient for a diagnosis of abuse or dependence.

    B. *Misuse* can be defined as use for a purpose not consistent with medical guidelines.

    C. Recurrent substance use in adolescents rarely leads to impaired functioning.

    D. The diagnosis of substance abuse requires evidence of a maladaptive pattern of substance use with clinically significant levels of impairment or distress.

    E. A substance dependence diagnosis requires that additional criteria, such as withdrawal, tolerance, and loss of control over use, be met.

The correct response is option A.

Recurrent substance use in adolescents results in an inability to meet major role obligations, leading to impaired functioning in one or more major areas of their life and an increase in the likelihood of legal problems due to possession, risk-taking behavior, and exposure to hazardous situations. Substance use per se is not sufficient for a diagnosis of abuse or dependence, even in adolescents.

Although not an official term, *misuse* can be defined as use for a purpose not consistent with medical guidelines (e.g., modifying dose, using to achieve euphoria, and/or using with other nonprescribed psychoactive substances [World Health Organization 2007]).

The diagnosis of *substance abuse* requires evidence of a maladaptive pattern of substance use with clinically significant levels of impairment or distress.

Substance dependence requires that the adolescent meet at least three criteria, including such symptoms as withdrawal, tolerance, and loss of control over use. **(pp. 241–242)**

> World Health Organization: Lexicon of Alcohol and Drug Terms Published by the World Health Organization. Geneva, Switzerland, World Health Organization. Available at: http://www.who.int/substance_abuse/terminology/who_lexicon/en/index.html. Accessed July 15, 2007.

17.2 Regarding the comorbidity of substance use disorder (SUD), all of the following statements are correct *except*

    A. In addiction treatment programs, more than 50% of adolescents with co-occurring mental illness have three or more co-occurring psychiatric disorders.

    B. The most common comorbid conditions are conduct problems, attention-deficit/hyperactivity disorder (ADHD), mood disorders, and trauma-related symptoms.

    C. Some studies of youth with SUD show that females exhibit more internalizing symptoms than males.

    D. Except for depression, the early symptoms of most psychiatric disorders generally emerge prior to the onset of substance use.

    E. The specific type of a comorbid psychiatric diagnosis predicts relapse risk.

The correct response is option E.

Rather than type of diagnosis, the total number of psychiatric symptoms may predict relapse risk (McCarthy et al. 2005).

More than half of adolescents in addictions treatment who have a co-occurring mental illness have three or more co-occurring psychiatric disorders (Dennis et al. 2003). The most commonly comorbid psychiatric disorders among youth in addictions treatment include conduct problems, attention-deficit/hyperactivity disorder, mood disorders (e.g., depression), and trauma-related symptoms (Grella et al. 2001). Some studies of youth with SUD have found that females are more likely to exhibit internalizing (e.g., depression, anxiety) symptoms and trauma syndromes compared with males (e.g., Clark et al. 1997).

The early symptoms of most psychiatric disorders, excluding depression, generally emerged prior to the onset of substance use; full criteria for a nonsubstance psychiatric disorder were typically met prior to SUD onset in adolescence (Costello et al. 1999). **(p. 244)**

Clark DB, Pollock N, Bukstein OG, et al: Gender and comorbid psychopathology in adolescents with alcohol dependence. J Am Acad Child Adolesc Psychiatry 36:1195–1203, 1997

Costello EJ, Erkanli A, Federman E, et al: Development of psychiatric comorbidity with substance abuse in adolescents: effects of timing and sex. J Clin Child Psychol 28:298–311, 1999

Dennis ML, Dawud-Noursi S, Muck RD, et al: The need for developing and evaluating adolescent treatment models, in Adolescent Substance Abuse Treatment in the United States: Exemplary Models From a National Evaluation Study. Edited by Stevens SJ, Morral AR. Binghamton, NY, Haworth Press, 2003, pp 3–34

Grella C, Hser YI, Joshi V, et al: Drug treatment outcomes for adolescents with comorbid mental and substance use disorders. J Nerv Ment Dis 189:384–392, 2001

McCarthy DM, Tomlinson KL, Anderson KG, et al: Relapse in alcohol- and drug-disordered adolescents with comorbid psychopathology: changes in psychiatric symptoms. Psychol Addict Behav 19:28–34, 2005

17.3 The "gateway" substances with which most adolescents start are

    A. Tobacco and alcohol.

    B. Inhalants.

    C. Marijuana and alcohol.

    D. Amphetamines.

    E. Over-the-counter cough and cold medicines.

The correct response is option A.

First experiences with substance use most often take place in a social context with the use of "gateway" substances, such as alcohol and cigarettes, which are legal for adults and readily available to minors (Kandel and Yamaguchi 2002). Initial use may occur because of adolescent curiosity or the availability of a substance. Progressively fewer adolescents advance to later and more serious levels of substance use. Although drug consumption frequently follows a predictable sequence (referred to as the "gateway hypothesis" [Kandel and Yamaguchi 2002]), the risk for and rate of progression to SUD are the same whether consumption begins with a legal or an illegal drug (Tarter et al. 2006). **(p. 245)**

Kandel D, Yamaguchi K: Stages of drug involvement in the U.S. population, in Stages and Pathways of Drug Involvement: Examining the Gateway Hypothesis. Edited by Kandel D. New York, Cambridge University Press, 2002, pp 65–89

Tarter R, Vanyukov M, Kirisci L, et al: Predictors of marijuana use in adolescent before and after illicit drug use: examination of the gateway hypothesis. Am J Psychiatry 163:2134–2140, 2006

17.4 All of the following statements regarding the validity of adolescent self-report of substance use are true *except*

    A. A majority of adolescents in drug clinics or schools provide temporally consistent reports.

    B. An "intake-discharge effect" is often observed, wherein the level of use reported at discharge is much lower than that endorsed at admission to a treatment program.

    C. The use of a structured interview may support or validate the self-report.

D. Urine drug screen (UDS) is associated with greater drug use disclosures.

E. The engagement and skillfulness of the assessment interviewer predict more valid self-report responses.

The correct response is option B.

Both clinicians and investigators have noted an "intake-discharge effect" in which the level of use reported at discharge and problems as well as SUDs are higher than those endorsed at admission to a treatment program (Stinchfield 1997). The possible causes of the intake-discharge effect include factors at intake such as denial, reluctance to self-disclose because of embarrassment, and the wish to avoid sanctions for use, as well as the ability of the adolescent in treatment to more carefully examine the extent of substance use.

Although the clinician should always question whether any self-report about substance use is truthful, the majority of adolescents in drug clinics or schools give temporally consistent reports of substance use (Winters et al. 1991). The use of structured interviews or standardized questionnaires may also serve to support or validate the self-report.

The use of toxicological methods such as UDS can validate self-report by testing for the use of a specific agent. The use of urine or other toxicology screens has been associated with greater drug use disclosures (Wish et al. 1997). The attitude and skill of the assessment interviewer are often the best promoters of the validity of self-report, with engagement with the adolescent predicting more valid responses. **(pp. 247–248)**

> Stinchfield R: Reliability of adolescent self-reported pretreatment alcohol and other drug use. Subst Use Misuse 32:63–76, 1997
>
> Winters KC, Stinchfield RD, Henly GA, et al: Validity of adolescent self-report of alcohol and other drug involvement. Int J Addict 25:1379–1395, 1991
>
> Wish ED, Hoffman JA, Nemes S: The validity of self-reports of drug use at treatment admission and at follow-up: comparisons with urinalysis and hair analysis. NIDA Res Monogr 167:200–226, 1997

17.5 The pretreatment factors that are associated with poorer outcomes of substance use and relapse include all of the following *except*

A. Co-occurring psychopathology.

B. Higher severity of substance use.

C. Nonwhite race.

D. Criminality.

E. Lower educational status.

The correct response is option C.

Pretreatment factors associated with poorer outcomes (usually substance use and relapse to use) are co-occurring psychopathology, nonwhite race, higher severity of substance use, criminality, and lower educational status.

Reviews of studies of adolescent treatment outcome have concluded that treatment is better than no treatment (Deas and Thomas 2001; Williams et al. 2000). In the year following treatment, adolescents report decreased heavy drinking, marijuana and other illicit drug use, and criminal involvement as well as improved psychological adjustment and school performance (Grella et al. 2001; Hser et al. 2001). Longer duration of treatment is associated with several favorable outcomes. **(p. 252)**

> Deas D, Thomas SE: An overview of controlled studies of adolescent substance abuse treatment. Am J Addict 10:178–189, 2001
>
> Grella C, Hser YI, Joshi V, et al: Drug treatment outcomes for adolescents with comorbid mental and substance use disorders. J Nerv Ment Dis 189:384–392, 2001
>
> Hser YI, Grella CE, Hubbard RL, et al: An evaluation of drug treatments for adolescents in four U.S. cities. Arch Gen Psychiatry 58:689–695, 2001
>
> Williams RJ, Chang SY, Addiction Centre Adolescent Research Group: A comprehensive and comparative review of adolescent substance abuse treatment outcome. Clinical Psychology: Science and Practice 7:138–166, 2000

Chapter 18

Depression and Dysthymia

Select the single best response for each question.

18.1 Which of the following epidemiological findings concerning depression in children and adolescents is *true?*

    A. The prevalence of major depressive disorder is approximately 4%–8% in children.

    B. The male-to-female ratio for depression in children is 1:2.

    C. The cumulative prevalence of depression by age 18 is approximately 10% in community samples.

    D. The risk for depression remains constant after puberty.

    E. Approximately 5%–10% of children and adolescents have subsyndromal symptoms of major depressive disorder.

The correct response is option E.

Approximately 5%–10% of children and adolescents have subsyndromal symptoms of major depressive disorder (MDD). These youth have considerable psychosocial impairment and high family loading for depression, and are at increased risk for suicide and for developing the full symptoms of depression (Birmaher et al. 1996).

    The prevalence of MDD is approximately 2% in children and 4%–8% in adolescents, with a male-to-female ratio of 1:1 during childhood and 1:2 during adolescence (Birmaher et al. 1996). The risk for depression increases by a factor of two to four after puberty, particularly in females, and the cumulative prevalence by age 18 is approximately 20% in community samples. The few epidemiological studies that include dysthymic disorder report a prevalence of 0.6%–1.7% in children and 1.6%–8.0% in adolescents (Birmaher et al. 1996). **(pp. 261–262)**

> Birmaher B, Ryan ND, Williamson DE, et al: Childhood and adolescent depression: a review of the past 10 years. Part I. J Am Acad Child Adolesc Psychiatry 35:1427–1439, 1996

18.2 Although most children and adolescents recover from their first depressive episode, longitudinal studies of clinical and community samples of depressed youth have shown that the probability of recurrence after 5 years is

    A. 10%.

    B. 20%.

    C. 30%.

    D. 50%.

    E. 70%.

The correct response is option E.

The median duration of a major depressive episode in clinically referred youth is about 8 months and in community samples is about 1–2 months. Although most children and adolescents recover from their first depressive episode, longitudinal studies of both clinical and community samples of depressed youth have shown that the probability of recurrence reaches 20%–60% by 1–2 years after remission and climbs to 70% after 5 years (Birmaher et al. 2002; Costello et al. 2002). Recurrences can persist throughout life, and a substantial proportion of children and adolescents with MDD will continue to suffer from MDD episodes as adults. **(p. 265)**

Birmaher B, Arbelaez C, Brent D: Course and outcome of child and adolescent major depressive disorder. Child Adolesc Psychiatr Clin North Am 11:619–637, 2002

Costello EJ, Pine DS, Hammen C, et al: Development and natural history of mood disorders. Biol Psychiatry 52:529–542, 2002

18.3   You elect to treat a depressed adolescent with psychotherapy. Which of the following psychotherapies has been shown to be efficacious in randomized controlled clinical trials?

A. Systemic behavioral family therapy.
B. Long-term psychodynamic psychotherapy.
C. Brief psychodynamic psychotherapy.
D. Interpersonal psychotherapy.
E. None of the above.

The correct response is option D.

Several types of psychotherapy are being used for the treatment of youth with depression. However, only cognitive-behavior therapy (CBT) and interpersonal psychotherapy (IPT) have evidence of efficacy from randomized clinical trials, particularly for depressed adolescents (Weisz et al. 2006).

Psychodynamic therapy is widely used in clinical practice despite lack of evidence for efficacy. Because family interaction is related to the onset and course of adolescent depression (Birmaher et al. 2000; Nomura et al. 2002; Pilowsky et al. 2006), the improvement of family interactions is a logical treatment target in adolescent depression. However, only one randomized clinical trial has examined the impact of family therapy and found that CBT was superior to a systemic behavioral family therapy in the short-term reduction of adolescent depression (Brent et al. 1997). **(pp. 268–269)**

Birmaher B, Brent DA, Kolko D, et al: Clinical outcome after short-term psychotherapy for adolescents with major depressive disorder. Arch Gen Psychiatry 57:29–36, 2000

Brent DA, Holder D, Kolko D, et al: A clinical psychotherapy trial for adolescent depression comparing cognitive, family, and supportive treatments. Arch Gen Psychiatry 54:877–885, 1997

Nomura Y, Wickramaratne PJ, Warner V, et al: Family discord, parental depression, and psychopathology in offspring: ten-year follow-up. J Am Acad Child Psychiatry 41:402–409, 2002

Pilowsky DJ, Wickramaratne P, Nomura Y, et al: Family discord, parental depression, and psychopathology in offspring: 20-year follow-up. J Am Acad Child Psychiatry 45:452–460, 2006

Weisz JR, McCarty CA, Valeri SM: Effects of psychotherapy for depression in children and adolescents: a meta-analysis. Psychol Bull 132:132–149, 2006

18.4   A meta-analysis of all published and unpublished pharmacological, randomized controlled trials (RCTs) for major depressive disorder (MDD) in youth showed a benefit of selective serotonin reuptake inhibitor (SSRI) antidepressants over placebo, yielding a risk difference of

A. 11%.
B. 19%.
C. 24%.
D. 30%.
E. 35%.

The correct response is option A.

A meta-analysis of all published and unpublished pharmacological RCTs for MDD in youth showed an average response of 61% (95% confidence interval [CI], 58%–63%) for the SSRI antidepressants and 50% (95% CI, 47%–53%) for placebo, yielding a risk difference of 11% (95% CI, 7%–15%) (Bridge et al. 2007). Using these data, the number needed to treat to get one response that is attributable to active treatment was 10 overall (95% CI, 7%–

15%). Several studies showed small or no differences between the SSRI and placebo, in part because the rates of placebo response were high. This was more obvious in depressed children than in adolescents. **(p. 270)**

> Bridge JA, Iyengar S, Salary CB, et al: Clinical response and risk for reported suicidal ideation and suicide attempts in pediatric antidepressant treatment: a meta-analysis of randomized controlled trials. JAMA 297:1683–1696, 2007

18.5   You wish to start your patient, a 13-year-old girl with depression, on a selective serotonin reuptake inhibitor (SSRI), but her parents express concern about the U.S. Food and Drug Administration (FDA) "black box" warning of an increased risk of suicide in youths receiving SSRIs. Being familiar with results from a meta-analysis that reanalyzed the FDA findings (Hammad et al. 2006) and a study that used more appropriate statistical analyses (Bridge et al. 2007), you respond by providing the following information:

A. Only about 5 in 100 youth exposed to antidepressants had a new or worsening spontaneously reported suicidal ideation or behavior.

B. Pharmacoepidemiological studies support a positive relationship between SSRI use and the reduction in the adolescent and young adult suicide rate.

C. The number needed to harm (NNH) that can be attributed to the active treatment for antidepressants was 10.

D. Evaluation of suicidal ideation and attempts ascertained through rating scales in 17 studies showed a modest increase in the onset and worsening of suicidality.

E. After the black box warning was imposed, the prescription of antidepressants declined and the rates of suicide increased.

The correct response is option E.

As stated by the FDA (Hammad et al. 2006), with the increase in use of SSRIs there has been a dramatic decline in adolescent suicide (Olfson et al. 2003). In contrast, after the black box warning for all antidepressants was imposed by the FDA, the prescription of antidepressants diminished (Libby et al. 2007) and, although not clearly caused by the reduction of antidepressants, the rates of suicide increased (Hamilton et al. 2007). Pharmacoepidemiological studies, although correlative rather than causal, support a positive relationship between SSRI use and the reduction in the adolescent and young adult suicide rate (Gibbons et al. 2006; Valuck et al. 2004).

Among the side effects of antidepressants, in addition to the rare risk of triggering hypomania in predisposed children, the most serious one is the small but statistically significant risk of onset or worsening of suicidal ideation and, more rarely, suicide attempts. A meta-analysis that reanalyzed the FDA analyses (Hammad et al. 2006), including more published and unpublished antidepressant RCTs and using more appropriate statistical analyses (Bridge et al. 2007), found that for major depressive disorder (MDD), obsessive-compulsive disorder (OCD), and non-OCD anxiety disorders, the pooled risk difference for new or increased spontaneously reported suicidal ideation or suicidal behaviors for all antidepressants (SSRIs, venlafaxine, and bupropion) was 0.7% (95% CI, 0.1%–1.3%). Thus, about 1 in 100 youth exposed to antidepressants had new or worsening *spontaneously reported* suicidal ideation or behavior. There were very few suicide attempts and *no completions*. Interestingly, when the analyses were done for each disorder separately, there were no significant differences between the antidepressants and placebo. For example, for MDD, the rates of suicidal ideation/attempts were 3% for those taking the antidepressants and 2% for those receiving placebo, yielding a risk difference of 1%. Using these data, the number of depressed subjects needed to treat to observe one adverse event (NNH) that could be attributed to the active treatment for antidepressants was 112 (Bridge et al. 2007).

In contrast to the analyses of *spontaneously reported* suicidal adverse events, evaluation of suicidal ideation and attempts ascertained through rating scales in 17 studies did not show significant onset or worsening of suicidality (Hammad et al. 2006). **(pp. 270–271)**

Bridge JA, Iyengar S, Salary CB, et al: Clinical response and risk for reported suicidal ideation and suicide attempts in pediatric antidepressant treatment: a meta-analysis of randomized controlled trials. JAMA 297:1683–1696, 2007

Gibbons RD, Hur K, Bhaumik DK, et al: The relationship between antidepressant prescription rates and rate of early adolescent suicide. Am J Psychiatry 163:1898–1904, 2006

Hamilton BE, Minino AM, Martin JA, et al: Annual summary of vital statistics: 2005. Pediatrics 119:345–360, 2007

Hammad TA, Laughren T, Racoosin J: Suicidality in pediatric patients treated with antidepressant drugs. Arch Gen Psychiatry 63:332–339, 2006

Libby AM, Brent DA, Morrato EH, et al: Decline in treatment of pediatric depression after FDA advisory on risk of suicidality with SSRIs. Am J Psychiatry 164:884–891, 2007

Olfson M, Shaffer D, Marcus SC, et al: Relationship between antidepressant medication treatment and suicide in adolescents. Arch Gen Psychiatry 60:978–982, 2003

Valuck RJ, Libby AM, Sills MR, et al: Antidepressant treatment and risk of suicide attempt by adolescents with major depressive disorder: a propensity-adjusted retrospective cohort study. CNS Drugs 18:1119–1132, 2004

Chapter 19

Bipolar Disorder

Select the single best response for each question.

19.1 Which of the following statements regarding the DSM-IV-TR (American Psychiatric Association 2000) definition of bipolar disorder is *false*?

    A. Manic episode must be present in bipolar I disorder.
    B. Depressive episode must be present in bipolar I disorder.
    C. Depressive episode must be present in bipolar II disorder.
    D. Hypomania must be present in bipolar II disorder.
    E. Cyclothymia presents with cycles of subsyndromal mania and depression.

The correct response is option B.

Bipolar disorder is defined by episodes of mania (bipolar I disorder); hypomania, characterized by briefer duration of manic symptoms with less impairment (bipolar II disorder); or manic symptoms of insufficient number and/or duration to meet mania or hypomania criteria (bipolar disorder not otherwise specified [NOS]). Depressive episodes, at all levels of severity and duration, need not occur in bipolar I disorder, but usually do. In bipolar II disorder, full major depression occurs with hypomania. *Cyclothymia* refers to cycles of subsyndromal mania and depression. **(p. 279)**

> American Psychiatric Association: Diagnostic and Statistical Manual of Mental Disorders, 4th Edition, Text Revision. Washington, DC, American Psychiatric Association, 2000

19.2 In bipolar disorder, what episode frequency defines "rapid cycling" according to DSM-IV-TR (American Psychiatric Association 2000)?

    A. One per month.
    B. Two or more per year.
    C. Four or more per year.
    D. Six or more per year.
    E. Once per season.

The correct response is option C.

According to DSM-IV-TR, bipolar disorder is further classified by how the manic and depressive symptoms and episodes relate to each other. When episodes of mania and depression follow each other without a well interval, the type is said to be "circular." Four or more episodes per year define "rapid cycling." If manic and depressive symptoms occur simultaneously during an episode, the episode is called "mixed." **(p. 279)**

> American Psychiatric Association: Diagnostic and Statistical Manual of Mental Disorders, 4th Edition, Text Revision. Washington, DC, American Psychiatric Association, 2000

19.3 All of the following statements regarding comorbidity of bipolar disorder are correct *except*

    A. The most common simultaneous comorbidities occurring during mania are attention-deficit/hyperactivity disorder (ADHD), oppositional defiant disorder (ODD), conduct disorder, and anxiety.

B. ADHD co-occurs with bipolar disorder more in prepubertal children than in adolescents.
C. The combination of externalizing disorders and bipolar disorder may represent a phenotype specific to adolescents.
D. About 20% of children with mania have a comorbid pervasive developmental disorder.
E. Early-onset bipolar disorder appears to increase the rate of substance abuse.

The correct response is option C.

The combination of externalizing disorders and bipolar disorder may represent a phenotype specific to prepubertal children (Biederman et al. 2000), not adolescents. Conduct disorder may precede or co-occur with bipolar disorder.

People who meet criteria for mania almost invariably meet criteria for at least one other disorder. The most common simultaneous comorbidities (ADHD, ODD, conduct disorder, anxiety) occur during mania and are difficult to distinguish from it without a good history.

ADHD, which begins prior to bipolar disorder and may co-occur with it, may be found in up to 90% of prepubertal children and about half of adolescents with bipolar disorder (Faraone et al. 1997; Tillman et al. 2003).

Bipolar disorder in children with developmental disorders is less well studied (see Gutkovich and Carlson 2008 for review). About 20% of children diagnosed with mania also had comorbid pervasive developmental disorder, but up to 60% of patients with mood disorders obtained parent ratings of autism spectrum behaviors in the "likely autism spectrum disorders" range.

Substance and alcohol abuse are common comorbidities in adolescents with bipolar disorder. ADHD and conduct disorder, which may be co-occurring in early-onset bipolar disorder, are both risk factors for the development of substance use disorder. However, early-onset bipolar disorder itself appears to increase rates of substance abuse over and above other externalizing disorders. **(pp. 283–284)**

Biederman J, Mick E, Faraone SV, et al: Pediatric mania: a developmental subtype of bipolar disorder? Biol Psychiatry 48:458–466, 2000

Faraone SV, Biederman J, Wozniak J, et al: Is comorbidity with ADHD a marker for juvenile-onset mania? J Am Acad Child Adolesc Psychiatry 36:1046–1055, 1997

Gutkovich ZA, Carlson GA: Medication treatment of bipolar disorder in developmentally disabled children and adolescents. Minerva Pediatr 60:69–85, 2008

Tillman R, Geller B, Bolhofner K, et al: Ages of onset and rates of syndromal and subsyndromal comorbid DSM-IV diagnoses in a prepubertal and early adolescent bipolar disorder phenotype. J Am Acad Child Adolesc Psychiatry 42:1486–1493, 2003

19.4 Functional magnetic resonance imaging (fMRI) studies of children with bipolar disorder suggest perturbations in prefrontal limbic circuitry. Findings from recent studies include all of the following *except*

A. Children detect greater hostility in emotionally neutral faces.
B. Children show elevated levels of fear when viewing faces.
C. Activation of the left amygdala-striatal-ventral prefrontal circuit is increased when rating face hostility.
D. Activation of the amygdala during emotional changes is decreased.
E. Probability of misinterpreting facial expression is increased.

The correct response is option D.

Recent fMRI studies suggest perturbations in prefrontal-limbic circuitry (Pavuluri et al. 2007): bipolar children detected greater hostility in emotionally neutral faces (Rich et al. 2006), as well as elevated levels of fear when viewing them, and exhibited increased activation of the left amygdala-striatal-ventral prefrontal circuit when rating face hostility.

Heightened activation of the amygdala during emotional challenges may interfere with attentional capacities among children with bipolar disorder, thus increasing the probability that they will misinterpret the nature of incoming stimuli (facial expression) and respond in an inappropriate manner. **(p. 284)**

Pavuluri MN, O'Connor MM, Harral E, et al: Affective neural circuitry during facial emotion processing in pediatric bipolar disorder. Biol Psychiatry 62:158–167, 2007

Rich BA, Vinton DT, Roberson-Nay R, et al: Limbic hyperactivation during processing of neutral facial expressions in children with bipolar disorder. Proc Natl Acad Sci U S A 103:8900–8905, 2006

19.5 All of the following statements regarding the onset, course, and prognosis of bipolar disorder are correct *except*

    A. Bipolar disorder often begins with depression or dysthymia.

    B. Early-onset bipolar disorder is characterized by slow response to treatment and persistent mood fluctuations.

    C. Bipolar disorder NOS has a faster response to treatment than bipolar I disorder or bipolar II disorder.

    D. About one-quarter of children with bipolar disorder NOS converted to bipolar I disorder or bipolar II disorder based on a 2-year follow-up study.

    E. Poor prognostic indicators may include nonadherence to prescribed medications, low socioeconomic status (SES), low maternal warmth, psychosis, comorbid anxiety, and rapid cycling.

The correct response is option C.

Children with bipolar disorder NOS suffer from a more chronic course of illness than youth with bipolar I or II disorder, with persistent subthreshold symptoms and slower response to acute treatment.

Bipolar disorder often begins with depression or dysthymia. Over a 2- to 4-year follow-up in U.S. samples, early-onset bipolar disorder (both broad and narrow phenotypes) is characterized by slow response to treatment, persistent mood fluctuations, elevated risk for suicide attempts, and severe psychosocial impairment.

Within 2 years of follow-up, one-quarter of individuals initially diagnosed with bipolar disorder NOS converted to bipolar I or II disorder (Birmaher et al. 2006).

Nonadherence to pharmacological treatment, low SES, low maternal warmth, psychosis, comorbid anxiety, and rapid cycling are poor prognostic indicators (Birmaher et al. 2006; DelBello et al. 2007; Geller et al. 2004). **(p. 285)**

Birmaher B, Axelson D, Strober M, et al: Clinical course of children and adolescents with bipolar spectrum disorders. Arch Gen Psychiatry 63:175–183, 2006

DelBello MP, Hanseman D, Adler CM, et al: Twelve-month outcome of adolescents with bipolar disorder following first hospitalization for a manic or mixed episode. Am J Psychiatry 164:582–590, 2007

Geller B, Tillman R, Craney JL, et al: Four-year prospective outcome and natural history of mania in children with a prepubertal and early adolescent bipolar disorder phenotype. Arch Gen Psychiatry 61:459–467, 2004

19.6 Which of the following medications has been approved by the U.S. Food and Drug Administration (FDA) for the treatment of mania in youth?

    A. Olanzapine.

    B. Divalproex.

    C. Carbamazepine.

    D. Ziprasidone.

    E. Aripiprazole.

The correct response is option E.

As of 2007, eight medications (lithium, divalproex, extended-release carbamazepine, olanzapine, quetiapine, risperidone, aripiprazole, and ziprasidone) have FDA approval in adults for the treatment of acute mania, and two (olanzapine plus fluoxetine combined [OFC] and quetiapine) have approval for bipolar depression. Two medications have approval for maintenance treatment; lithium is approved for prevention of mania, and lamotrigine for bipolar depression. In young people, lithium has been approved for adolescent mania, and risperidone and aripiprazole have been approved to treat mania in children as young as age 10. **(p. 289)**

Chapter 20

Generalized Anxiety Disorder, Specific Phobia, Panic Disorder, Social Phobia, and Selective Mutism

Select the single best response for each question.

20.1 Which of the following childhood-onset disorders has a chronic waxing and waning course and may remit spontaneously in one-third of lifetime cases?

    A. Generalized anxiety disorder.
    B. Specific phobia.
    C. Panic disorder.
    D. Social phobia.
    E. Selective mutism.

The correct response is option A.

Generalized anxiety disorder is a chronic condition with a waxing and waning course. One-third of lifetime cases have a spontaneous remission (Wittchen et al. 1994).

Childhood phobias are relatively stable over time (Ollendick et al. 2002), and their symptoms tend to decline with age (Muris et al. 1999).

The age at onset for panic disorder is late adolescence and early adulthood (American Psychiatric Association 2000). It is less common in younger children.

Social phobia is a relatively stable problem and is likely to persist over time if left untreated. It usually begins between early and middle adolescence but occurs in children as young as 8 years (Beidel et al. 1999).

Selective mutism has its onset between 3 and 5 years of age. It is characterized by persistent difficulty in speaking situations and a chronic course of mutism. Children who do not improve prior to adolescence may have a more persistent form of selective mutism (Cohan et al. 2006). **(pp. 300, 307 [Table 20–9])**

American Psychiatric Association: Diagnostic and Statistical Manual of Mental Disorders, 4th Edition, Text Revision. Washington, DC, American Psychiatric Association, 2000

Beidel DC, Turner SM, Morris TL: Psychopathology of childhood social phobia. J Am Acad Child Adolesc Psychiatry 38:643–650, 1999

Cohan SL, Price JM, Stein MB: Suffering in silence: why a developmental psychopathology perspective on selective mutism is needed. J Dev Behav Pediatr 27:341–355, 2006

Muris P, Schmidt H, Merckelbach H: The structure of specific phobia symptoms among children and adolescents. Behav Res Ther 37:863–868, 1999

Ollendick TH, King NJ, Muris P: Fears and phobias in children: phenomenology, epidemiology and aetiology. Child and Adolescent Mental Health 7:98–106, 2002

Wittchen H-U, Zhao S, Kessler RC, et al: DSM-III-R generalized anxiety disorder in the National Comorbidity Survey. Arch Gen Psychiatry 51:355–364, 1994

20.2   In regard to common biological influences on the development of childhood anxiety, which of the following statements is *true?*

   A. Children with anxiety disorders show less autonomic reactivity in response to stress.
   B. State anxiety has demonstrated more evidence for genetic influences when compared with trait anxiety.
   C. Behavioral inhibition in children is associated with the development of anxiety.
   D. Children at risk for anxiety disorders are less likely to have irregularities in sleeping and eating patterns.
   E. Longitudinal studies have failed to demonstrate a link between anxiety sensitivity and the development of panic disorder.

The correct response is option C.

Behavioral inhibition in children (e.g., the tendency toward being shy, timid, quiet, and initially avoidant of novel and uncertain stimuli) is associated with the development of anxiety (Kagan 1988).

Children with anxiety disorders show greater autonomic reactivity in response to stress (Kagan 1988) and have different patterns of cortisol dysregulation (Feder et al. 2004).

Trait anxiety, a more stable personality characteristic guiding responses to anxiety-provoking situations, has demonstrated more evidence for genetic influences when compared with *state anxiety*, a transitory pattern of anxiety symptoms in response to stressors (Lau et al. 2006).

Children at risk for anxiety disorders display gastrointestinal distress in response to stressors (Campo et al. 2003) and are more likely to have irregularities in sleeping and eating patterns (Ong et al. 2006).

Anxiety sensitivity, a tendency to ascribe negative consequences to physiological responses typically associated with anxiety (e.g., shortness of breath, increased heart rate, trembling) is common among children at risk for anxiety disorders (Reiss 1991). Longitudinal studies show specific links between anxiety sensitivity and the development of panic disorder (e.g., Weems et al. 2002). **(pp. 306, 308 [Table 20–10])**

Campo JV, Dahl RE, Williamson DE, et al: Gastrointestinal distress to serotonergic challenge: a risk marker for emotional disorder. J Am Acad Child Adolesc Psychiatry 42:1221–1226, 2003

Feder A, Coplan JD, Goetz RR, et al: Twenty-four hour cortisol secretion patterns in prepubertal children with anxiety or depressive disorders. Biol Psychiatry 53:198–204, 2004

Kagan J: Biological bases of childhood shyness. Science 240:167–171, 1988

Lau JY, Eley TC, Stevenson J: Examining the state-trait anxiety relationship: a behavioural genetic approach. J Abnorm Child Psychol 34:19–27, 2006

Ong SH, Wickramaratne P, Tang M, et al: Early childhood sleep and eating problems as predictors of adolescent and adult mood and anxiety disorders. J Affect Disord 96:1–8, 2006

Reiss S: Expectancy model of fear, anxiety, and panic. Clin Psychol Rev 11:141–153, 1991

Weems CF, Hayward C, Killen J, et al: A longitudinal investigation of anxiety sensitivity in adolescence. J Abnorm Psychol 111:471–477, 2002

20.3   Which of the following parenting behaviors is associated with higher levels of anxiety in children?

   A. High levels of parental control.
   B. High levels of parental warmth.
   C. High levels of parental sensitivity.
   D. Lower levels of parental rejection.
   E. Lower levels of parental criticism.

The correct response is option A.

High levels of parental control (overprotective/overcontrolling parenting) are thought to encourage children's dependence on parents, lower their sense of mastery and control in difficult situations, and thus contribute to higher levels of anxiety (Chorpita and Barlow 1998).

Low levels of parental warmth and sensitivity and higher levels of parental rejection and criticism are thought to influence children's ability to regulate their own emotions and tolerate negative affect, including their experiences of anxiety (Lieb et al. 2000).

By modeling anxious responses to potentially threatening situations, parents may reinforce the child's own anxious coping responses, reducing the likelihood of learning effective strategies to reduce anxiety. **(pp. 306, 308 [Table 20–10])**

Chorpita BF, Barlow DH: The development of anxiety: the role of control in the early environment. Psychol Bull 124:3–21, 1998
Lieb R, Wittchen HU, Höfler M, et al: Parental psychopathology, parenting styles, and the risk of social phobia in offspring: a prospective-longitudinal community study. Arch Gen Psychiatry 57:859–866, 2000

20.4   Which of the following psychotherapies has received the most empirical support from randomized controlled studies for efficacy in the treatment of anxiety disorders in children and adolescents?

   A. Interpersonal psychotherapy (IPT).
   B. Cognitive-behavioral therapy (CBT).
   C. Dialectical behavioral therapy.
   D. Psychodynamic psychotherapy.
   E. Supportive psychotherapy.

The correct response is option B.

Among the psychotherapies, exposure-based CBT has received the most empirical support from randomized controlled studies for the treatment of anxiety disorders in children and adolescents and is currently the psychotherapy of choice for this population (reviewed in Compton et al. 2004; In-Albon and Schneider 2007). CBT has been shown to reduce anxiety symptoms and is superior to waitlist control; however, relative efficacy and effectiveness versus alternative psychotherapeutic interventions have not been investigated.

CBT is a diverse group of interventions that are administered by trained clinicians in a flexible manner for the patient presenting with one disorder or comorbid disorders (Compton et al. 2004). Behavioral therapies are grounded in conditioning and social learning models and have guided interventions used to treat specific phobia and social phobia (Graczyk et al. 2005). CBT for childhood anxiety disorders consists of several components: psychoeducation, somatic management, cognitive restructuring, problem solving, exposure, and relapse prevention (Velting et al. 2004).

Psychoanalysis and psychodynamic psychotherapy have been used in the clinical treatment of anxiety disorders in children and adolescents, but empirical evidence regarding efficacy or effectiveness is very limited (In-Albon and Schneider 2007; King et al. 2005). **(pp. 312–314)**

Compton SN, March JS, Brent D, et al: Cognitive-behavioral psychotherapy for anxiety and depressive disorders in children and adolescents: an evidence-based medicine review. J Am Acad Child Adolesc Psychiatry 43:930–959, 2004
Graczyk PA, Connolly SD, Corapci F: Anxiety disorders in children and adolescents: theory, treatment, and prevention, in Handbook of Adolescent Behavior Problems: Evidence-Based Approaches to Prevention and Treatment. Edited by Gullotta TP, Adams GR. New York, Springer, 2005, pp 131–157
In-Albon T, Schneider S: Psychotherapy of childhood anxiety disorders: a meta-analysis. Psychother Psychosom 76:15–24, 2007
King NJ, Muris P, Ollendick TH: Childhood fears and phobias: assessment and treatment. Child and Adolescent Mental Health 10:50–56, 2005
Velting ON, Setzer NJ, Albano AM: Update on and advances in assessment and cognitive-behavioral treatment of anxiety disorders in children and adolescents. Professional Psychology: Research and Practice 35:42–54, 2004

20.5   Which of the following agents is considered the first-line treatment for anxiety disorders in children?

   A. Serotonin-norepinephrine reuptake inhibitors (SNRIs).
   B. Atypical antipsychotics.
   C. Tricyclic antidepressants.
   D. Benzodiazepines.
   E. Selective serotonin reuptake inhibitors (SSRIs).

The correct response is option E.

A developing evidence base suggests that SSRIs should be considered the first-line pharmacological treatment for pediatric anxiety disorders (Seidel and Walkup 2006). Several randomized, placebo-controlled trials with SSRIs have established the short-term efficacy of SSRIs for the treatment of childhood anxiety disorders (Table 20–1; corresponds to Table 20–12 in the Textbook).

SSRIs have generally been well tolerated by children with anxiety disorders. Common side effects reported in clinical trials include gastrointestinal symptoms, headache, increased motor activity, and insomnia. Often these side effects are mild and transient and medication treatment can continue. Less common side effects such as disinhibition and more severe forms of behavioral activation such as agitation or reactive aggression need to be monitored as well. **(pp. 314–315; Table 20–12)**

Seidel L, Walkup JT: Selective serotonin reuptake inhibitor use in the treatment of pediatric non-obsessive-compulsive disorder anxiety disorders. J Child Adolesc Psychopharmacol 16:171–179, 2006

Berney T, Kolvin I, Bhate SR, et al: School phobia: a therapeutic trial with clomipramine and short-term outcome. Br J Psychiatry 138:110–118, 1981

Bernstein GA, Garfinkel BD, Borchardt CM: Comparative studies of pharmacotherapy for school refusal. J Am Acad Child Adolesc Psychiatry 29:773–781, 1990

Birmaher B, Axelson DA, Monk K, et al: Fluoxetine for the treatment of childhood anxiety disorders. J Am Acad Child Adolesc Psychiatry 42:415–423, 2003

Black B, Uhde TW: Treatment of elective mutism with fluoxetine: a double-blind, placebo-controlled study. J Am Acad Child Adolesc Psychiatry 33:1000–1006, 1994

Gittelman-Klein R, Klein DF: School phobia: controlled imipramine treatment. Calif Med 115(3):42, 1971

Graae F, Milner J, Rizzotto L, et al: Clonazepam in childhood anxiety disorders. J Am Acad Child Adolesc Psychiatry 33:372–376, 1994

Klein RG, Koplewicz HS, Kanner A: Imipramine treatment in children with separation anxiety disorder. J Am Acad Child Adolesc Psychiatry 31:21–28, 1992

Research Units on Pediatric Psychopharmacology Anxiety Study Group: Fluvoxamine for the treatment of anxiety disorders in children and adolescents. N Engl J Med 344:1279–1285, 2001

Rynn MA, Siqueland L, Rickels K: Placebo-controlled trial of sertraline in the treatment of children with generalized anxiety disorder. Am J Psychiatry 158:2008–2014, 2001

Rynn MA, Riddle MA, Yeung PP, et al: Efficacy and safety of extended-release venlafaxine in the treatment of generalized anxiety disorder in children and adolescents: two placebo-controlled trials. Am J Psychiatry 164:290–300, 2007

Simeon JG, Ferguson HB, Knott V, et al: Clinical, cognitive, and neurophysiological effects of alprazolam in children and adolescents with overanxious and avoidant disorders. J Am Acad Child Adolesc Psychiatry 31:29–33, 1992

Wagner KD, Berard R, Stein MB, et al: A multicenter, randomized, double-blind, placebo-controlled trial of paroxetine in children and adolescents with social anxiety. Arch Gen Psychiatry 61:1153–1162, 2004

Walkup JT, Albano AM, Piacentini J, et al: Cognitive-behavioral therapy, sertraline, or a combination in childhood anxiety. N Engl J Med 359:2753–2766, 2008

Table 20–1. Placebo-controlled pharmacological treatment studies[a]

Author	Treatment	Demographics	Diagnoses	Results
Serotonin reuptake inhibitors				
Black and Uhde 1994 [rdb]	Fluoxetine (12–27 mg/day), 12 weeks	N = 15, ages 6–11	SM plus SoP or AD	Fluoxetine > Pbo
Research Units on Pediatric Psychopharmacology Anxiety Study Group 2001 [rct]	Fluvoxamine (50–250 mg/day child, max 300 mg/day adolescent), 8 weeks	N = 128, ages 6–17	SoP, SAD, GAD	Fluvoxamine > Pbo
Rynn et al. 2001 [rdb]	Sertraline (50 mg/day), 9 weeks	N = 22, ages 5–17	GAD	Sertraline > Pbo
Birmaher et al. 2003 [rdb]	Fluoxetine (20 mg/day), 12 weeks	N = 74, ages 7–17	GAD, SoP, SAD	Fluoxetine > Pbo / Fluoxetine = Pbo
Wagner et al. 2004 [rdb]	Paroxetine (10–50 mg/day), 16 weeks	N = 322, ages 8–17	SoP	Paroxetine > Pbo
Walkup et al. 2008 [rdb]	Sertraline (25–200 mg/day), 12 weeks	N = 209, ages 7–17	SoP, SAD, GAD	Sertraline > Pbo
Other antidepressants				
Gittelman-Klein and Klein 1971 [rdb]	Imipramine (100–200 mg/day)	N = 35, ages 6–14	School phobia with anxiety disorders	Imipramine > Pbo
Berney et al. 1981 [rdb]	Clomipramine (40–75 mg/day)	N = 51, ages 9–14	School refusal	Clomipramine = Pbo
Klein et al. 1992 [rdb]	Imipramine (75–275 mg/day)	N = 21, ages 6–15	SAD with or without school phobia	Imipramine = Pbo
Rynn et al. 2007 [rdb]	Venlafaxine ER (37.5–225 mg/day), 8 weeks	N = 320, ages 6–17 (two studies combined)	GAD	Venlafaxine ER > Pbo (study 1) / Venlafaxine ER = Pbo (study 2)
Benzodiazepines				
Bernstein et al. 1990 [rdb]	Alprazolam (0.75–4.0 mg/day) vs. imipramine (50–175 mg/day)	N = 24, ages 7–18	School refusal, SAD	Alprazolam = imipramine = Pbo
Simeon et al. 1992 [rdb]	Alprazolam (0.5–3.5 mg/day)	N = 30, ages 8–17	OAD, AD	Alprazolam = Pbo
Graae et al. 1994 [rdb]	Clonazepam (0.5–2.0 mg/day)	N = 15, ages 7–13	SAD	Clonazepam = Pbo

Note. AD = avoidant disorder; ER = extended release; GAD = generalized anxiety disorder; OAD = overanxious disorder; OCD = obsessive-compulsive disorder; Pbo = placebo; rct = randomized controlled trial; rdb = randomized double-blind trial; SAD = separation anxiety disorder; SM = selective mutism; SoP = social phobia.
[a]Data reported in this table reflect medication arm of multimodal study only.

Chapter 21

Separation Anxiety Disorder and School Refusal

Select the single best response for each question.

21.1 All of the following statements regarding separation anxiety disorder (SAD) are correct *except*

    A. SAD is the only anxiety disorder in DSM-IV-TR (American Psychiatric Association 2000) that is included under the category of disorders usually first diagnosed in infancy, childhood, or adolescence.

    B. Separation anxiety can be a developmentally appropriate response.

    C. Separation anxiety typically declines between 7 and 9 years of age.

    D. SAD only occurs when the child shows developmentally inappropriate and excessive anxiety associated with separation from a primary caregiver.

    E. A child may experience anxiety prior to, during, and/or in anticipation of the separation.

The correct response is option C.

Separation anxiety typically declines between 3 and 5 years of age as a result of the child's cognitive maturation that allows the child to comprehend that separation from a caregiver is temporary.

SAD is the only anxiety disorder in DSM-IV-TR (American Psychiatric Association 2000) that is included under the category of disorders usually first diagnosed in infancy, childhood, or adolescence. The onset of the disorder is prior to 18 years of age, and it is not typically diagnosed in adulthood.

Separation anxiety is a developmentally appropriate response in young children upon separation from their primary caregivers. This is normal from 6 to 30 months of age and usually intensifies between 13 and 18 months of age (Kearney et al. 2003).

SAD occurs when the child demonstrates developmentally inappropriate distress associated with separation from a primary caregiver (American Psychiatric Association 2000). The child's anxiety may be present prior to, during, and/or in anticipation of the separation. **(p. 325)**

    American Psychiatric Association: Diagnostic and Statistical Manual of Mental Disorders, 4th Edition, Text Revision. Washington, DC, American Psychiatric Association, 2000

    Kearney CA, Sims KE, Pursell CR, et al: Separation anxiety disorder in young children: a longitudinal and family analysis. J Clin Child Adolesc Psychol 32:593–598, 2003

21.2 Which of the following statements regarding the epidemiology and comorbidity of separation anxiety disorder (SAD) is *false*?

    A. Prevalence rates of SAD range between 3% and 5%.

    B. Several studies show higher prevalence rates of SAD in girls than in boys.

    C. Fifty percent of a community sample of 8-year-old children exhibited subclinical levels of separation anxiety.

    D. Children with SAD are more likely to have a comorbid mood disorder compared with children with generalized anxiety disorder (GAD) or social phobia (SP).

    E. Children with SAD are more likely to have a sleep terror disorder compared with children with GAD or SP.

The correct response is option D.

Verduin and Kendall (2003) compared comorbidity rates in 199 children (8–13 years) with a primary diagnosis of GAD, SAD, or SP. Children with SAD were the least likely to have a comorbid mood disorder and most likely to be diagnosed with sleep terror disorder.

The prevalence rate of SAD in youth typically ranges between 3% and 5% (Black 1995; Shear et al. 2006). SAD is more prevalent in children compared with adolescents (Breton et al. 1999). Several studies have demonstrated higher prevalence rates of SAD in females compared with males (e.g., Ehringer et al. 2006); however, other studies have not found significant gender differences (e.g., Costello et al. 1996; Last et al. 1992). Many youth exhibit subclinical levels of separation anxiety but do not meet diagnostic criteria for SAD. Kashani and Orvaschel (1990) found a prevalence rate of approximately 50% for subclinical symptoms of SAD among a community sample of 8-year-old children. **(p. 326)**

Black B: Separation anxiety disorder and panic disorder, in Anxiety Disorders in Children and Adolescents. Edited by March JS. New York, Guilford, 1995, pp 212–234

Breton JJ, Bergeron L, Valla JP, et al: Quebec child mental health survey: prevalence of DSM-III-R mental health disorders. J Child Psychol Psychiatry 40:375–384, 1999

Costello EJ, Angold A, Burns BJ, et al: The Great Smoky Mountains Study of Youth: goals, design, methods, and the prevalence of DSM-III-R disorders. Arch Gen Psychiatry 53:1129–1136, 1996

Ehringer MA, Rhee SH, Young S, et al: Genetic and environmental contributions to common psychopathologies of childhood and adolescence: a study of twins and their siblings. J Abnorm Child Psychol 34:1–17, 2006

Kashani JH, Orvaschel H: A community study of anxiety in children and adolescents. Am J Psychiatry 147:313–318, 1990

Last CG, Perrin S, Hersen M, et al: DSM-III-R anxiety disorders in children: sociodemographic and clinical characteristics. J Am Acad Child Adolesc Psychiatry 31:1070–1076, 1992

Shear K, Jin R, Ruscio AM, et al: Prevalence and correlates of estimated DSM-IV child and adult separation anxiety disorder in the National Comorbidity Survey Replication. Am J Psychiatry 163:1074–1083, 2006

Verduin TL, Kendall PC: Differential occurrence of comorbidity within childhood anxiety disorders. J Clin Child Adolesc Psychol 32:290–295, 2003

21.3 According to the American Academy of Child and Adolescent Psychiatry (AACAP) practice parameter (2007), effective treatment of children with separation anxiety disorder (SAD) often includes all of the following *except*

  A. Psychoeducation.
  B. School consultation.
  C. Cognitive-behavioral therapy (CBT).
  D. Selective serotonin reuptake inhibitors (SSRIs).
  E. Psychoanalytical psychotherapy.

The correct response is option E.

Psychoanalytical psychotherapy is not recommended for separation anxiety disorder.

The AACAP practice parameter for youth diagnosed with an anxiety disorder recommends that treatment planning consider a multimodal approach (American Academy of Child and Adolescent Psychiatry 2007). Effective treatment of children with SAD often includes child and parent psychoeducation, school consultation, CBT, and SSRIs. **(p. 329)**

American Academy of Child and Adolescent Psychiatry: Practice parameter for the assessment and treatment of children and adolescents with anxiety disorders. J Am Acad Child Adolesc Psychiatry 46:267–283, 2007

21.4 All of the following statements regarding school refusal are correct *except*

    A. It is an anxiety disorder listed in DSM-IV-TR (American Psychiatric Association 2000).

    B. It is associated with separation anxiety disorder (SAD), generalized anxiety disorder (GAD), social phobia (SP), depression, and oppositional defiant disorder (ODD).

    C. It presents as having trouble attending school.

    D. Separation anxiety and school phobia have also been used to describe school refusal.

    E. School refusal does not usually include children who do not attend school because of truancy, antisocial behaviors, or conduct disorders.

The correct response is option A.

Unlike SAD, school refusal is not a DSM-IV-TR diagnosis; it is a symptom associated with several diagnoses, including SAD, GAD, social phobia, major depression, and ODD. *School refusal* is often defined as difficulty attending school associated with emotional distress, especially anxiety and depression (King and Bernstein 2001). Terms such as *separation anxiety* and *school phobia* have been used synonymously with school refusal. However, the term *school refusal* is favored because it is descriptive and inclusive and does not imply etiology (King and Bernstein 2001). School refusal does not typically include youth who are not attending school because of truancy, antisocial features, or conduct disorder. **(p. 331)**

American Psychiatric Association: Diagnostic and Statistical Manual of Mental Disorders, 4th Edition, Text Revision. Washington, DC, American Psychiatric Association, 2000

King NJ, Bernstein GA: School refusal in children and adolescents: a review of the past 10 years. J Am Acad Child Adolesc Psychiatry 40:197–205, 2001

21.5 All of the following statements regarding evaluation of school refusal are correct *except*

    A. Evaluation should follow consensus guidelines.

    B. Multimodal assessment with multiple informants should be used.

    C. Comprehensive evaluation may include clinical interviews, semistructured diagnostic interview, examining contributing factors.

    D. Psychoeducational and language evaluations can be helpful.

    E. The School Refusal Assessment Scale can be used.

The correct response is option A.

There are no specific consensus guidelines for the assessment and treatment of school refusal. Because school refusal is often associated with anxiety, guidelines developed for childhood anxiety disorders (American Academy of Child and Adolescent Psychiatry 2007) are helpful.

    Youth with school refusal vary in their clinical presentation; therefore, it is most beneficial to use a multimodal assessment with multiple informants (e.g., youth, parents, school personnel) (King and Bernstein 2001; Ollendick and King 1998). Based on the vulnerabilities and symptoms associated with school refusal, a comprehensive evaluation may include several of the following components: clinical interview, semistructured diagnostic interview, examination of factors contributing to the school refusal, self-ratings and parent and teacher ratings of symptoms of anxiety and depression, evaluation of family functioning, and review of school attendance. It may also be helpful to complete a psychoeducational and language evaluation to rule out learning and language deficits that could be contributing to the school refusal behaviors.

    The School Refusal Assessment Scale (SRAS; parent and child versions) was developed to assess the primary function of school refusal behavior (Kearney 2002; Kearney and Silverman 1993). The SRAS assesses the strength of four functional conditions that often maintain school refusal behavior: avoidance of school-related stimuli that trigger negative affect, escape from negative social and/or evaluative situations, getting attention from others, and/or receipt of tangible reinforcements when not in school. This assessment tool may be helpful in planning effective treatment for youth with school refusal. **(pp. 333–334)**

American Academy of Child and Adolescent Psychiatry: Practice parameter for the assessment and treatment of children and adolescents with anxiety disorders. J Am Acad Child Adolesc Psychiatry 46:267–283, 2007

Kearney CA: Identifying the function of school refusal behavior: a revision of the School Refusal Assessment Scale. Journal of Psychopathology and Behavioral Assessment 24:235–245, 2002

Kearney CA, Silverman WK: Measuring the function of school refusal behavior: the School Refusal Assessment Scale. Journal of Clinical Child Psychology 22:85–96, 1993

King NJ, Bernstein GA: School refusal in children and adolescents: a review of the past 10 years. J Am Acad Child Adolesc Psychiatry 40:197–205, 2001

Ollendick TH, King NJ: Assessment practices and issues with school-refusing children. Behaviour Change: Journal of the Australian Behaviour Modification Association 15:16–30, 1998

Chapter 22

Posttraumatic Stress Disorder

Select the single best response for each question.

22.1 A variety of risk factors have been identified in the development of posttraumatic stress disorder (PTSD) after a disaster. Which of the following is one of those risk factors?

   A. Experiencing sleep disturbance immediately after the event.
   B. The presence of a predisaster personality disorder.
   C. Increased media viewing of the disaster.
   D. Having an immediate evacuation.
   E. None of the above.

The correct response is option C.

A variety of risk factors have been identified for developing PTSD after disaster exposure and include increased media viewing of the disaster (Pfefferbaum et al. 1999), experiencing panic symptoms in the immediate aftermath of the disaster (Pfefferbaum et al. 2006; Thienkrua et al. 2006), having a delayed evacuation, having felt one's own or a family's member's life was in danger (Thienkrua et al. 2006), and presence of a predisaster anxiety disorder (LaGreca et al. 1998). PTSD is more common among girls than boys. Preliminary evidence suggests that youth with poorer performance on neurocognitive tests prior to trauma exposure are more vulnerable to developing PTSD (Parslow and Jorm 2007). **(p. 340)**

> La Greca AM, Silverman WK, Wasserstein SB: Children's predisaster functioning as a predictor of posttraumatic stress symptoms following Hurricane Andrew. J Consult Clin Psychol 66:883–892, 1998
>
> Parslow RA, Jorm AF: Pretrauma and posttrauma neurocognitive functioning and PTSD symptoms in a community sample of young adults. Am J Psychiatry 164:509–515, 2007
>
> Pfefferbaum B, Nixon SJ, Krug RS, et al: Clinical needs assessment of middle and high school students following the 1995 Oklahoma City bombing. Am J Psychiatry 156:1069–1074, 1999
>
> Pfefferbaum B, Stuber J, Galea S, et al: Panic reactions to terrorist attacks and probably PTSD in adolescents. J Trauma Stress 19:217–228, 2006
>
> Thienkrua W, Cardozo BL, Chakkraband ML, et al: Symptoms of PTSD and depression among children in tsunami-affected areas in southern Thailand. JAMA 296:549–559, 2006

22.2 In childhood samples, the psychiatric disorders most often comorbid with posttraumatic stress disorder (PTSD) are

   A. Attention-deficit/hyperactivity disorder (ADHD) or oppositional/conduct disorders.
   B. Psychotic disorders.
   C. Depressive disorders.
   D. Substance use disorders.
   E. None of the above.

The correct response is option C.

Comorbidity appears to be the rule rather the exception in child cohorts with PTSD. These children commonly have depressive, other anxiety, and/or behavioral problems. Some child samples have shown comorbidity of up to 60% with depressive disorders; this is consistent with adult PTSD cohorts. Externalizing symptoms are common as well; comorbid conditions may include ADHD or oppositional or conduct disorders. Older children and adolescents may engage in substance use or abuse. These behaviors may represent attempts to avoid trauma reminders or may be signs of an independent substance use disorder. Dialogue is ongoing regarding whether youth develop "complex PTSD" and if so how the clinical manifestations of this differ from the combination of PTSD and existing comorbid conditions (Briere and Spinazzola 2005). **(p. 340)**

Briere J, Spinazzola J: Phenomenology and psychological assessment of complex posttraumatic states. J Trauma Stress 18:401–412, 2005

22.3   The most evidence for treatment of childhood posttraumatic stress disorder (PTSD) exists for which of the following treatments?

   A. Brief psychodynamic psychotherapy.
   B. Trauma-focused psychotherapy.
   C. Selective serotonin reuptake inhibitor (SSRI) antidepressants.
   D. Interpersonal psychotherapy.
   E. Atypical antipsychotics.

The correct response is option B.

Among the available treatments for childhood PTSD, there is more evidence for trauma-focused psychotherapies (i.e., therapies that specifically address and focus on children's traumatic experiences) than for pharmacotherapies. Therefore, in most cases clinicians should provide children with evidence-based psychotherapy prior to starting medication unless there is a compelling reason to do otherwise. In some cases, there may be justification for starting medication immediately; for example, there may be a comorbid condition for which there is a proven pharmacological treatment, the child may be so dysregulated or dangerous that a medication is required for immediate safety, or the child is unable to function without the immediate addition of medication for another reason (e.g., sleep is severely impaired and the condition has not responded to reasonable psychosocial interventions). **(p. 343)**

22.4   Which of the following medications has been found beneficial in treating childhood posttraumatic stress disorder (PTSD)?

   A. Olanzapine.
   B. Lorazepam.
   C. Clonidine.
   D. Monoamine oxidase inhibitors (MAOIs).
   E. All of the above.

The correct response is option C.

Small open trials have suggested the potential benefit of selective serotonin reuptake inhibitors (e.g., Seedat et al. 2002), propranolol (Famularo et al. 1988), and clonidine (Harmon and Riggs 1996; Perry 1994) for treating childhood PTSD. **(p. 345)**

Famularo R, Kinscherff R, Fenton T: Propranolol treatment for childhood posttraumatic stress disorder, acute type: a pilot study. Am J Dis Child 142:1244–1247, 1988

Harmon RJ, Riggs PD: Clonidine for posttraumatic stress disorder in preschool children. J Am Acad Child Adolesc Psychiatry 35:1247–1249, 1996

Perry BD: Neurobiological sequelae of childhood trauma: PTSD in children, in Catecholamine Function in Post-traumatic Stress Disorder: Emerging Concepts. Edited by Murburg MM. Washington, DC, American Psychiatric Press, 1994, pp 223–255

Seedat S, Stein DJ, Ziervogel C, et al: Comparison of response to selective serotonin reuptake inhibitor in children, adolescents, and adults with PTSD. J Child Adolesc Psychopharmacol 12:37–46, 2002

22.5   Which of the following newer treatments has been found effective in decreasing posttraumatic stress disorder (PTSD) symptoms in children?

    A. Restricting movement through binding.
    B. Eye movement desensitization and reprocessing (EMDR).
    C. Restricting nutritional intake.
    D. "Rebirthing" techniques.
    E. None of the above.

The correct response is option B.

EMDR is effective in decreasing PTSD symptoms in adults (Chemtob et al. 2000). It has been adapted for children and tested in one well-controlled trial that showed that children receiving EMDR demonstrated more improvement in reexperiencing symptoms—but not in avoidance or hyperarousal symptoms—than a waitlist control group (Ahmad and Sundelin-Wahlsten 2008). Debate is ongoing regarding the mechanism of efficacy for EMDR; these authors noted that their adaptation was effective for children due to its similarity to cognitive therapy.

Unproven techniques, such as severely restricting movement through binding, restricting nutritional intake, or using "rebirthing" interventions, are sometimes used for traumatized children. These interventions have led to serious complications, including death. Professional organizations, including the American Academy of Child and Adolescent Psychiatry (www.aacap.org) and the American Professional Society on the Abuse of Children (www.apsac.org), recommend that these interventions not be used. **(p. 346)**

Ahmad A, Sundelin-Wahlsten V: Applying EMDR on children with PTSD. Eur Child Adolesc Psychiatry 17:127–132, 2008

Chemtob CM, Tolin DF, van der Kolk BA, et al: Eye movement desensitization and reprocessing, in Effective Treatments for PTSD. Edited by Foa EB, Keane TM, Friedman MJ. New York, Guilford, 2000, pp 139–154

Chapter 23

Obsessive-Compulsive Disorder

Select the single best response for each question.

23.1 Unique characteristics of pediatric obsessive-compulsive disorder (OCD) relative to adult-onset OCD include all of the following *except*

    A. Pediatric OCD is male predominant.
    B. Pediatric OCD is more familial and has a better prognosis than OCD beginning in adulthood.
    C. Pediatric OCD frequently manifests with obsessions without well-defined compulsions.
    D. Religious and sexual obsessions are overrepresented in adolescents.
    E. Hoarding is seen more often in children than in adolescents and adults.

The correct response is option C.

Children with OCD frequently display compulsions without well-defined obsessions and symptoms other than typical washing or checking rituals (e.g., blinking and breathing rituals) (Rettew et al. 1992).

OCD in childhood is distinct in important ways from the disorder seen in adults. Pediatric OCD generally has a prepubertal age at onset and is male predominant (3:2 male to female). Boys may have an earlier onset than girls. Pediatric OCD is more highly familial and has a generally better prognosis than OCD beginning in adulthood.

Geller et al. (2001) found that religious and sexual obsessions were overrepresented in adolescents compared with children and adults. Only hoarding was seen more often in children than in adolescents and adults. **(pp. 349–351)**

> Geller D, Biederman J, Agranat A, et al: Developmental aspects of obsessive compulsive disorder: findings in children, adolescents and adults. J Nerv Ment Dis 189:471–477, 2001
> Rettew DC, Swedo SE, Leonard HL, et al: Obsessions and compulsions across time in 79 children and adolescents with obsessive-compulsive disorder. J Am Acad Child Adolesc Psychiatry 31:1050–1056, 1992

23.2 Which of the following statements regarding pathophysiology and risk factors of obsessive-compulsive disorder (OCD) is *true*?

    A. Frontal cortico-striatal-thalamic circuits are involved.
    B. Imaging studies detected structural abnormalities in the cingulate cortex, basal ganglia, and thalami.
    C. Magnetic resonance spectroscopy (MRS) studies show a significant reduction in *N*-acetylaspartate (NAA)/choline level in the medial thalami region.
    D. In a single photon emission computed tomography (SPECT) study, early-onset cases showed decreased cerebral blood flow in the right thalamus, left anterior cingulate cortex, and bilateral inferior prefrontal cortex compared with late-onset ones.
    E. All of the above.

The correct response is option E.

Several frontal cortico-striatal-thalamic circuits have been implicated in the pathophysiology of OCD, and several neurotransmitter systems modulate this feedback loop, including the excitatory amine glutamate as well as dopamine- and serotonin-containing neurons (Rosenberg and Keshavan 1998). Pediatric imaging studies appear similar to those in adults, detecting structural abnormalities in the cingulate cortex, basal ganglia, and thalami of pediatric OCD patients (Rosenberg and Keshavan 1998).

Fitzgerald et al. (2000) used MRS imaging in pediatric OCD patients and matched control subjects and found a significant reduction in NAA/choline and NAA/creatine/phosphocreatine levels bilaterally in the medial thalami of affected children compared with control subjects.

In a SPECT study of 13 adults with early-onset (<10 years) versus later-onset OCD and 22 healthy control subjects, early-onset cases showed decreased cerebral blood flow in the right thalamus, left anterior cingulate cortex, and bilateral inferior prefrontal cortex relative to late-onset subjects (Busatto et al. 2001). **(pp. 352–353)**

Busatto GF, Buchpiguel CA, Zamignani DR, et al: Regional cerebral blood flow abnormalities in early-onset obsessive-compulsive disorder: an exploratory SPECT study. J Am Acad Child Adolesc Psychiatry 40:347–354, 2001

Fitzgerald KD, Moore GJ, Paulson LA, et al: Proton spectroscopic imaging of the thalamus in treatment-naive pediatric obsessive compulsive disorder. Biol Psychiatry 47:174–182, 2000

Rosenberg DR, Keshavan MS: AE Bennett Research Award. Toward a neurodevelopmental model of obsessive-compulsive disorder. Biol Psychiatry 43:623–640, 1998

23.3 Which of the following statements regarding genetics and environmental factors in obsessive-compulsive disorder (OCD) is *false?*

A. The concordance rates for monozygotic twins are much higher than those for dizygotic twins.
B. Childhood-onset OCD demonstrates higher genetic and familial risks.
C. A genome-wide linkage study found susceptibility loci on several chromosomes.
D. Studies support the possibility that a single gene is responsible for OCD.
E. Nonheritable etiological factors of OCD are at least as important as genetic factors.

The correct response is option D.

It is highly likely that there are several genes that are important for the expression of this complex disorder.

The contribution of genetic factors to the development of OCD has been explored in twin, family-genetic, and segregation analysis studies (Hanna et al. 2005; Nestadt et al. 2000; Pauls et al. 1995). The concordance rates for monozygotic twins are significantly higher than for dizygotic twins (van Grootheest et al. 2005). Although family studies consistently demonstrate that OCD is familial (Lenane et al. 1990; Pauls et al. 1995), the risk of OCD in first-degree relatives appears to be greater for index cases with a childhood onset.

A genome-wide linkage scan for OCD showed evidence for susceptibility loci on chromosomes 3q, 7p, 1q, 15q, and 6q (Shugart et al. 2006).

Nonheritable etiological factors are as great as or greater than genetic factors for risk of developing OCD. In fact, many if not most cases of OCD arise *without* a positive family history of the disorder—so-called sporadic cases. Although sporadic occurrences do not rule out a genetic etiology (for example, because of spontaneous mutations), familial and sporadic "subtypes" of OCD repeatedly have been identified (Hanna et al. 2005; Nestadt et al. 2000; Pauls et al. 1995), leading to speculation about the differing impact of environmental and genetic factors on familial and nonfamilial forms of the disorder. Information regarding environmental triggers of the disorder may be especially relevant for the sporadic form because the OCD cannot be explained by the presence of an affected relative. **(pp. 353–354)**

Hanna G, Himle JA, Curtis GC, et al: A family study of obsessive-compulsive disorder with pediatric probands. Am J Med Genet A 134:13–19, 2005

Lenane MC, Swedo SE, Leonard H, et al: Psychiatric disorders in first degree relatives of children and adolescents with obsessive compulsive disorder. J Am Acad Child Adolesc Psychiatry 29:407–412, 1990

Nestadt G, Samuels J, Riddle M, et al: A family study of obsessive-compulsive disorder. Arch Gen Psychiatry 57:358–363, 2000

Pauls DL, Alsobrook JP 2nd, Goodman W, et al: A family study of obsessive-compulsive disorder. Am J Psychiatry 152:76–84, 1995

Shugart YY, Samuels J, Willour VL, et al: Genomewide linkage scan for obsessive-compulsive disorder: evidence for susceptibility loci on chromosomes 3q, 7p, 1q, 15q, and 6q. Mol Psychiatry 11:763–770, 2006

van Grootheest DS, Cath DC, Beekman AT, et al: Twin studies on obsessive-compulsive disorder: a review. Twin Res Hum Genet 8:450–458, 2005

23.4 Which of the following statements regarding the Children's Yale-Brown Obsessive-Compulsive Scale (CY-BOCS) is *true?*

    A. It is a 10-item anchored ordinal scale (0–4) that rates the clinical severity of the disorder.

    B. The scores include the time occupied, degree of life interference, subjective distress, internal resistance, and degree of control.

    C. It includes a checklist of more than 60 symptoms of obsessions and compulsions.

    D. Scores of 8–15 represent mild cases, 16–23 moderate cases, and ≥24 severe cases.

    E. All of the above.

The correct response is option E.

The CY-BOCS is a 10-item anchored ordinal scale (0–4) that rates the clinical severity of the disorder by scoring amount of time occupied (0 = no time, 4 = more than 8 hours per day), degree of life interference (0 = none, 4 = extreme), subjective distress (0 = none, 4 = extreme), internal resistance (0 = always, 4 = none), and degree of control (0 = excellent, 4 = none) for both obsessions and compulsions. The CY-BOCS also includes a checklist of more than 60 symptoms of obsessions and compulsions categorized by the predominant theme involved, such as contamination, hoarding, washing, checking, and so on. Scores of 8–15 are considered to represent mild illness; 16–23, moderate illness; and 24 or greater, severe illness. **(p. 355)**

23.5 Which of the following is the first-line treatment of choice for mild to moderate cases of obsessive-compulsive disorder (OCD) in children?

    A. Behavioral modification.

    B. Family therapy.

    C. Psychoeducation.

    D. Cognitive-behavioral therapy (CBT).

    E. Clomipramine.

The correct response is option D.

CBT is the first-line treatment for mild to moderate cases of OCD in children. Since the publication of a CBT treatment manual that operationalized and systematized this method (March and Mulle 1998), numerous studies have consistently shown its acceptability and efficacy (March et al. 2001; Piacentini et al. 2003). **(p. 356)**

March JS, Mulle K: OCD in Children and Adolescents: A Cognitive-Behavioral Treatment Manual. New York, Guilford, 1998

March JS, Franklin M, Nelson A, et al: Cognitive-behavioral psychotherapy for pediatric obsessive-compulsive disorder. J Clin Psychol 30:8–18, 2001

Piacentini J, Bergman RL, Keller M, et al: Functional impairment in children and adolescents with obsessive compulsive disorder. J Child Adolesc Psychopharmacol 13 (suppl):61–69, 2003

23.6 Which of the following are U.S. Food and Drug Administration (FDA)–approved medications for treating pediatric obsessive-compulsive disorder (OCD)?

    A. Clomipramine.

    B. Fluoxetine.

    C. Fluvoxamine.

D. Sertraline.

E. All of the above.

The correct response is option E.

Clomipramine was the first agent approved for use in pediatric populations with OCD, in 1989. Subsequent multisite randomized controlled trials, many of which were industry-sponsored, have demonstrated significant efficacy of the selective serotonin reuptake inhibitors compared with placebo, including sertraline (March et al. 1998), fluvoxamine (Riddle et al. 2001), fluoxetine (Geller et al. 2001), and paroxetine (Geller et al. 2002). No comparative treatment studies have yet been performed, and there is little to guide clinicians in the choice of therapeutic agents. Although not approved by the FDA for pediatric use, paroxetine and citalopram are also used. **(p. 357)**

Geller D, Hoog SL, Heiligenstein JH, et al: Fluoxetine treatment for obsessive-compulsive disorder in children and adolescents: a placebo-controlled clinical trial. J Am Acad Child Adolesc Psychiatry 40:773–779, 2001

Geller D, Wagner KD, Emslie GJ, et al: Efficacy of paroxetine in pediatric OCD: results of a multicenter study. Paper presented at the 155th annual meeting of the American Psychiatric Association Meeting, Philadelphia, PA, May 2002

March JS, Biederman J, Wolkow R, et al: Sertraline in children and adolescents with obsessive-compulsive disorder: a multicenter randomized control trial. JAMA 280:1752–1756, 1998

Riddle MA, Reeve EA, Yaryura-Tobias JA, et al: Fluvoxamine for children and adolescents with obsessive-compulsive disorder: a randomized, controlled, multicenter trial. J Am Acad Child Adolesc Psychiatry 40:222–229, 2001

Chapter 24

Early-Onset Schizophrenia

Select the single best response for each question.

24.1 All of the following statements regarding early-onset schizophrenia (EOS) are correct *except*

A. EOS is defined as schizophrenia with onset prior to age 16 years.
B. Childhood-onset schizophrenia (COS) refers to schizophrenia with onset prior to age 13 years.
C. EOS is considered to be continuous with adult-onset schizophrenia (AOS).
D. COS appears to be rare.
E. EOS, especially COS, appears more often in males.

The correct response is option A.

EOS is defined as schizophrenia with onset prior to age 18 years, with COS referring to schizophrenia with onset prior to age 13 years. EOS is considered to be continuous with AOS. Onset prior to age 13 years appears to be rare (American Academy of Child and Adolescent Psychiatry 2001). EOS, especially COS, appears more often in males (American Academy of Child and Adolescent Psychiatry 2001). **(pp. 367, 368)**

American Academy of Child and Adolescent Psychiatry: Practice parameter for the assessment and treatment of children and adolescents with schizophrenia. J Am Acad Child Adolesc Psychiatry 40:4S–23S, 2001

24.2 All of the following statements regarding the etiology of early-onset schizophrenia (EOS)/childhood-onset schizophrenia (COS) are correct *except*

A. Schizophrenia is viewed as a heterogeneous disorder with multiple etiologies.
B. Based on genetic studies, causal relationships between the illness and candidate genes are established.
C. Youth with COS appear to have a higher rate of cytogenetic abnormalities than adults.
D. Environmental exposures may mediate disease risk.
E. Based on imaging studies, age-specific gray matter reduction was found.

The correct response is option B.

Research based on the "common disease–common allele" model has identified multiple candidate regions and candidate genes (Harrison and Weinberger 2005; Owen et al. 2004) for schizophrenia. However, causal relationships between the illness and candidate genes are difficult to establish, and associations are often not replicable.

Schizophrenia is viewed as a heterogeneous disorder with multiple etiologies. To date, no single set of causes of the disorder has been identified. The current evidence suggests that the development of schizophrenia is best explained by a multifactorial neurodevelopmental model, in which multiple genetic and environmental exposures play a role.

Youth with COS appear to have a higher rate of cytogenetic abnormalities than reported in adults with schizophrenia, including 22q11 deletion syndrome (Gothelf et al. 2007; Lewandowski et al. 2007; Maynard et al. 2003).

Environmental exposures may mediate disease risk via a number of different mechanisms, including direct neurological damage, gene-environment interactions, epigenetic effects, and/or de novo mutations (McClellan et al. 2006).

The National Institute of Mental Health COS study has demonstrated significant gray matter volumetric reductions in their cohort. Longitudinal studies have shown a more rapid progressive loss of gray matter (3%–4% per year in COS versus 1%–2% in controls), which occurs in a parietal-to-frontal pattern during adolescence (Thompson et al. 2001). Follow-up studies show that cortical thinning in COS may plateau in early adulthood, when it becomes similar to the schizophrenic adult regional pattern (Greenstein et al. 2006; Sporn et al. 2003). These changes appear specific to COS because they occur in medication-naive patients (Narr et al. 2005a, 2005b) and are not found in those with transient psychosis (Gogtay et al. 2004) nor in studies of adults (Greenstein et al. 2006; Sporn et al. 2003). (pp. 368–369)

Gogtay N, Sporn A, Clasen LS, et al: Comparison of progressive cortical gray matter loss in childhood-onset schizophrenia with that in childhood-onset atypical psychoses. Arch Gen Psychiatry 61:17–22, 2004

Gothelf D, Feinstein C, Thompson T, et al: Risk factors for the emergence of psychotic disorders in adolescents with 22q11.2 deletion syndrome. Am J Psychiatry 164:663–669, 2007

Greenstein D, Lerch J, Shaw P, et al: Childhood onset schizophrenia: cortical brain abnormalities as young adults. J Child Psychol Psychiatry 47:1003–1012, 2006

Harrison PJ, Weinberger DR: Schizophrenia genes, gene expression, and neuropathology: on the matter of their convergence. Mol Psychiatry 10:40–68, 2005

Lewandowski KE, Shashi V, Berry PM, et al: Schizophrenic-like neurocognitive deficits in children and adolescents with 22q11 deletion syndrome. Am J Med Genet B Neuropsychiatr Genet 144:27–36, 2007

Maynard TM, Haskell GT, Peters AZ, et al: A comprehensive analysis of 22q11 gene expression in the developing and adult brain. Proc Natl Acad Sci U S A 100:14433–14438, 2003

McClellan J, Susser E, King MC: Maternal famine, de novo mutations, and schizophrenia. JAMA 296:582–584, 2006

Narr KL, Bilder RM, Toga AW, et al: Mapping cortical thickness and gray matter concentration in first episode schizophrenia. Cereb Cortex 15:708–719, 2005a

Narr KL, Toga AW, Szeszko P, et al: Cortical thinning in cingulate and occipital cortices in first episode schizophrenia. Biol Psychiatry 58:32–40, 2005b

Owen MJ, Williams NM, O'Donovan MC: The molecular genetics of schizophrenia: new findings promise new insights. Mol Psychiatry 9:14–27, 2004

Sporn AL, Greenstein DK, Gogtay N, et al: Progressive brain volume loss during adolescence in childhood-onset schizophrenia. Am J Psychiatry 160:2181–2189, 2003

Thompson PM, Vidal C, Giedd JN, et al: Mapping adolescent brain change reveals dynamic wave of accelerated gray matter loss in very early onset schizophrenia. Proc Natl Acad Sci U S A 98:11650–11655, 2001

24.3 In regard to differences between early-onset schizophrenia (EOS) and adult-onset schizophrenia (AOS), all of the following statements are correct *except*

A. EOS is diagnosed using the same criteria as for adults.
B. Negative symptoms appear to be the most specifically associated with EOS.
C. Catatonia occurs more frequently in EOS.
D. Thought disorder in EOS is generally characterized by loose associations and illogical thinking.
E. The majority of youth with EOS have histories of premorbid problems.

The correct response is option C.

Hallucinations, disordered thought, and affective flattening are common in EOS, whereas complex delusions and catatonia occur less frequently (Green et al. 1992; Werry et al. 1991).

In DSM-IV-TR (American Psychiatric Association 2000), EOS is diagnosed using the same criteria as for adults (Table 24–1). Among youth with a variety of psychotic illnesses, negative symptoms appear to be the most specifically associated with EOS (McClellan et al. 2002). Thought disorder in EOS is generally characterized by loose associations and illogical thinking (Caplan et al. 1989). The majority of youth with EOS have histories of premorbid problems, including cognitive delays, learning problems, behavioral difficulties, and social withdrawal or oddities. (pp. 369–371; Table 24–1)

Table 24–1. DSM-IV-TR diagnostic criteria for schizophrenia

A. *Characteristic symptoms:*   Two (or more) of the following, each present for a significant portion of time during a 1-month period (or less if successfully treated):

(1) delusions

(2) hallucinations

(3) disorganized speech (e.g., frequent derailment or incoherence)

(4) grossly disorganized or catatonic behavior

(5) negative symptoms, i.e., affective flattening, alogia, or avolition

   Note: Only one Criterion A symptom is required if delusions are bizarre or hallucinations consist of a voice keeping up a running commentary on the person's behavior or thoughts, or two or more voices conversing with each other.

B. *Social/occupational dysfunction:*   For a significant portion of the time since the onset of the disturbance, one or more major areas of functioning such as work, interpersonal relations, or self-care are markedly below the level achieved prior to the onset (or when the onset is in childhood or adolescence, failure to achieve expected level of interpersonal, academic, or occupational achievement).

C. *Duration:*   Continuous signs of the disturbance persist for at least 6 months. This 6-month period must include at least 1 month of symptoms (or less if successfully treated) that meet Criterion A (i.e., active-phase symptoms) and may include periods of prodromal or residual symptoms. During these prodromal or residual periods, the signs of the disturbance may be manifested by only negative symptoms or two or more symptoms listed in Criterion A present in an attenuated form (e.g., odd beliefs, unusual perceptual experiences).

D. *Schizoaffective and mood disorder exclusion:*   Schizoaffective disorder and mood disorder with psychotic features have been ruled out because either (1) no major depressive, manic, or mixed episodes have occurred concurrently with the active-phase symptoms; or (2) if mood episodes have occurred during active-phase symptoms, their total duration has been brief relative to the duration of the active and residual periods.

E. *Substance/general medical condition exclusion:*   The disturbance is not due to the direct physiological effects of a substance (e.g., a drug of abuse, a medication) or a general medical condition.

F. *Relationship to a pervasive developmental disorder:*   If there is a history of autistic disorder or another pervasive developmental disorder, the additional diagnosis of schizophrenia is made only if prominent delusions or hallucinations are also present for at least a month (or less if successfully treated).

Classification of longitudinal course (can be applied only after at least 1 year has elapsed since the initial onset of active-phase symptoms):

Episodic with interepisode residual symptoms (episodes are defined by the reemergence of prominent psychotic symptoms); *also specify if:*   **With prominent negative symptoms**

Episodic with no interepisode residual symptoms

Continuous (prominent psychotic symptoms are present throughout the period of observation); *also specify if:*   **With prominent negative symptoms**

Single episode in partial remission; *also specify if:*   **With prominent negative symptoms**

Single episode in full remission

Other or unspecified pattern

Source.   Reprinted from American Psychiatric Association: *Diagnostic and Statistical Manual of Mental Disorders*, 4th Edition, Text Revision. Washington, DC, American Psychiatric Association, 2000, pp. 312–313. Used with permission. Copyright © 2000 American Psychiatric Association.

American Psychiatric Association: Diagnostic and Statistical Manual of Mental Disorders, 4th Edition, Text Revision. Washington, DC, American Psychiatric Association, 2000

Caplan R, Guthrie D, Fish B, et al: The Kiddie Formal Thought Disorder Rating Scale: clinical assessment, reliability, and validity. J Am Acad Child Adolesc Psychiatry 28:408–416, 1989

Green WH, Padron-Gayol M, Hardesty AS, et al: Schizophrenia with childhood onset: a phenomenological study of 38 cases. J Am Acad Child Adolesc Psychiatry 31:968–976, 1992

McClellan J, McCurry C, Speltz ML, et al: Symptom factors in early onset psychotic disorders. J Am Acad Child Adolesc Psychiatry 41:791–798, 2002

Werry JS, McClellan JM, Chard L: Childhood and adolescent schizophrenic, bipolar, and schizoaffective disorders: a clinical and outcome study. J Am Acad Child Adolesc Psychiatry 30:457–465, 1991

24.4   All of the following statements regarding differential diagnosis of early-onset schizophrenia (EOS) are correct *except*

  A. Both psychotic and nonpsychotic disorders can present with psychosis.
  B. Psychosis caused by medical conditions is often associated with delirium.
  C. Both legal and illegal drugs can provoke psychosis.
  D. Research supports that prolonged episodes of substance abuse are the environmental stimulus for the expression of schizophrenia.
  E. Most children reporting apparent psychotic symptoms do not have a true psychotic disorder.

The correct response is option D.

Chronic psychotic states produced by substance abuse are similar in character to schizophrenia. There is continued debate as to whether these prolonged episodes represent independent drug effects or an environmental stimulus for the expression of schizophrenia in a vulnerable individual.

Other syndromes and conditions that present with psychotic symptoms need to be differentiated from EOS. Psychotic and nonpsychotic disorders can present with reports of psychosis.

Numerous medical conditions can result in symptoms of psychosis. Psychosis caused by an underlying medical condition is often associated with delirium, a condition associated with significantly increased morbidity and mortality.

Both legal and illegal drugs can result in psychosis. Prescription drugs associated with psychosis, especially when taken inappropriately, include corticosteroids, anesthetics, anticholinergics, antihistamines, amphetamines, and dextromethorphan. Drugs of abuse that can result in psychosis include dextromethorphan, lysergic acid diethylamide (LSD), hallucinogenic mushrooms, psilocybin, peyote, cannabis, stimulants, salvia, and inhalants.

Many children report symptoms suggestive of hallucinations and delusions yet do not present with other evidence of psychosis, such as disorganization in thought and bizarre behavior. Most children reporting apparent psychotic symptoms do not have a true psychotic disorder (Garralda 1984). **(pp. 371–373; see also Table 24–2)**

> Garralda ME: Hallucinations in children with conduct and emotional disorders, II: the follow-up study. Psychol Med 14:597–604, 1984

24.5   All of the following statements regarding the treatment of early-onset schizophrenia (EOS) are correct *except*

  A. A comprehensive integrated approach is required.
  B. Risperidone and aripiprazole have been approved by the U.S. Food and Drug Administration (FDA) for the treatment of adolescents with schizophrenia.
  C. Clozapine was found to be superior in treating youth with treatment-resistant schizophrenia.
  D. To avoid risks of side effects, rapid increases in dose should be avoided.
  E. There is a strong empirical evidence for psychosocial interventions in EOS.

The correct response is option E.

Empirical evidence for psychosocial interventions in EOS is limited. However, clinical consensus suggests that children and adolescents will most likely benefit from comprehensive intervention strategies that focus on behavioral and family functioning and medication compliance.

Treatment of EOS requires a comprehensive, integrated approach combining medication therapies with psychosocial interventions.

Risperidone and aripiprazole have been approved by the FDA for the treatment of adolescents with schizophrenia. Clozapine was found to be superior to both haloperidol (Kumra et al. 1996) and olanzapine (Shaw et al. 2006) in youth with treatment-resistant schizophrenia. However, clozapine's side-effect profile limits its use to patients who have failed other antipsychotic agents.

Rapid increases in dose can result in greater likelihood of side effects and increases the use of high doses that generally do not hasten recovery. **(pp. 374–375)**

Kumra S, Frazier JA, Jacobsen LK, et al: Childhood-onset schizophrenia: a double-blind clozapine-haloperidol comparison. Arch Gen Psychiatry 53:1090–1097, 1996

Shaw P, Sporn A, Gogtay N, et al: Childhood-onset schizophrenia: a double-blind, randomized clozapine-olanzapine comparison. Arch Gen Psychiatry 63:721–730, 2006

Chapter 25

Obesity

Select the single best response for each question.

25.1 A child is considered obese when his or her body mass index (BMI) is at or above what percentile?

   A. 80th percentile.
   B. 85th percentile.
   C. 90th percentile.
   D. 95th percentile.
   E. 99th percentile.

The correct response is option D.

BMI is calculated by dividing weight in kilograms by the square of height in meters (kg/m^2). In youth, BMI percentiles for age and gender are based on the Centers for Disease Control and Prevention growth charts. A child with a BMI within the 85th to 95th percentiles is considered overweight, a child with a BMI at or above the 95th percentile is considered obese, and a child with a BMI at or above the 99th percentile is considered to have severe childhood obesity (Barlow and Expert Committee 2007). **(p. 383)**

> Barlow SE, Expert Committee: Expert committee recommendations regarding the prevention, assessment, and treatment of child and adolescent overweight and obesity: summary report. Pediatrics 120:S164–S192, 2007

25.2 Which of the following genetic syndromes is associated with obesity?

   A. Prader-Willi syndrome.
   B. Laurence-Moon/Bardet-Biedl syndrome.
   C. Borjeson-Forssman-Lehmann syndrome.
   D. Cohen syndrome.
   E. All of the above.

The correct response is option E.

Medical conditions or syndromes are thought to be responsible for less than 10% of all cases of childhood obesity. However, when present, these disorders can have substantial effects. Certain genetic syndromes have been linked with obesity, including Prader-Willi, Laurence-Moon/Bardet-Biedl, Alstrom, Borjeson-Forssman-Lehmann, Cohen, and Turner syndromes. **(p. 385)**

25.3 According to the Barlow and Expert Committee report, all of the following play important roles in hunger, satiety, and fat distribution *except*

   A. Gamma-aminobutyric acid (GABA).
   B. Leptin.
   C. Ghrelin.
   D. Adiponectin.
   E. Insulin.

The correct response is option A.

GABA does not play a role in hunger and satiety.

The mechanisms responsible for hunger, eating, and energy storage are complex and appear to be interconnected. Examination of appetite in human and animal studies has demonstrated the connection between efferent and afferent signals in the brain and periphery to influence eating. Leptin, ghrelin, adiponectin, plasma glucose, and insulin all have important roles in hunger, satiety, and fat distribution (Barlow and Expert Committee 2007; Zametkin et al. 2004). **(p. 386)**

Barlow SE, Expert Committee: Expert committee recommendations regarding the prevention, assessment, and treatment of child and adolescent overweight and obesity: summary report. Pediatrics 120:S164–S192, 2007

Zametkin AJ, Zoon CK, Klein HW, et al: Psychiatric aspects of child and adolescent obesity: a review of the past 10 years. J Am Acad Child Adolesc Psychiatry 43:134–150, 2004

25.4 True statements regarding risk factors for obesity include all of the following *except*

    A. Maternal or gestational diabetes are linked with later development of child obesity.
    B. Birth weight >97th percentile predicts a higher future body mass index (BMI).
    C. Breast-feeding predicts a higher future BMI.
    D. Early adiposity rebound predicts future overweight.
    E. Up to 80% of overweight adolescents become obese adults.

The correct response is option C.

Results of research examining the effect of breast-feeding on weight status are mixed (Barlow and Expert Committee 2007).

Multiple risk factors, or critical periods, across development have been associated with child and adolescent obesity. Prenatal factors including maternal diabetes or gestational diabetes have been linked with later development of child obesity. Infant birth weight greater than the 97th percentile has been shown to have a positive correlation with future BMI. Up to 80% of overweight teens become obese adults (Daniels et al. 2005), highlighting the need for early intervention. **(p. 386)**

Barlow SE, Expert Committee: Expert committee recommendations regarding the prevention, assessment, and treatment of child and adolescent overweight and obesity: summary report. Pediatrics 120:S164–S192, 2007

Daniels SR, Arnett DK, Eckel RH, et al: Overweight in children and adolescents: pathophysiology, consequences, prevention, and treatment. Circulation 111:1999–2012, 2005

25.5 According to the Barlow and Expert Committee report, what is the primary goal of obesity treatment?

    A. Weight loss.
    B. Weight maintenance.
    C. Body mass index (BMI) maintenance.
    D. Long-term physical health through permanent healthy lifestyle habits.
    E. Food intake reduction.

The correct response is option D.

According to the Expert Committee, "the primary goal of obesity treatment is improvement of long-term physical health through permanent healthy lifestyle habits" (Barlow and Expert Committee 2007, p. S181).

Weight loss is not listed as a goal. For some children, because of their ongoing growth, weight maintenance may be a more realistic goal because stable weight with increasing height will result in lower BMI. Even small decreases in BMI may be accompanied by improvements in physical health, such as significant improvements in blood pressure, total cholesterol, low-density lipoprotein cholesterol, triglycerides, insulin, and aerobic fitness. Decreased food intake is not a primary goal. **(p. 389)**

Barlow SE, Expert Committee: Expert committee recommendations regarding the prevention, assessment, and treatment of child and adolescent overweight and obesity: summary report. Pediatrics 120:S164–S192, 2007

25.6 Which of the following pairs of medications has been approved by the U.S. Food and Drug Administration (FDA) for use in youth with obesity?

    A. Topiramate and bupropion.
    B. Metformin and modafinil.
    C. Sibutramine and orlistat.
    D. Methylphenidate and dextroamphetamine.
    E. Adderall and lisdexamfetamine.

The correct response is option C.

As is the case with most pharmacological development, weight loss medications have been much more extensively studied in adults than youth. However, two medications have now been approved by the FDA. Sibutramine has been approved for use in patients age 16 years and older. Orlistat has been approved by the FDA for use in patients age 12 years and older. **(pp. 392–393)**

Chapter 26

Anorexia Nervosa and Bulimia Nervosa

Select the single best response for each question.

26.1 In a study examining the relative rates of eating disorder diagnoses in an adolescent clinical sample, what was the most common diagnosis?

    A. Anorexia nervosa.
    B. Bulimia nervosa.
    C. Eating disorder not otherwise specified (EDNOS).
    D. Body dissatisfaction disorder.
    E. None of the above.

The correct response is option C.

If strict DSM-IV-TR (American Psychiatric Association 2000) definitions are applied, most adolescents with disturbed eating behaviors are categorized as having EDNOS. In the only study examining relative rates of eating disorder diagnoses in an adolescent clinical sample, 57% in a cohort of 281 adolescents were categorized as having EDNOS (Eddy et al. 2008). In this sample, individuals with EDNOS constituted a heterogeneous group, with eating disorder presentations ranging from subthreshold anorexia nervosa to binge-eating disorder. This finding may indicate that EDNOS is an imprecise diagnosis that consequently does not shed much light on relevant treatment decisions. A broader view of the features that are common to all eating disorders (i.e., a "transdiagnostic" perspective) may lead to a more comprehensive understanding of eating difficulties (Fairburn et al. 2003). **(p. 400)**

American Psychiatric Association: Diagnostic and Statistical Manual of Mental Disorders, 4th Edition, Text Revision. Washington, DC, American Psychiatric Association, 2000

Eddy K, Celio Doyle A, Hoste R, et al: Eating disorder not otherwise specified (EDNOS): an examination of EDNOS presentations in adolescents. J Am Acad Child Adolesc Psychiatry 47:156–164, 2008

Fairburn CG, Cooper Z, Shafran R: Cognitive-behavioral therapy for eating disorders: a "transdiagnostic" theory and treatment. Behav Res Ther 41:509–528, 2003

26.2 In a recent national comorbidity survey, the lifetime prevalence rate of binge-eating disorder (BED) among women was

    A. 0.5%.
    B. 0.9%.
    C. 1.5%.
    D. 2.0%.
    E. 3.5%.

The correct response is option E.

Research on the epidemiology of BED is considered preliminary, but a recent national comorbidity survey indicated lifetime prevalence rates of 3.5% among women and 2% among men (Hudson et al. 2007). Rates of BED are as high as 20%–30% among specific populations, including overweight and obese individuals seeking weight loss treatment (Spitzer et al. 1992, 1993). Among overweight treatment-seeking youth, rates of BED are estimated to be up to 10% (Eddy et al. 2007), while less frequent binge eating and associated distress are more common (e.g., Eddy et al. 2007; Tanofsky-Kraff et al. 2004).

A recent national comorbidity survey including a representative sample of individuals 18 and older indicated that the lifetime prevalence of anorexia nervosa is 0.9% among females and 0.3% among males (Hudson et al. 2007). Notably, however, in most clinical samples, 90%–95% of those with anorexia nervosa are female. Anorexia nervosa is most common among adolescent females (point prevalence in adults of 0.5%) with a typical onset during mid- to late adolescence (American Psychiatric Association 2000).

The national comorbidity survey indicated that the lifetime prevalence of bulimia nervosa is 1.5% among females and 0.5% among males (Hudson et al. 2007), although, as with anorexia nervosa, females predominate in clinical samples of patients with bulimia nervosa. Rates of bulimia nervosa are likely to be increased among certain populations (e.g., college females). **(p. 401)**

American Psychiatric Association: Practice guidelines for the treatment of patients with eating disorders (revision). Am J Psychiatry 157 (suppl):1–39, 2000

Eddy K, Tanofsky-Kraff M, Thompson-Brenner H, et al: Eating disorder pathology among overweight treatment-seeking youth: clinical correlates and cross-sectional risk modeling. Behav Res Ther 45:2360–2371, 2007

Hudson JI, Hiripi E, Pope HG Jr, et al: The prevalence and correlates of eating disorders in the National Comorbidity Survey Replication. Biol Psychiatry 61:348–358, 2007

Spitzer RL, Devlin MJ, Walsh BT, et al: Binge eating disorder: a multisite field trial for the diagnostic criteria. Int J Eat Disord 11:191–203, 1992

Spitzer RL, Yanovski S, Wadden T, et al: Binge eating disorder: its further validation in a multisite trial. Int J Eat Disord 13:137–153, 1993

Tanofsky-Kraff M, Yanovski SZ, Wilfley DE, et al: Eating disordered behaviors, body fat, and psychopathology in overweight and normal-weight children. J Consult Clin Psychol 72:53–61, 2004

26.3   The mortality rate in young women with anorexia nervosa is how many times higher than in young women in the general population?

    A. 2 times.
    B. 4 times.
    C. 6 times.
    D. 8 times.
    E. 12 times.

The correct response is option E.

Mortality in anorexia nervosa is estimated to be 0.56% per year, which is a 12-fold increase over that expected for young women in the general population (Herzog et al. 2000; Sullivan 1995). Suicide is particularly increased and accounts for at least half of the deaths in those with anorexia nervosa (Franko et al. 2004; Steinhausen 2002). **(p. 404)**

Franko DL, Keel PK, Dorer DJ, et al: What predicts suicide attempts in women with eating disorders? Psychol Med 34:843–853, 2004

Herzog DB, Greenwood DN, Dorer DJ, et al: Mortality in eating disorders: a descriptive study. Int J Eat Disord 28:20–26, 2000

Steinhausen HC: The outcome of anorexia nervosa in the 20th century. Am J Psychiatry 159:1284–1293, 2002

Sullivan PF: Mortality in anorexia nervosa. Am J Psychiatry 152:1073–1074, 1995

26.4   The National Institute for Health and Clinical Excellence (NICE) in the United Kingdom summarized guidelines for adult and adolescent eating disorders based on a comprehensive review of the literature. NICE graded treatment modalities using an A to C grade. Which of the following treatments received an A grade?

    A. Interpersonal psychotherapy for adolescents with anorexia nervosa.
    B. Cognitive-behavioral therapy (CBT) for adults with bulimia nervosa.
    C. Family intervention for adolescent anorexia nervosa.
    D. Selective serotonin reuptake inhibitors (SSRIs) for adults with anorexia nervosa.
    E. Dialectical behavioral therapy for adolescents with bulimia nervosa.

The correct response is option B.

Currently, there are relatively few clinical treatment guidelines for eating disorders. It was therefore particularly timely when NICE (National Collaborating Centre for Mental Health 2004) in the United Kingdom took a first step in summarizing guidelines for adult and adolescent eating disorders based on a comprehensive review of the literature. NICE recommends that treatment modalities be graded A to C. Grade A implies strong empirical support from several well-conducted randomized trials, whereas grade C implies expert consensus. By far the majority of the more than 100 recommendations that were made received only a grade C. There were two exceptions: CBT for adults with bulimia nervosa received an A, whereas family intervention for adolescent anorexia nervosa, with a focus on the eating disorder, received a B. No specific recommendation was made for adolescents with bulimia nervosa. **(p. 407)**

> National Collaborating Centre for Mental Health: Eating Disorders: Core Interventions in the Treatment and Management of Anorexia Nervosa, Bulimia Nervosa and Related Eating Disorders. London, UK, British Psychological Society and Gaskell, 2004

26.5   Which of the following findings have been reported about the efficacy of using medications to treat bulimia nervosa?

    A. In adults with bulimia nervosa, antidepressants are no different than placebo in reducing binge frequency.
    B. Weight and shape concerns in patients with bulimia nervosa are unaffected by medication compared with placebo.
    C. When added to psychological treatments of bulimia nervosa, medications greatly improved treatment outcomes.
    D. Mood disturbance in patients with bulimia nervosa is unaffected by medication compared with placebo.
    E. None of the above.

The correct response is option E.

Randomized, controlled pharmacological clinical trials in adults with bulimia nervosa have largely indicated that antidepressants are superior to placebo in reduction of binge frequency (Walsh et al. 1997). Further, weight and shape concerns and mood disturbance also seem to demonstrate increased improvement with medication compared with placebo (Mitchell et al. 1993). However, controlled studies in adults directly evaluating the relative and combined effectiveness of CBT and antidepressant medication (Walsh et al. 1997) have suggested that when added to psychological treatments (e.g., CBT or interpersonal psychotherapy), medications did not generally improve treatment outcomes. Taken together, these data suggest that the use of antidepressants in adults with bulimia nervosa offers only a marginal advantage over CBT alone. **(p. 411)**

> Mitchell JE, Raymond N, Specker S: A review of the controlled trials of pharmacotherapy and psychotherapy in the treatment of bulimia nervosa. Int J Eat Disord 14:229–247, 1993
> Walsh BT, Wilson GT, Loeb KL, et al: Medication and psychotherapy in the treatment of bulimia nervosa. Am J Psychiatry 154:523–531, 1997

Chapter 27

Tic Disorders

Select the single best response for each question.

27.1 Characteristics of tics include all of the following *except*

    A. Tics are sudden, quick, and repetitive stereotyped movements occurring in any part of the body.

    B. Tics may wax and wane.

    C. Tics are totally involuntary.

    D. Unlike other movement disorders, tics may occur during sleep.

    E. Tics can be categorized as either simple or complex.

The correct response is option C.

Tics are best understood as "relatively involuntary." They may be suppressed successfully for minutes to hours, but they cannot be constrained indefinitely.

Tics are repetitive, brief, sudden, stereotyped movements that can occur in any voluntary muscle. Tics affect the same muscles over days and hours but also migrate to different parts of the body and spread to include more regions over months and years. Specific tics appear and disappear or reappear after a long hiatus. Generally, tics appear in the face (e.g., eye blinks, grimaces) first and then progress to more caudal muscles in the neck, shoulders, arms, trunk, back, and legs.

Tics characteristically show variable frequency and intensity throughout the day, across months, and through years. This waxing and waning is not random. Tics occur in clusters and bundles of clusters that have been described as "bouts" and "bouts of bouts" (Peterson and Leckman 1998). Tics may also occur during sleep, unlike other movement disorders (Kostanecka-Endress et al. 2003).

Tics are often categorized as either simple or complex. *Simple* tics are those confined exclusively to one or a few muscle groups and are very brief, such as a grimace, shoulder shrug, a cough, or a sniff sound. *Complex* tics involve multiple muscle groups and integrated actions, such as thrusting one arm forward while slapping the contralateral thigh with the corresponding hand or repeatedly uttering the first line of a jingle. **(pp. 417–418)**

> Kostanecka-Endress T, Banaschewski T, Kinkelbur J, et al: Disturbed sleep in children with Tourette syndrome: a polysomnographic study. J Psychosom Res 55:23–29, 2003
>
> Peterson BS, Leckman JF: The temporal dynamics of tics in Gilles de la Tourette syndrome. Biol Psychiatry 44:1337–1348, 1998

27.2 Comorbid diagnoses common with Tourette's disorder include all of the following *except*

    A. Attention-deficit/hyperactivity disorder (ADHD).

    B. Obsessive-compulsive disorder (OCD).

    C. Anxiety disorder.

    D. Major depression.

    E. Schizophrenia.

The correct response is option E.

Schizophrenia is not a common comorbid diagnosis with Tourette's disorder.

In nonclinic populations with Tourette's disorder, ADHD has been observed in 40%–60% (Kadesjo and Gillberg 2000; Kurlan et al. 2002; Sheppard et al. 1999), and 10%–80% have OCD (Apter et al. 1993; Kurlan et al. 2002). Among those with Tourette's disorder seeking clinical care, 30% have comorbid anxiety disorders (Coffey et al. 2000), and 10%–75% have major depression (Robertson et al. 2006). **(p. 420)**

Apter A, Pauls DL, Bleich A, et al: An epidemiologic study of Gilles de la Tourette's syndrome in Israel. Arch Gen Psychiatry 50:734–738, 1993

Coffey BJ, Biederman J, Smoller JW, et al: Anxiety disorders and tic severity in juveniles with Tourette's disorder. J Am Acad Child Adolesc Psychiatry 39:562–568, 2000

Kadesjo B, Gillberg C: Tourette's disorder: epidemiology and comorbidity in primary school children. J Am Acad Child Adolesc Psychiatry 39:548–555, 2000

Kurlan R, Como PG, Miller B, et al: The behavioral spectrum of tic disorders: a community-based study. Neurology 59:414–420, 2002

Robertson MM, Williamson F, Eapen V: Depressive symptomatology in young people with Gilles de la Tourette Syndrome: a comparison of self-report scales. J Affect Disord 91:265–268, 2006

Sheppard DM, Bradshaw JL, Purcell R, et al: Tourette's and comorbid syndromes: obsessive compulsive and attention deficit hyperactivity disorder. A common etiology? Clin Psychol Rev 19:531–552, 1999

27.3 Which of the following statements regarding the neuroanatomy and neurophysiology of tics is *true?*

A. Association between tics and abnormal functioning in cortico-striatal-thalamo-cortical (CSTC) loop circuits was not found.
B. Circuits originating in motor and dorsolateral cortex are least important for tics.
C. Dopamine plays an important role in producing tics.
D. Disorganizing thalamic discharges lead to decreased activation in the frontal cortex.
E. None of the above.

The correct response is option C.

At the cellular level in the striatum, medium spiney neurons and dopamine play a key role in producing tics.

Tics are associated with abnormal functioning in CSTC loop circuits (Parent and Hazrati 1995). Circuits originating in the motor and dorsolateral cortex are considered to be the most important for tic disorders.

A current theory (Leckman et al. 2006) suggests that the normal relationship between striatum and thalamus is disrupted by malfunctioning "pacemaker" firings of matrisomes in the striatum. Disorganizing thalamic discharges (Leckman et al. 2006) subsequently lead to excessive activation in the frontal cortex (Leckman et al. 2006) or excessive disorganized intercommunication between motor and orbitofrontal CSTC loops (Jeffries et al. 2002), leading to motor, premonitory, and emotional symptoms (Leckman et al. 2006). **(p. 422)**

Jeffries KJ, Schooler C, Schoenbach C, et al: The functional neuroanatomy of Tourette's syndrome: an FDG PET study III: functional coupling of regional cerebral metabolic rates. Neuropsychopharmacology 27:92–104, 2002

Leckman JF, Vaccarino FM, Kalanithi PS, et al: Annotation: Tourette syndrome: a relentless drumbeat—driven by misguided brain oscillations. J Child Psychol Psychiatry 47:537–550, 2006

Parent A, Hazrati LN: Functional anatomy of the basal ganglia, I: the cortico-basal ganglia-thalamo-cortical loop. Brain Res Brain Res Rev 20:91–127, 1995

27.4 All of the following statements regarding treatment recommendations for tics are correct *except*

A. Behavioral interventions can reduce the severity and frequency of tics.
B. Dopamine antagonists are the mainstay of treatment for moderate to severe tics.
C. Clonidine can be used in the treatment of mild to moderate tics.
D. Selective serotonin reuptake inhibitors (SSRIs) with cognitive-behavior therapy (CBT) are recommended for patients with obsessive-compulsive disorder (OCD) plus a family history of tic disorders.
E. Stimulants are indicated in children with tics and Tourette's disorder.

The correct response is option E.

Case reports (Erenberg 2005; Robertson 2006) have led some experts to recommend against the use of stimulants in patients with ADHD and Tourette's disorder and the U.S. Food and Drug Administration (FDA) to assert that stimulants are contraindicated in children with tics and Tourette's disorder. However, longitudinal studies have reported that tics did not increase with methylphenidate or dextroamphetamine treatment, or that increases were clinically trivial (Erenberg 2005; Kurlan 2003; Roessner et al. 2006). Thus, current guidelines are equivocal regarding the first-line agents for ADHD in Tourette's (Gilbert 2006).

There is growing evidence that recently developed behavioral interventions can reduce the severity and frequency of tics.

The mainstay of treatment for moderate to severe tics is medications that block dopamine. These medications are the most studied for the tic disorders and provide the most consistent, robust, and positive results.

The more benign side-effect profile of clonidine has led some authorities to consider it the first-line pharmacological agent for treatment of mild to moderate tics (Gilbert 2006; Gilbert and Singer 2001; Swain et al. 2007).

In OCD, there is good evidence that obsessions and compulsions in persons with a personal or family history of tic disorders may not respond as well to behavioral or pharmacological treatment as those without such a history. First-line intervention using CBT or a combination of SSRIs with CBT is recommended. **(pp. 424–428)**

Erenberg G: The relationship between Tourette syndrome, attention deficit hyperactivity disorder, and stimulant medication: a critical review. Semin Pediatr Neurol 12:217–221, 2005

Gilbert D: Treatment of children and adolescents with tics and Tourette syndrome. J Child Neurol 21:690–700, 2006

Gilbert D, Singer HS: Risperidone was as effective as pimozide for Tourette's disorder. Evid Based Ment Health 4:75, 2001

Kurlan R: Tourette's syndrome: are stimulants safe? Curr Neurol Neurosci Rep 3:285–288, 2003

Robertson MM: Attention deficit hyperactivity disorder, tics and Tourette's syndrome: the relationship and treatment implications. A commentary. Eur Child Adolesc Psychiatry 15:1–11, 2006

Roessner V, Robatzek M, Knapp G, et al: First-onset tics in patients with attention-deficit-hyperactivity disorder: impact of stimulants. Dev Med Child Neurol 48:616–621, 2006

Swain JE, Scahill L, Lombroso PJ, et al: Tourette syndrome and tic disorders: a decade of progress. J Am Acad Child Adolesc Psychiatry 46:947–968, 2007

27.5 In regard to the genetics of tic disorders, all of the following statements are correct *except*

A. Twin and family studies support evidence that Tourette's disorder is fundamentally a genetic condition.
B. The twin concordance rate for Tourette's is 53%–56% for monozygotic pairs and 8% in dizygotic siblings.
C. The prevalence of Tourette's disorder in families of European origin in first-degree relatives is between 15% and 53%.
D. Rates of obsessive-compulsive disorder (OCD) symptoms among relatives of Tourette's probands are 5–10 times the general population prevalence.
E. There is evidence for genetic susceptibility for chromosomes 2, 3, 4, 5, 6, 8, 13, 14, and 21.

The correct response is option D.

Family studies found rates of OCD and obsessive-compulsive symptoms among relatives of Tourette's probands that are 10–20 times the general population prevalence (Bloch et al. 2006; Pauls et al. 1991; Walkup et al. 1996).

Twin and family studies provide sturdy evidence that Tourette's and chronic tic disorders (CTDs) are fundamentally genetic conditions. The twin concordance rate for Tourette's disorder is 53%–56% for monozygotic pairs and 8% in dizygotic siblings (Hyde et al. 1992; Price et al. 1985).

In families of European origin, ascertained by the presence of a Tourette's proband, the prevalence of Tourette's disorder or CTD in first-degree relatives ranges from 15% to 53%. When these rates are compared with the general population prevalence of Tourette's disorder or CTD of 1%–1.8%, the 10- to 50-fold difference strongly suggests a genetic contribution.

Whole genome scans have identified candidate genes that await further specification and replication. There is evidence for genetic susceptibility for chromosomes 2, 3, 4, 5, 6, 8, 13, 14, and 21. **(pp. 420, 422)**

Bloch MH, Peterson BS, Scahill L, et al: Adulthood outcome of tic and obsessive-compulsive symptom severity in children with Tourette syndrome. Arch Pediatr Adolesc Med 160:65–69, 2006

Hyde TM, Aaronson BA, Randolph C, et al: Relationship of birth weight to the phenotypic expression of Gilles de la Tourette's syndrome in monozygotic twins. Neurology 42:652–658, 1992

Pauls DL, Raymond CL, Stevenson JM, et al: A family study of Gilles de la Tourette syndrome. Am J Hum Genet 48:154–163, 1991

Price RA, Kidd KK, Cohen DJ, et al: A twin study of Tourette syndrome. Arch Gen Psychiatry 42:815–820, 1985

Walkup JT, Rosenberg LA, Brown J, et al: The validity of instruments measuring tic severity in Tourette's syndrome. J Am Acad Child Adolesc Psychiatry 31:472–477, 1992

Chapter 28

Elimination Disorders

Select the single best response for each question.

28.1 Which of the following comorbid psychiatric disorders is most common in children with secondary enuresis?

    A. Attention-deficit/hyperactivity disorder (ADHD).
    B. Major depressive disorder.
    C. Generalized anxiety disorder.
    D. Panic disorder.
    E. Social phobia.

The correct response is option A.

Children with secondary enuresis are more apt to present with comorbid psychiatric disorders than those with primary enuresis (von Gontard et al. 1999). A major area of investigation has been with regard to comorbid ADHD (Baeyens et al. 2004; Biederman et al. 1995). These studies support the hypothesis that the enuresis is comorbid with the ADHD and is not secondarily related to the ADHD. Other than the association with ADHD, the primary finding has been that behavioral disorders in children with enuresis are nonspecific (Mikkelsen et al. 1980). This is consistent with a number of studies that link enuresis with a generalized developmental delay in maturation (Touchette et al. 2005). **(pp. 436–437)**

> Baeyens D, Roeyers H, Hoebeke P, et al: Attention deficit/hyperactivity disorder in children with nocturnal enuresis. J Urol 171:2576–2579, 2004
> Biederman J, Santangelo SL, Faraone SV: Clinical correlates of enuresis in ADHD and non-ADHD children. J Child Psychol Psychiatry 36:865–877, 1995
> Mikkelsen EJ, Rapoport JL: Enuresis: psychopathology, sleep stage, and drug response. Urol Clin North Am 7:361–377, 1980
> Touchette E, Petit D, Paquet J, et al: Bed-wetting and its association with developmental milestones in early childhood. Arch Pediatr Adolesc Med 159 (suppl):1129–1134, 2005
> von Gontard A, Mauer-Mucke K, Pluck J, et al: Clinical behavioral problems in day- and night-wetting children. Pediatr Nephrol 13:662–667, 1999

28.2 Which of the following medications is most frequently used as a first-line treatment for enuresis?

    A. Imipramine.
    B. Amitriptyline.
    C. Desmopressin acetate (DDAVP).
    D. Selective serotonin reuptake inhibitors (SSRIs).
    E. Atypical antipsychotics.

The correct response is option C.

Treatment of enuresis with DDAVP has largely supplanted the use of imipramine. Initially, DDAVP was administered by nasal inhalation, although an oral formulation was later developed. Moffatt et al. (1993) published a review article that identified 18 randomized, controlled studies including 689 subjects. Many of these subjects had not responded to prior treatment. The range of efficacy, as measured by the decrease in frequency of enuretic events, was from 10% to 91%. In most subjects, wetting resumed after the DDAVP was discontinued; only 5.7% were reported to maintain continence after discontinuation of the DDAVP.

The first era of pharmacological treatment followed MacLean's observation that imipramine was an effective treatment. His initial report in 1960 (MacLean 1960) was subsequently supported by multiple double-blind studies (Mikkelsen and Rapoport 1980). The treatment was generally found to be safe, although there were some tragic reports of fatal overdoses in children who thought that if taking a few pills would make the enuresis go away for a night, than taking the whole bottle would completely cure them. Treatment with imipramine does require cardiac monitoring and periodic blood levels to guard against toxicity. Imipramine is still used for children who are refractory to other methods of treatment, either as an adjunctive or stand-alone treatment. **(pp. 439–440)**

MacLean RE: Imipramine hydrochloride (Tofranil) and enuresis. Am J Psychiatry 117:551, 1960

Mikkelsen EJ, Rapoport JL: Enuresis: psychopathology, sleep stage, and drug response. Urol Clin North Am 7:361–377, 1980

Moffatt ME, Harlos S, Kirshen AJ, et al: Desmopressin acetate and nocturnal enuresis: how much do we know? Pediatrics 92:420–425, 1993

28.3   In a large longitudinal study, researchers found that the most effective treatment of enuresis, in terms of degree of relapse after the cessation of active treatment, was

  A. Imipramine.
  B. Fluid restriction.
  C. Desmopressin acetate (DDAVP).
  D. Nighttime awakening to urinate.
  E. Bell and pad method of conditioning.

The correct response is option E.

In a large longitudinal study, Monda and Husmann (1995) compared the results of observation only with treatment with imipramine, DDAVP, or the bell and pad method. The length of follow-up was 12 months. However, treatment was weaned after 6 months, so that the response at 6 months represents the effects of active treatment and the 12-month data represent the frequency with which continence was maintained after cessation of active treatment. These results clearly indicate the superiority of the bell and pad method of treatment with regard to the degree of relapse after the cessation of active treatment. A subsequent systematic review of the literature involving the alarm, imipramine, and DDAVP confirmed this finding (Glazener and Evans 2002).

A number of behavioral strategies have been reported, including retention control training, evening fluid restriction, reward systems, and nighttime awakening to urinate. A thorough review of the published literature regarding these interventions (Glazener and Evans 2004) indicated that the methodology and small sample size of these reports precluded a rigorous meta-analysis. **(pp. 440–441)**

Glazener CM, Evans JH: Desmopressin for nocturnal enuresis in children. Cochrane Database Syst Rev (3):CD002112, 2002

Glazener CM, Evans JH: Simple behavioural and physical interventions for nocturnal enuresis in children. Cochrane Database Syst Rev (2):CD003637, 2004

Monda JM, Husmann DA: Primary nocturnal enuresis: a comparison among observation, imipramine, desmopressin acetate and bed-wetting alarm systems. J Urol 154:745–748, 1995

28.4   Which of the following epidemiological findings concerning encopresis is *false?*

  A. Male to female ratio of 3:1.
  B. More prevalent than enuresis.
  C. Prevalence rate in children between 7 and 8 years of age is approximately 1.5%.
  D. Prevalence decreases as children age.
  E. None of the above.

The correct response is option B.

Encopresis is less prevalent than enuresis. Unfortunately, the sampling strategy and frequency of encopretic episodes vary considerably in large, cross-sectional studies. However, there is enough consistency to warrant comparison. The first large study (Bellman 1966) found a prevalence of 1.5% among a cohort of 8,863 children between 7 and 8 years of age. The male-to-female ratio was 3:1, and as with enuresis, the prevalence decreases as the child ages. Subsequent epidemiological studies have been generally consistent with these initial findings (Heron et al. 2008; van der Wal et al. 2005). **(pp. 441–442)**

Bellman M: Studies on encopresis. Acta Paediatr Scand Suppl 170, 1966

Heron J, Joinson C, Croudace T, et al: Trajectories of daytime wetting and soiling in a United Kingdom 4- to 9-year-old population birth cohort study. J Urol 179 (suppl):1970–1975, 2008

van der Wal MF, Benninga MA, Hirasing RA: The prevalence of encopresis in a multicultural population. J Pediatr Gastroenterol Nutr 40 (suppl):345–348, 2005

28.5   Which of the following statements concerning encopresis is *true?*

A. Two subtypes of encopresis are recognized in DSM-IV-TR (American Psychiatric Association 2000): voluntary and involuntary.
B. Nonretentive encopresis has been more extensively studied than retentive encopresis.
C. The most accepted treatment of encopresis is imipramine.
D. The natural history of encopresis is to move toward continence.
E. None of the above.

The correct response is option D.

A distinction is not made in DSM-IV-TR for whether the encopresis is involuntary or voluntary. As with enuresis, a distinction is made between *primary* and *secondary* encopresis, with the latter term referring to those who achieve continence and then relapse.

The natural history of encopresis is to move toward continence. However, the natural history and rate of spontaneous remission is not as well understood as that of enuresis.

There are two primary subtypes of encopresis: *retentive,* which involves constipation and related overflow incontinence, and *nonretentive* encopresis. Retentive encopresis has been more extensively studied with regard to physiology and treatment. The most accepted form of treatment is a protocol that contains educational, psychological, behavioral, and physiological components. **(pp. 441, 444–445)**

American Psychiatric Association: Diagnostic and Statistical Manual of Mental Disorders, 4th Edition, Text Revision. Washington, DC, American Psychiatric Association, 2000

Chapter 29

Sleep Disorders

Select the single best response for each question.

29.1   The most dramatic developmental changes in sleep architecture and sleep requirements occur during

    A. The first 6 months.
    B. The first year.
    C. The first 5 years.
    D. The first 12 years.
    E. The first 18 years.

The correct response is option B.

Sleep and circadian rhythms develop from infancy into adult expression as a reflection of central nervous system maturation. The most dramatic changes in sleep architecture and sleep requirements occur during the first year of life. **(p. 449)**

29.2   Which of the following questionnaire or scales uses eight subscales that reflect the major domains of behavioral and medical sleep disorders?

    A. The Pediatric Sleep Questionnaire (PSQ).
    B. The Children's Sleep Habits Questionnaire (CSHQ).
    C. The Sleep Disorders Inventory for Students (SDIS).
    D. The Epworth Sleepiness Scale.
    E. A sleep log/sleep diary.

The correct response is option B.

Several questionnaires have been developed and validated to assess for the most common sleep problems in children and adolescents. The CSHQ yields eight subscales that reflect the major domains of behavioral and medical sleep disorders and a total score indicating the extent and severity of sleep related problems (Owens et al. 2000).

The PSQ has been validated for the assessment of sleep-disordered breathing, daytime sleepiness, snoring, and behavioral problems like hyperactivity, impulsivity, and inattention in children 2–18 years of age (Chervin et al. 2000).

The SDIS is a validated parent- and self-report questionnaire for children ages 2–10 years of age (SDIS-C) and for adolescents ages 11–18 years (SDIS-A) that can be used for screening of sleep disorders in a variety of clinical and school settings.

The Epworth Sleepiness Scale is a clinical tool recently modified for use with children and adolescents (Drake et al. 2003) that is very helpful for screening of subjective propensity to fall asleep in certain situations and for measuring treatment outcome.

A sleep log/sleep diary is a valuable tool that provides nightly information on the child's bedtime, sleep-onset time, rise time, and number of nocturnal awakenings, which is usually to be completed for a period of 2 weeks. **(p. 451)**

Chervin R, Hedger K, Dillon JE, et al: Pediatric Sleep Questionnaire (PSQ): validity and reliability of scales for sleep-disordered breathing, snoring, sleepiness, and behavioral problems. Sleep Med 1:21–32, 2000

Drake C, Nickel C, Burduvali E, et al: The Pediatric Daytime Sleepiness Scale (PDSS): sleep habits and school outcomes in middle-school children. Sleep 26:455–458, 2003

Owens J, Spirito A, McGuinn M: The Children's Sleep Habits Questionnaire (CSHQ): psychometric properties of a survey instrument for school-aged children. Sleep 23:1043–1051, 2000

29.3   Which of the following statements correctly describes nocturnal polysomnography (PSG)?

A. PSG is the gold standard procedure to study sleep-disordered breathing and other types of intrinsic sleep disorders in children.

B. PSG records electroencephalogram (EEG), electro-oculogram, airflow, respiratory and abnormal efforts, oxygen saturation, end-tidal carbon dioxide (ET CO_2), and limb muscle activity.

C. PSG is indicated for the diagnosis of obstructive sleep apnea, central apnea, alveolar hypoventilation, snoring, and upper airway resistance syndrome in youth.

D. PSG is used for diagnosing periodic limb movement disorder (PLMD) and for evaluating nocturnal seizures and parasomnias.

E. All of the above.

The correct response is option E.

Nocturnal PSG is currently the gold standard procedure to study sleep-disordered breathing and other types of intrinsic sleep disorders in children. It includes recordings of EEG, electro-oculogram, electromyogram, airflow, respiratory and abdominal efforts, oxygen saturation, ET CO_2, and limb muscle activity.

PSG is indicated for the diagnosis of obstructive sleep apnea, central apnea, alveolar hypoventilation, snoring, and upper airway resistance syndrome in children. PSG is also used to establish the diagnosis of PLMD and to evaluate for nocturnal seizures and parasomnias, such as rapid eye movement (REM) sleep behavior disorder. **(p. 451)**

29.4   According to recent studies, attention-deficit/hyperactivity disorder (ADHD) is strongly associated with which of the following sleep disorders?

A. Kleine-Levin syndrome (KLS).
B. Narcolepsy.
C. Obstructive sleep apnea (OSA).
D. Restless legs syndrome (RLS) and periodic limb movement disorder (PLMD).
E. Circadian rhythm sleep disorder.

The correct response is option D.

Because RLS and PLMD have been more extensively studied, the association between these disorders and ADHD in children has become evident (Cortese et al. 2005). Many children with ADHD have been found to have RLS/PLMD and vice versa. A strong association among RLS, PLMD, and ADHD was shown in a number of studies, with 26%–64% of children with ADHD meeting criteria for PLMD on polysomnography (Picchietti et al. 1998, 1999) and over 44% of children with PLMD having a clinical diagnosis of ADHD (Crabtree et al. 2003).

KLS, a rare and complex neurological disorder with typical onset during adolescence, is characterized by periods of excessive amounts of sleep and altered behavior. The exact prevalence of KLS is unknown, especially in the pediatric population.

Narcolepsy is a rare neurological disorder characterized by daytime sleepiness, cataplexy (sudden loss of muscle tone triggered by emotional arousal such as laughter), hypnagogic hallucinations, and sleep paralysis. The classic tetrad of narcolepsy including all of the above symptoms is rare in children. Most pediatric patients present with excessive daytime sleepiness and sleep attacks often masked by behavioral and emotional symptoms such as irritability, hyperactivity, inattention, and increased sleep needs at younger age.

Although habitual snoring has been reported in as many as 12% of children, the general prevalence of pediatric OSA is approximately 1%–3% (Marcus 2001). The prevalence rates are much higher among children with neuromuscular and craniofacial abnormalities, with rates approaching 85% in some children with genetic syndromes (Brooks 2002).

Circadian rhythm sleep disorders are the disruption of the internal body rhythms that regulate sleep-wakefulness and are characterized by normal sleep that occurs at the "wrong" time relative to social demands. It is estimated that circadian rhythm sleep disorders affect over 10% of children. **(pp. 453–456, 457, 458)**

> Brooks LJ: Genetic syndromes affecting breathing during sleep in children, in Sleep Medicine. Edited by Lee-Chiong TL, Sateia MJ, Carskadon MA. Philadelphia, PA, Hanley & Belfus, 2002, pp 305–314
> Cortese S, Konofal E, Lecendreux M, et al: Restless legs syndrome and attention-deficit/hyperactivity disorder: a review of the literature. Sleep 28:1007–1013, 2005
> Crabtree VM, Ivanenko A, O'Brien LM, et al: Periodic limb movement disorder of sleep in children. J Sleep Res 12:73–81, 2003
> Marcus CL: Sleep-disordered breathing in children. Am J Respir Crit Care Med 164:16–30, 2001
> Picchietti D, England SJ, Walters AS, et al: Periodic limb movement disorder and restless legs syndrome in children with attention-deficit hyperactivity disorder. J Child Neurol 13:588–594, 1998
> Picchietti D, Underwood DJ, Farris WA, et al: Further studies on periodic limb movement disorder and restless legs syndrome in children with attention-deficit hyperactivity disorder. Mov Disord 14:1000–1007, 1999

29.5 Many psychiatric disorders are associated with significant comorbid sleep problems. In which of the following disorders are sleep complaints among adolescents most prevalent?

    A. Attention-deficit/hyperactivity disorder (ADHD).
    B. Mood disorders.
    C. Autism spectrum disorders.
    D. Substance abuse disorders.
    E. Anxiety disorders.

The correct response is option D.

Sleep complaints are highly prevalent among adolescents using illicit drugs, alcohol, and cigarettes. The most common sleep-related symptoms in adolescents abusing substances are excessive daytime sleepiness, insomnia, and delayed sleep phase syndrome.

There is a large body of literature indicating high prevalence of sleep disorders in children with ADHD, based on subjective parental and self-reports and objective instrumental assessments of sleep.

Problems with sleep initiation, sleep maintenance, and hypersomnia are some of the most prevalent symptoms among children and adolescents with depressive disorders.

Sleep difficulties are estimated to occur in 44%–86% of children with autism or autism spectrum disorders (Richdale 1999; Stores and Wiggs 1998).

Anxiety and sleep problems are closely tied together, especially during childhood. A longitudinal study of sleep and behavioral and emotional problems revealed that the presence of sleep problems at age 4 years is significantly correlated with the development of depression and anxiety by age 15 years (Gregory and O'Connor 2002). **(pp. 458–459)**

> Gregory AM, O'Connor TG: Sleep problems in childhood: a longitudinal study of developmental change and association with behavioral problems. J Am Acad Child Adolesc Psychiatry 41:964–971, 2002
> Richdale AL: Sleep problems in autism: prevalence, cause and intervention. Dev Med Child Neurol 41:60–66, 1999
> Stores G, Wiggs L: Abnormal sleep patterns associated with autism. Autism 2:157–169, 1998

29.6 All of the following statements regarding treatment of primary insomnia are correct *except*

    A. Nonpharmacological interventions are the first choice of treatment.
    B. Behavioral interventions can be useful.
    C. Sleeping environment should be controlled.
    D. Cognitive therapy can be used especially for older children and adolescents.
    E. The U.S. Food and Drug Administration (FDA) has approved two agents for use in pediatric insomnia.

The correct response is option E.

There are no well-designed controlled studies of sedative-hypnotics in children, and there are no FDA-approved pharmacological agents for use in pediatric insomnia.

Nonpharmacological interventions are the first choice of treatment. Behavioral interventions include parental education, "sleep hygiene," extinction, graduated extinction, scheduled awakenings, and positive bedtime routines and cognitive-behavioral therapy (Kuhn and Elliott 2003; Mindell 1999). The sleeping environment should be controlled to exclude television, video games, computer, and so on. Cognitive therapy has been implemented successfully to treat insomnia in older children and adolescents. **(pp. 453–454)**

> Kuhn BR, Elliott AJ: Treatment efficacy in behavioral pediatric sleep medicine. J Psychosom Res 54:587–597, 2003
>
> Mindell JA: Empirically supported treatments in pediatric psychology: bedtime refusal and night wakings in young children. J Pediatr Psychol 24:465–481, 1999

Chapter 30

Evidence-Based Practices

Select the single best response for each question.

30.1 Which of the following sources would be likely to offer the most complete information regarding the efficacy of a specific medication in the treatment of adolescents, based on randomized controlled clinical trials?

    A. PubMed.
    B. PsycINFO, which uses a Medical Index Subject Heading (MeSH).
    C. Cochrane Library Systematic Reviews database.
    D. Cochrane Library Clinical Trials database.
    E. None of the above.

The correct response is option D.

The Cochrane Library's two most relevant databases are Clinical Trials (also called CENTRAL), which is composed of individual controlled trials, and Systematic Reviews. The Clinical Trials site strives to be complete, with over 350,000 registered controlled trials; importantly, it includes controlled trials and published trials only. Its advantage over a search for randomized controlled trials (RCTs) at the PubMed site is that Clinical Trials is more complete.

PubMed supplies over 17 million citations from MEDLINE and other life science journals. PubMed is the public site where the database MEDLINE can be accessed, but commercial vendors also support access through their standard interface. MEDLINE uses MeSHs to categorize journal articles. Most importantly, MEDLINE, accessed at the PubMed site, has a sophisticated Clinical Queries site that is extremely useful in searching for information from only RCTs. If a question primarily concerns the efficacy or potential harm of a therapy or medication, begin at this Clinical Queries site. Here, software enables the user to create a highly specific search that will retrieve only RCTs.

PsycINFO is a database of the American Psychological Association. Over 2,000 journals, 98% peer-reviewed, make up 78% of the database. Books and book chapters and selected dissertations from Dissertation Abstracts International each make up 11%. This database includes abstracts for articles published after 1994. Rather than using MeSH, each abstract is indexed using the Thesaurus of Psychological Index Terms, available online, with over 7,900 controlled terms. **(pp. 466–467)**

30.2 Clinicians seeking information about a specific disorder and its treatment would do well to apply which of the following search strategies?

    A. Start narrow and then go broad.
    B. Tailor the search to the question.
    C. Reject transparency.
    D. Avoid consensus-driven guidelines such as the *Cochrane Handbook for Systematic Reviews of Interventions.*
    E. None of the above.

The correct response is option B.

Skills for accessing and summarizing the literature efficiently are essential to implementing evidence-based practices. In conducting strategic searches of the literature, the following strategies are useful:

- *Define what you want to know and what resources and time are available.* Start with knowing what databases are available and whether they include full-text articles. Tailor the search to the question.
- *Start broad and then go narrow.* Cast a wide net initially—a broad, "sensitive" search retrieving far more references than could be actually read—then tighten the search using explicit "limits" that eliminate some references and retain others.
- *Use transparent methods.* A search is transparent if the reader can use the description to achieve the same results at each step. Transparency is highly desirable because it increases credibility and makes redoing searches easy. To create transparency, describe the results for each search term, and then combine sets of references using Boolean operators. Software at search sites can save how many "hits" (retrieved references) resulted at each stage, as well as the effects of combining sets and of adding each limit. Avoid adding multiple limits simultaneously, because the effect of each limit is then less transparent.
- *Consider using Cochrane Library guidelines.* The *Cochrane Handbook for Systematic Reviews of Interventions* (2008) contains the methodology used by authors of Cochrane's systematic reviews to search for evidence. This transparent, well-defined, consensus-driven methodology is useful for more definitive searches if time and resources permit.

(pp. 467–468)

Cochrane Handbook for Systematic Reviews of Interventions Version 5.0.0 [updated February 2008]. The Cochrane Collaboration, 2008. Available at: http://www.cochrane.org/resources/handbook. Accessed January 6, 2008.

30.3   Which of the following integrates consensus and evidence into prescriptive decision trees?

    A. Practice guidelines.
    B. Treatment algorithms.
    C. Systematic reviews.
    D. Expert consensus statements.
    E. None of the above.

The correct response is option B.

Treatment algorithms represent a particularly convenient form of practice guideline that integrate consensus and evidence into prescriptive decision trees or process flow charts (Chorpita et al. 2005; Kashner et al. 2003).

Many professional organizations publish practice guidelines. The American Academy of Child and Adolescent Psychiatry, the American Psychiatric Association, and the National Institute for Health and Clinical Excellence in the United Kingdom all publish guidelines on the Internet.

By definition, a systematic review uses transparent methodology designed to minimize multiple sources of bias. An expert consensus statement differs from a systematic review in that it often includes expert opinion rather than drawing conclusions almost exclusively from published data. **(p. 469)**

Chorpita BF, Daleiden EL, Weisz JR: Modularity in the design and application of therapeutic interventions. Appl Prev Psychol 21:1–16, 2005

Kashner TM, Carmody TJ, Suppes T, et al: Catching up on health outcomes: the Texas Medication Algorithm Project. Health Serv Res 38:311–331, 2003

30.4   Which of the following qualities characterizes organizations that are effective at implementing innovation?

    A. Strong leadership.
    B. Openness to experimentation.
    C. Effective monitoring.
    D. Knowledge sharing.
    E. All of the above.

The correct response is option E.

Organizations effective at implementing innovations tend to have cultures that include knowledge sharing, strong leadership with a clear strategic vision, visionary staff in key positions, openness to experimentation and risk taking, available "extra" resources, staff training and coaching, and effective monitoring and feedback systems (Fixsen et al. 2005; Greenhalgh et al. 2004). **(p. 470)**

> Fixsen D, Naoom SF, Blase KA, et al: Implementation Research: A Synthesis of the Literature (FMHI Publication #231). Tampa, FL, University of South Florida, Louis de la Parte Florida Mental Health Institute, The National Implementation Research Network, 2005
> Greenhalgh T, Robert G, Bate P, et al: How to spread good ideas: a systematic review of the literature on diffusion, dissemination, and sustainability of innovations in health service delivery and organisation, 2004. Available at: http://www.sdo.nihr.ac.uk/files/project/38-final-report.pdf. Accessed April 21, 2009.

30.5   A set of protocols that share common features or mechanisms of action is called

    A. Treatment family.
    B. Specific protocol.
    C. Common practices within a protocol.
    D. Core component method.
    E. Distillation and matching.

The correct response is option A.

A critical element of evidence-based initiatives is whether treatments are defined at the level of treatment families, specific protocols, or practices within protocols:

- A *treatment family* is a set of protocols that share common features or mechanisms of action, similar to a class of medications.
- *Specific protocols* describe the treatment activities (e.g., procedures, sequence, and dosage) that were actually tested in research studies: this is the familiar "manualized" approach to a specific disorder.
- A common practices approach analyzes specific protocols into more elementary components of practice and then aggregates these components across studies to identify common elements. This *core component method*, or *distillation and matching*, is so called because the common core components effective in many different manualized treatments for the same class of problems have been "distilled" to choose only those elements proven to be present in many of the manuals with demonstrated efficacy for that class of problems.

(p. 471)

Chapter 31

Child Abuse and Neglect

Select the single best response for each question.

31.1 Correct statements regarding the epidemiology of child abuse and neglect include all of the following *except*

    A. Sexual abuse still appears to be underreported.
    B. Between 1993 and 2001, the overall number of victimized children declined.
    C. More children experience physical abuse than experience neglect or sexual abuse.
    D. Young age (under 3 years) and male gender are risk factors for fatalities caused by maltreatment.
    E. Some studies report that up to 25% of girls are sexually abused in some manner before age 18 years.

The correct response is option C.

According to a report issued by the National Child Abuse and Neglect Data System of the U.S. Department of Health and Human Services (2001a, 2001b), almost 60% of all child abuse victims experienced neglect, 21.3% experienced physical abuse, and 11.3% were sexually abused.

The work of Kempe et al. (1962), who first described the battered child syndrome, led to recognition of child abuse as a major pediatric, psychiatric, and social problem. However, sexual abuse still appears to be significantly underreported.

The overall number of victimized children has continued to decrease since 1993 (U.S. Department of Health and Human Services 2001a, 2001b). Reasons for this decline are not well understood. The number of child fatalities caused by maltreatment remains unchanged, with younger children at greatest risk, especially those younger than 3 years (Kaplan et al. 1999) and boys.

Some studies report that 10%–25% of girls are sexually victimized in some manner before age 18 (Fergusson et al. 1996). The most common age of initial sexual abuse is between 8 and 11 years. **(p. 480)**

Fergusson DM, Horwood LJ, Lynskey MT: Childhood sexual abuse and psychiatric disorder in young adulthood, II: psychiatric outcomes of childhood sexual abuse. J Am Acad Child Adolesc Psychiatry 34:1365–1374, 1996

Kaplan SJ, Pelcovitz D, Labruna V: Child and adolescent abuse and neglect research: a review of the past 10 years, part I: physical and emotional abuse and neglect. J Am Acad Child Adolesc Psychiatry 38:1214–1222, 1999

Kempe CH, Silverman FN, Steele BF, et al: The battered child syndrome. JAMA 181:17–24, 1962

U.S. Department of Health and Human Services: HHS reports new child abuse and neglect statistics. HHS News, April 2, 2001a

U.S. Department of Health and Human Services: Trends in the Well-Being of America's Children and Youth 2001. Washington, DC, Office of the Assistant Secretary for Planning and Evaluation, 2001b, pp 142–143

31.2 Risk factors for child abuse include which of the following?

    A. Single-parent and stepfamilies.
    B. Unstable families and personality disorder in the parents.
    C. Parental mental illness, substance abuse, poverty, minority ethnicity.
    D. Child's prematurity, mental retardation, and physical handicaps.
    E. All of the above.

The correct response is option E.

Most experts believe that physical and sexual abuse results from a combination of factors within both parents and children, in conjunction with their specific environment, with youth from single-parent and stepfamilies having higher rates of victimization.

Child abuse tends to occur in multiproblem families with significant instability and characerological or personality disorder in the parents. Other risk factors include parental mental illness, substance abuse, lack of social support, poverty, minority ethnicity, lack of acculturation, presence of four or more children in a family, young parental age, stressful events, and exposure to family violence.

Child-specific risk factors include prematurity, mental retardation, and physical handicaps (Cicchetti and Toth 1995). **(pp. 480–481)**

Cicchetti D, Toth SL: A developmental psychopathology perspective on child abuse and neglect. J Am Acad Child Adolesc Psychiatry 34:541–565, 1995

31.3 Which of the following tests should be the first-line imaging investigation of a suspected brain or head injury?

A. Magnetic resonance imaging (MRI).
B. Computed tomography (CT).
C. Ultrasound.
D. Functional MRI (fMRI).
E. Single photon emission computed tomography (SPECT).

The correct response is option B.

In the event of suspected brain or head injury, a CT scan is the first-line imaging investigation, with its sensitivity to intraparenchymal, subarachnoid, subdural, and epidural hemorrhage and also to mass effect.

Because of its relative insensitivity to subarachnoid blood and fractures, an MRI study is considered complementary to a CT scan and ideally should be obtained 2–3 days later if possible. Because MRI may fail to detect acute bleeding, its use should be delayed for 5–7 days in acutely ill children (American Academy of Pediatrics Section on Radiology 2000; Cheung 1999). Both MRI and CT scans can assist in determining when the injuries occurred and can also substantiate repeated injuries by documenting changes in the chemical states of hemoglobin in affected areas. Ultrasound may also be indicated to identify epiphyseal injury. **(pp. 481–483)**

American Academy of Pediatrics Section on Radiology: Diagnostic imaging of child abuse. Pediatrics 105:1345–1348, 2000

Cheung KK: Identifying and documenting findings of physical child abuse and neglect. J Pediatr Health Care May/June:142–143, 1999

31.4 Which of the following findings is considered to be a definitive confirmation of sexual activity in or sexual abuse of a child?

A. Bruising or scarring of perianal area.
B. Presence of HIV.
C. Presence of chlamydia.
D. Presence of anogenital condylomata acuminata.
E. Pregnancy or the presence of semen.

The correct response is option E.

Definitive findings confirming sexual activity include pregnancy or the presence of semen. Pregnancy in an adolescent should always lead to an inquiry as to the possibility of sexual abuse.

Specific findings such as a dilated hymen or anus, bruising, scarring, or perianal tearing are important findings to discern and to document appropriately (American Academy of Child and Adolescent Psychiatry Working

Group on Quality Issues 1999). The presence of sexually transmitted diseases may or may not confirm the occurrence of sexual activity or abuse.

The presence of HIV, chlamydia, or anogenital condylomata acuminata should raise suspicion for sexual abuse but still may not represent diagnostic certainty. **(p. 482)**

American Academy of Child and Adolescent Psychiatry Working Group on Quality Issues: Practice parameters for the assessment and treatment of children and adolescents who are sexually abusive of others. J Am Acad Child Adolesc Psychiatry 38 (12 suppl):55S–76S, 1999

31.5   All of the following are guidelines outlined by the American Academy of Pediatrics Committee on Child Abuse and Neglect for performing a physical examination of sexual abuse victims *except*

   A. Careful explanation of every step.
   B. Particular attention given to the examination of the mouth, genitals, perineal region, anus, buttocks, and thighs.
   C. Presence of a supportive adult and a nursing chaperone.
   D. Use of sedation is contraindicated.
   E. Thorough documentation and appropriate agency reporting.

The correct response is option D.

The American Academy of Pediatrics Committee on Child Abuse and Neglect (1999) has outlined comprehensive guidelines for the necessary physical examination after sexual abuse; among them are the following:

- If collection of forensic samples is imperative and the child is unable to cooperate, use of sedation should be considered.
- Careful explanation of every step should precede the examination.
- Particular attention needs to be given to examination of the mouth, genitals, perineal region, anus, buttocks, and thighs.
- A supportive adult known to the child as well as a nursing chaperone should be present.
- Appropriate agency reporting and thorough documentation of findings, including the child's statements and behavior, are essential.

(p. 483)

American Academy of Pediatrics Committee on Child Abuse and Neglect: Guidelines for the evaluation of sexual abuse of children: subject review. Pediatrics 103:186–191, 1999

Chapter 32

HIV and AIDS

Select the single best response for each question.

32.1   Which of the following epidemiological findings regarding HIV/AIDS in adolescents/young adults living in the United States is *true*?

A. The number of adolescents/young adults living with HIV/AIDS in the United States has remained constant since 2000.
B. In adolescents between the ages of 13 and 19 years, females account for 40% of the cases.
C. For males, heterosexual contact accounts for 75% of new HIV/AIDS infections.
D. Latino youth are the minority population most affected by HIV/AIDS.
E. None of the above.

The correct response is option B.

Females account for nearly 40% of the infections in adolescents ages 13–19 years, and most were infected through heterosexual contact, whereas male-to-male sexual contact accounts for three-quarters of the infections among adolescent males (Centers for Disease Control and Prevention 2007).

HIV infection among adolescents, especially those in minority communities, is increasing. There has been a 40% increase in adolescents/young adults living with HIV/AIDS in the United States since 2000.

Black or African American youth account for nearly 70% of the infections for adolescents. **(p. 495)**

Centers for Disease Control and Prevention: HIV/AIDS Surveillance in Adolescents and Young Adults (Through 2005). Atlanta, GA, Centers for Disease Control and Prevention, 2007. Available at: http://www.cdc.gov/ hiv/topics/surveillance/resources/slides/adolescents/. Accessed July 16, 2007.

32.2   The leading cause of new HIV infection in adolescents and young adults in the United States is

A. Intravenous drug abuse.
B. Medical procedures.
C. Blood transfusions.
D. Sexual intercourse.
E. None of the above.

The correct response is option D.

Transmission of HIV typically occurs by sexual behaviors, perinatal transmission, and injection substance abuse. Other routes of infection include exposure to HIV during medical procedures or blood transfusions. Among adolescents and young adults in the United States, sexual intercourse is the leading cause of new, nonperinatal HIV infection (Grant et al. 2006). **(p. 496)**

Grant AM, Jamieson DJ, Elam-Evans LD, et al: Reasons for testing and clinical and demographic profile of adolescents with nonperinatally acquired HIV infection. Pediatrics 117:e468–e475, 2006

32.3 Which of the following mechanisms of HIV-induced neurotoxicity is believed to produce cognitive impairment?

    A. Direct neuronal injury by virus proteins.
    B. Products of macrophage activation.
    C. Neuroreceptor blockade.
    D. Antibody-mediated cellular toxicity.
    E. All of the above.

The correct response is option E.

The mechanism of HIV-associated cognitive impairment is not completely understood. Mechanisms of neurotoxicity implicated include direct neuronal injury by virus proteins (Tat, gp120), products of macrophage activation (proinflammatory cytokines and chemokines interleukin 1, interleukin 6, tumor necrosis factor alpha, interferon gamma, monocyte chemoattractant protein 1, macrophage inflammatory proteins 1alpha and 1beta), neuroreceptor blockade, autoimmunity, and antibody-mediated cellular toxicity (Goodkin 2006, Shapshak et al. 1999, 2004). **(p. 497)**

> Goodkin K: Virology, immunology, transmission, and disease stage, in Psychiatric Aspects of HIV/AIDS. Edited by Fernandez F, Ruiz P. Philadelphia, PA, Lippincott Williams & Wilkins, 2006, pp 11–22
>
> Shapshak P, Segal DM, Crandall KA, et al: Independent evolution of HIV type 1 in different brain regions. AIDS Res Human Retroviruses 15:811–820, 1999
>
> Shapshak P, Duncan R, Minagar A, et al: Elevated expression of INF-gamma in the HIV-1 infected brain. Front Biosci 1:1073–1081, 2004

32.4 Which of the following statements concerning the cognitive effects of HIV infection in children and adolescents is *true?*

    A. Receptive language is significantly more impaired than expressive language.
    B. Impairment is more cortical than subcortical.
    C. Visuomotor skills are frequently spared.
    D. Spatial learning and memory are frequently impaired.
    E. The Folstein Mini-Mental State Examination is more sensitive than the HIV Dementia Scale for detecting cognitive impairment in HIV-infected adults and adolescents.

The correct response is option D.

Visuomotor skills and spatial learning and memory are frequently impaired in children with HIV infection (Frank et al. 1997; Keller et al. 2004). Wechsler Intelligence Scale for Children scores and academic achievement scores of older HIV-infected children have also been shown to be below average.

Studies assessing cognitive status in HIV-infected children show that expressive language is significantly more impaired than receptive language. Screening for HIV cognitive impairment is influenced by the fact that it is more subcortical than cortical, and therefore clinical symptoms tend to involve motor functions, memory, mood (with flattening of emotional range), apathy, and coarsening of personality.

For adolescents and adults, the HIV Dementia Scale is more sensitive to subcortical deficits than the Folstein Mini-Mental State Examination, which is directed mostly at cortical deficits and may not detect impairment until very late in the course of HIV cognitive decline. **(pp. 497–498)**

> Frank EG, Foley GM, Kuchuk A: Cognitive functioning in school-age children with HIV. Percept Mot Skills 85:267–272, 1997
>
> Keller MA, Venkatraman TN, Thomas A, et al: Altered neurometabolite development in HIV-infected children: correlation with neuropsychological tests. Neurology 62:1810–1817, 2004

32.5   In studies of HIV-infected adolescents, which of the following has been reported?

   A. High rates of depression on screening measures.
   B. Significant psychosocial stresses.
   C. Half continue to have unprotected sex.
   D. Approximately 85% had at least one DSM diagnosis.
   E. All of the above.

The correct response is option E.

Youth with HIV can present with a wide spectrum of psychiatric illnesses. Studies of HIV-infected adolescents in medical care (sample sizes between 200 and 300) have found that most adolescents report significant psychosocial stresses, nearly half report high levels of depression on screening measures, and nearly half continue to have unprotected sex (Murphy et al. 2000, 2001). In one study using structured diagnostic interviews with a small number of HIV-infected adolescents, 44% presented with current major depression, 85% had at least one DSM diagnosis, and 53% had a history of psychiatric disorders prior to HIV infection (Pao et al. 2000). **(p. 498)**

Murphy DA, Moscicki AB, Vermund SH, et al: Psychological distress among HIV-positive adolescents in the REACH study: effects of life stress, social support and coping. J Adolesc Health 27:391–398, 2000

Murphy DA, Durako SJ, Moscicki A, et al: No change in health risk behaviors over time among HIV infected adolescents in care: role of psychological distress. J Adolesc Health 29:57–63, 2001

Pao M, Lyon M, D'Angelo LJ, et al: Psychiatric diagnoses in HIV seropositive adolescents. Arch Pediatr Adolesc Med 154:240–244, 2000

Chapter 33

Bereavement and Traumatic Grief

Select the single best response for each question.

33.1 According to Worden (1996) and Wolfelt (1996), a typical task facing children who experience uncomplicated bereavement is

A. Accepting the reality of the death.
B. Fully experiencing the pain of the death.
C. Adjusting to an environment and self-identity without the deceased.
D. Converting the relationship with the deceased from one of interaction to one of memory.
E. All of the above.

The correct response is option E.

Although Kübler-Ross described grief reactions as occurring in stages, we now understand uncomplicated child-hood grief as consisting of typical tasks that may be accomplished over varying periods of time. These tasks do not necessarily occur in sequential order; children may return to a previous task while working through a later one. Worden (1996) and Wolfelt (1996) described the following tasks of uncomplicated child bereavement:

1. Accepting the reality of the death.
2. Fully experiencing the pain of the death.
3. Adjusting to an environment and self-identity without the deceased.
4. Converting the relationship with the deceased from one of interaction to one of memory.
5. Finding meaning in the deceased's death.
6. Experiencing a continued supportive relationship with adults in the future.

(p. 510)

> Wolfelt AD: Healing the Bereaved Child: Grief Gardening, Growth Through Grief and Other Touchstones for Caregivers. Fort Collins, CO, Companion Press, 1996
> Worden JW: Children and Grief: When a Parent Dies. New York, Guilford, 1996

33.2 All of the following statements regarding uncomplicated bereavement are correct *except*

A. Bereavement is the condition of having had someone close die.
B. Grief is the intense emotion that one feels upon having someone close die.
C. Mourning encompasses the religious, ethnic, community, and/or cultural practices associated with bereavement.
D. In contrast to adults, children often show more constant and prolonged grief.
E. Uncomplicated bereavement in children resembles depression in many ways.

The correct response is option D.

The terms *bereavement, grief,* and *mourning* are often used interchangeably, but they have different meanings. In contrast to adults, children often show these symptoms intermittently and may seem perfectly normal at other times, being able to play or laugh even during very solemn times such as at memorial services or when the rest of the family is crying.

Bereavement is the condition of having had someone close die. *Grief* is the intense emotion that one feels upon having someone close die. *Mourning* encompasses the religious, ethnic, community, and/or cultural practices associated with bereavement. Uncomplicated bereavement in children resembles depression in many ways, sharing great sadness or grief, crying, withdrawing from others, not wanting to eat, being unable to sleep or pay attention in school, losing interest in normal activities, and perhaps (especially in younger children) searching or asking for the deceased person. **(p. 509)**

33.3   There is little empirical information on the interventions for uncomplicated bereavement. Peer support groups have been providing services to bereaved children. All of the following descriptions of the Dougy model are correct *except*

    A. Groups are facilitated by adult volunteers.
    B. Providers conceptualize the group activities as therapeutic interventions.
    C. Providers do not regard child attendees as having pathological responses.
    D. Many providers do not believe in the existence of "traumatic grief" in children.
    E. Peer support is well accepted by families and children.

The correct response is option B.

Providers of children's support groups do not conceptualize these groups as "therapy," nor do they regard child attendees as having pathological responses. Rather, they view almost all responses to grief as being normal; for this reason, many do not believe in the existence of "traumatic grief" in children (Schurmann 2006).

Little is known about empirical outcomes for children in peer support groups because these have not been studied systematically. However, for children with uncomplicated bereavement, peer support is well accepted by families and children who access these services.

Most bereaved children in the United States receive no mental health interventions; for those children who do receive services, the most commonly provided appear to be bereavement peer support groups such as those developed by the Dougy Center (www.dougy.org). The Dougy model consists of peer support groups facilitated by adult volunteers. **(p. 511)**

Schurmann D: Childhood traumatic grief, in Plenary. Edited by Lurier A, Cohen J, Goodman R, et al. Presented at the 10th National Symposium on Children's Grief Support, Chicago, IL, June 2006

33.4   All of the following statements regarding the differences between uncomplicated bereavement and childhood traumatic grief (CTG) are correct *except*

    A. The nature of the death is often qualitatively different in cases of CTG.
    B. Not all causes of death lead to CTG.
    C. Core posttraumatic stress disorder (PTSD) symptoms are less typical in uncomplicated bereavement.
    D. In CTG, PTSD symptoms impinge on children's abilities to resolve bereavement tasks.
    E. Children with CTG demonstrate a certain degree of functional impairment.

The correct response is option B.

Any cause of death can lead to CTG if the child subjectively experiences it as traumatic. Deaths from anticipated causes can be frightening or shocking to children if they witness severe cyanosis, gasping for air, attempts at resuscitation, excessive bleeding, or similar events.

CTG is different from uncomplicated bereavement in several ways. First, the nature of the death is often (but not always) qualitatively different in cases of CTG, with these deaths typically being from sudden, unexpected, gory, and/or violent causes such as suicide, homicide, accidents, war, terrorism, and disasters.

Some PTSD symptoms, including sleep difficulties, loss of interest in usual activities, and trouble concentrating, are expected in bereaved children (American Psychiatric Association 2000). However, core PTSD symptoms such as intrusive reexperiencing of the deceased's death and persistent avoidance of death reminders are less typical of uncomplicated bereavement.

A diagnosis of CTG requires not only that PTSD symptoms are present but also that these symptoms are impinging on children's abilities to resolve bereavement tasks.

Children with CTG have some degree of functional impairment, whether in school, with friends, with family, or in their ability to accomplish their tasks of daily living, such as playing or doing homework. (pp. 511–512)

American Psychiatric Association: Diagnostic and Statistical Manual of Mental Disorders, 4th Edition, Text Revision. Washington, DC, American Psychiatric Association, 2000

33.5   All of the following treatment approaches have been used for childhood traumatic grief (CTG). Which one of the approaches has been supported as a randomized clinical trial (RCT) for young children experiencing domestic violence?

   A. Traumatic grief–cognitive-behavioral therapy (TG-CBT).
   B. UCLA traumatic grief program for adolescents.
   C. Grief and trauma intervention for elementary-age children.
   D. Child-parent psychotherapy (CPP) for traumatic grief in early childhood.
   E. None of the above.

The correct response is option D.

CPP is a relationship-based treatment for infants and preschoolers exposed to domestic violence. CPP has been supported in a RCT for young children experiencing domestic violence, including some children whose primary caretaker died as a result of this violence (Lieberman and Van Horn 2005). To date, the CTG adaptation of the CPP model has not been evaluated empirically as a separate model.

TG-CBT is derived from trauma-focused cognitive-behavioral therapy, an evidence-based treatment for posttraumatic stress disorder (PTSD). TG-CBT has been tested in two open trials and a small RCT. The two open trials (Cohen et al. 2004, 2006) included children with CTG secondary to various causes of death. Children receiving TG-CBT experienced significant improvement in CTG, PTSD, and other symptoms.

The trauma/grief-focused group psychotherapy model (Layne et al. 2001) is provided in groups for adolescents and has been adopted for youth as young as 11 years of age. The UCLA traumatic grief program for adolescents has been tested in two open studies: in Bosnian adolescents postwar and in adolescents exposed to community violence in Los Angeles (Layne et al. 2001; Saltzman et al. 2001). Both studies demonstrated that participants experienced significant improvement in CTG and PTSD symptoms as well as improved adaptive functioning (e.g., in academic achievement).

Salloum et al. (2001) described a pilot group model for adolescent survivors of homicide victims (grief and trauma intervention for elementary age children). Salloum (2004) subsequently adapted this model for adolescents exposed to other traumatic experiences. The goals of this model include reducing traumatic reactions associated with the traumatic death, providing education about trauma and grief, and offering a safe environment for children to share thoughts and feelings. It also addresses bereavement tasks of self-protection, acceptance/reworking, and identity/development. (pp. 512–515)

Cohen JA, Mannarino AP, Knudsen K: Treating childhood traumatic grief: a pilot study. J Am Acad Child Adolesc Psychiatry 43:1225–1233, 2004

Cohen JA, Mannarino AP, Staron VR: Modified cognitive behavioral therapy for childhood traumatic grief (CBT-CTG): a pilot study. J Am Acad Child Adolesc Psychiatry 45:1465–1473, 2006

Layne CM, Pynoos RS, Saltzman WS, et al: Trauma/grief-focused group psychotherapy: school-based post-war intervention with traumatized Bosnian adolescents. Group Dynamics: Theory, Research, and Practice 5:277–290, 2001

Lieberman AF, Van Horn P: Don't Hit My Mommy! A Manual for Child-Parent Psychotherapy With Young Witnesses of Family Violence. Washington, DC, Zero to Three Press, 2005

Salloum A: Group Work With Adolescents After Violent Death: A Manual for Practitioners. Philadelphia, PA, Brunner Routledge, 2004

Salloum A, Avery L, McClain RP: Group psychotherapy for adolescent survivors of homicide victims: a pilot study. J Am Acad Child Adolesc Psychiatry 40:1261–1267, 2001

Saltzman WR, Pynoos RS, Layne CM, et al: Trauma- and grief-focused intervention for adolescents exposed to community violence: results of a school-based screening and group treatment protocol. Group Dynamics: Theory, Research, and Practice 5:291–303, 2001

Chapter 34

Ethnic, Cultural, and Religious Issues

Select the single best response for each question.

34.1 According to the Committee on Cultural Psychiatry for the Group for the Advancement of Psychiatry, which concept is accurately defined by the description "It encompasses one's identity with a group of people sharing common origins, history, customs, and beliefs"?

    A. Culture.
    B. Ethnicity.
    C. Race.
    D. Cultural psychiatry.
    E. Religion.

The correct response is option B.

Ethnicity encompasses one's identity with a group of people sharing common origins, history, customs, and beliefs.

The Committee on Cultural Psychiatry for the Group for the Advancement of Psychiatry (2002) defines *culture* as "a set of meaning, behavioral norms, and values used by members of a particular society as they construct their unique view of the world. These…include social relationships, language, nonverbal expression of thoughts and emotions, religious beliefs, moral thought, technology, and financial philosophy" (pp. 6–7). Culture is dynamic, shapes and is shaped by individuals, and evolves over time as it is passed on to succeeding generations.

Race refers to physical, biological, and genetic qualities of humans, particularly as these features lend themselves to categorization of visible similarities or differences.

Cultural psychiatry is the discipline concerned with matters of culture, ethnicity, and race as they affect description, assessment, diagnosis, biopsychosocial formulation, treatment planning, and training in all aspects of psychiatric practice (Group for the Advancement of Psychiatry 2002; Ton and Lim 2006).

Religion and spirituality can be considered as a subset or category of culture. The unique role of religion and spirituality in virtually all cultures and their pervasive influences on mental health and illness merit special consideration. **(pp. 518, 523)**

> Group for the Advancement of Psychiatry, Committee on Cultural Psychiatry: Cultural Assessment in Clinical Psychiatry. Washington DC, American Psychiatric Publishing, 2002
>
> Ton H, Lim RF: The assessment of culturally diverse individuals, in Clinical Manual of Cultural Psychiatry. Edited by Lim RF. Washington, DC, American Psychiatric Publishing, 2006, pp 3–31

34.2 The term *cultural-bound syndromes* was introduced in 1967 and is currently included in Appendix I of DSM-IV-TR (American Psychiatric Association 2000). Which of the following characteristics accurately describes the disorders under this category?

    A. Are discrete and well-defined.
    B. Are accepted as specific disorders in the country of origin.
    C. Occur in response to specific precipitants in that culture.
    D. Occur much more frequently in the home culture than in other cultures.
    E. All of the above.

The correct response is option E.

The term *culture-bound syndromes* was introduced in 1967 to describe disorders that are 1) discrete and well-defined, 2) accepted as a specific disorder in the country of origin, 3) a response to specific precipitants in that culture, and 4) found to occur much more in the home culture than in other cultures (Guarnaccia and Rogler 1999; Levine and Gaw 1995). **(p. 519)**

American Psychiatric Association: Diagnostic and Statistical Manual of Mental Disorders, 4th Edition, Text Revision. Washington, DC, American Psychiatric Association, 2000

Guarnaccia PJ, Rogler LH: Research on culture-bound syndromes: new directions. Am J Psychiatry 156:1322–1327, 1999

Levine RE, Gaw AC: Culture-bound syndromes. Psychiatr Clin North Am 18:523–536, 1995

34.3   Which of these terms is accurately defined by the statement "the biological processes of drug absorption, distribution, metabolism, and excretion?"

    A. Pharmacokinetics.
    B. Pharmacodynamics.
    C. Pharmacogenetics.
    D. Ethnopsychopharmacology.
    E. None of the above.

The correct response is option A.

Cultural psychopharmacology is truly one of the most multidisciplinary fields in medicine today, encompassing psychiatry, pharmacology, genetics, pediatrics, neurology, toxicology, epidemiology, and molecular physiology.

For decades psychiatrists have detected variability among ethnic groups regarding *pharmacokinetics*, the biological processes of drug absorption, distribution, metabolism, and excretion; and *pharmacodynamics*, the physiological and biochemical effects of medications at sites in the human body. Differences in therapeutic drug doses, efficacy, half-lives, drug-drug interactions, tolerability, and short- and long-term side effects have been well-documented among different races and ethnic groups. Interest in this topic has soared with the growth of *pharmacogenetics*, the study of genetic influences on drug responses. Especially relevant to ethnopsychopharmacology is the discovery of genetic polymorphisms of the cytochrome P450 (CYP) liver enzymes responsible for oxidative metabolism of many psychotropic medications (Gaw 2001). **(p. 521)**

Gaw AC: Concise Guide to Cross-Cultural Psychiatry. Washington, DC, American Psychiatric Publishing, 2001

34.4   There are numerous cytochrome P450 (CYP) liver enzymes responsible for oxidative metabolism of many psychotropic medications. Which of the following CYP enzymes is the least significant in ethnopsychopharmacology?

    A. CYP2D6.
    B. CYP2C19.
    C. CYP2C9.
    D. CYP3A4.
    E. CYP1A2.

The correct response is option C.

CYP2C9 is the least significant enzyme in ethnopsychopharmacology.

The four most significant CYP enzymes at this time appear to be CYP2D6, CYP2C19, CYP3A4, and CYP1A2. The majority of antidepressants, antipsychotics, benzodiazepines, mood stabilizers, and several other neuropsychiatrically active substances serve as substrates for these four CYP enzymes. **(p. 521)**

34.5   The screening mnemonic FICA (Puchalski and Romer 2000) is a useful tool for beginning a discussion of patients' past religious and spiritual experiences. Which of the following questions is *not* included in the FICA screen?

     A. Is religious faith part of your day-to-day life?
     B. How has faith influenced your life, past and present?
     C. Are you currently part of a religious or spiritual community?
     D. What kind of religion are you practicing?
     E. What are the spiritual needs you would like to have addressed?

The correct response is option D.

"What kind of religion are you practicing?" is not a question included in the FICA screening tool.

The screening mnemonic FICA is simple and easy to use and remember and is a good tool for obtaining basic information.

Although primarily developed for adult populations, the mnemonic can be employed with parents and older children, provided that developmentally appropriate language is used by the interviewer. These questions serve as a starting point for discussion of past religious and spiritual experiences, current practices, satisfaction with religious and spiritual elements of life, and supportive resources (Caraballo et al. 2006; Puchalski and Romer 2000). **(pp. 526–527; see also Table 34–3)**

Caraballo A, Hamid H, Lee JR, et al: A resident's guide to the cultural formulation, in Clinical Manual of Cultural Psychiatry. Edited by Lim RF. Washington, DC, American Psychiatric Publishing, 2006, pp 243–269

Puchalski C, Romer AL: Taking a spiritual history allows clinicians to understand patients more fully. J Palliat Med 3:129–137, 2000

C h a p t e r   3 5

Youth Suicide

Select the single best response for each question.

35.1   All of the following definitions of suicide-related behaviors are correct *except*

    A. *Suicide* refers to a fatal, self-inflicted destructive act with explicit or implicit intent to die.

    B. *Suicide attempt* refers to a nonfatal, self-inflicted destructive act that leads to injury and that involves an explicit or implicit intent to die.

    C. *Suicidal ideation* refers to thoughts of harming or killing oneself.

    D. *Suicidality* refers to all suicide-related behaviors and thoughts.

    E. *Nonsuicidal self-injurious behavior* refers to any self-inflicted destructive act performed without intent to die.

The correct response is option B.

A *suicide attempt* is a nonfatal, self-inflicted destructive act that does not necessarily result in injury.

In an effort to correct a history of inconsistent and unclear terminology regarding suicide-related behavior, O'Carroll et al. (1996) developed the following set of terms:

- *Suicide*—Fatal, self-inflicted, destructive act with explicit or implicit intent to die.
- *Suicide attempt*—Nonfatal, self-inflicted, destructive act (not necessarily resulting in injury) with explicit or implicit intent to die.
- *Suicidal ideation*—Thoughts of harming or killing oneself.
- *Suicidality*—All suicide-related behaviors and thoughts.
- *Nonsuicidal self-injurious behavior*—Any self-inflicted destructive act performed without intent to die but with full intent of inflicting physical harm to oneself (viewed as distinct from suicidal behavior).

(p. 532 [Table 35–1])

        O'Carroll PW, Berman AL, Maris RW, et al: Beyond the Tower of Babel: a nomenclature for suicidology. Suicide Life Threat Behav 26:237–252, 1996

35.2   Which of the following statements regarding the characteristics of youth suicide is *false?*

    A. The rates of suicide increase with age.

    B. Suicidal behavior is rare in preschool-aged children.

    C. The rate of completed suicide among youth is higher for males than females.

    D. Females endorse similar rates of specific ideations and suicide attempt rates compared with males.

    E. Increased suicide risk is associated with lower socioeconomic status except for young African American males.

The correct response is option D.

Females endorse much higher rates of specific suicidal ideation (6% versus 2%) and have higher suicide attempt rates than males (10% versus 4%) (Lewinsohn et al. 1996).

The rates of attempted and completed suicide increase dramatically with age throughout childhood into adolescence.

Suicidal behavior is rare in preschool-age children; when present in this age group, physical and/or sexual abuse is common (Rosenberg et al. 1987).

The rate of completed suicide among youth is significantly higher for males than females, with a ratio of nearly 6:1 in 2001 (Anderson and Smith 2003).

With regard to socioeconomic status, in the United States increased suicide risk is conveyed by lower socioeconomic status—with the exception of young African American males, for whom completed suicide is associated with higher socioeconomic status (Gould et al. 1996). **(p. 532)**

> Anderson RN, Smith BL: Deaths: leading causes for 2001. Natl Vital Stat Rep 52:1–85, 2003
> Gould MS, Fisher P, Parides M, et al: Psychosocial risk factors of child and adolescent completed suicide. Arch Gen Psychiatry 53:1155–1162, 1996
> Lewinsohn PM, Rohde P, Seeley JR: Adolescent suicidal ideation and attempts: prevalence, risk factors, and clinical implications. Clinical Psychology: Science and Practice 3:25–46, 1996
> Rosenberg ML, Smith JC, Davidson LE, et al: The emergence of youth suicide: an epidemiologic analysis and public health perspective. Annu Rev Public Health 8:417–440, 1987

35.3   Which of the following groups of psychiatric disorders is most closely linked to suicidal behavior in youth?

  A. Mood disorders.
  B. Anxiety disorders.
  C. Disruptive behavioral and conduct disorders.
  D. Substance use disorders.
  E. None of the above.

The correct response is option A.

The overwhelming majority—nearly 90%—of youth who die by suicide have evidence of serious psychopathology (Brent et al. 1988). Youth who attempt suicide also demonstrate high rates of psychopathology, in the range of 60% (Gould et al. 1998). Mood disorders convey the most potent risk, with over 80% of attempters and 60% of completers meeting criteria for at least one major mood disorder (Brent 1993; Gould et al. 1998). Unipolar depression and bipolar disorder are most closely linked to suicidal behavior in youth (Brent et al. 1988).

Other psychiatric conditions frequently associated with youth suicide and suicide attempt include disruptive behavior, anxiety, and substance use disorders. Comorbidity is the rule rather than the exception among youth who attempt and complete suicide, with up to 70% of suicidal youth meeting criteria for multiple psychiatric conditions (Lewinsohn et al. 1996).

Although conduct disorder and related disruptive disorders are more likely to eventuate in suicide and suicidal behavior when comorbid with substance use, disruptive disorders also independently contribute to suicide risk (Fergusson et al. 1995). **(p. 533)**

> Brent DA: Depression and suicide in children and adolescents. Pediatr Rev 14:380–388, 1993
> Brent DA, Perper JA, Goldstein CE, et al: Risk factors for adolescent suicide: a comparison of adolescent suicide victims with suicidal inpatients. Arch Gen Psychiatry 45:581–588, 1988
> Fergusson DM, Horwood LJ, Lynskey MT: The stability of disruptive childhood behaviors. J Abnorm Child Psychol 23:379–396, 1995
> Gould MS, King R, Greenwald S, et al: Psychopathology associated with suicidal ideation and attempts among children and adolescents. J Am Acad Child Psychiatry 37:915–923, 1998
> Lewinsohn PM, Rohde P, Seeley JR: Adolescent suicidal ideation and attempts: prevalence, risk factors, and clinical implications. Clinical Psychology: Science and Practice 3:25–46, 1996

35.4 A promising approach to treatment of youth suicidality is

    A. Safety planning.
    B. Means restriction.
    C. Dialectical behavior therapy (DBT).
    D. Developmental group therapy.
    E. All of the above.

The correct response is option E.

All of the approaches above show promise in the treatment of suicidal behavior in youth.

Approaches to the treatment of youth suicidality that show promise include clinical interventions like safety planning, means restriction, and hospitalization, as well as psychosocial treatment packages that involve cognitive, emotion regulation, and interpersonal approaches.

A safety plan is a hierarchically arranged list of strategies that the patient agrees to employ in the event of a suicidal crisis. The development of a safety plan is considered one of the most critical parts of the assessment and treatment of suicidal youth, and involves collaboration between the clinician, patient, and family.

Few studies have been conducted to evaluate the effectiveness of restriction of access to lethal means.

DBT, a treatment that focuses on the development of mindfulness, emotional regulation, distress tolerance, and interpersonal skills, has been shown to reduce recurrent suicidal and self-harm behavior in personality disordered adults. It was modified for use with suicidal adolescents by decreasing the length of treatment and incorporating family members into treatment (Miller et al. 2006).

Developmental group therapy is a skills-based approach focused on family conflict, problem solving, interpersonal relationships, anger management, school problems, depression, and hopelessness. Wood et al. (2001) compared 6-session skills-based developmental group therapy plus usual care with usual care alone in adolescents who had engaged in at least two episodes of self-harm within the past year. As compared with usual care, the experimental treatment group showed an overall reduction in conduct and school problems as well as repeated self-harm episodes. **(pp. 535–538)**

Miller AL, Rathus JH, Linehan MM: Dialectical Behavior Therapy With Suicidal Adolescents. New York, Guilford, 2006

Wood A, Trainor G, Rothwell J, et al: Randomized trial of group therapy for repeated deliberate self-harm in adolescents. J Am Acad Child Adolesc Psychiatry 40:1246–1253, 2001

35.5 All of the following statements regarding pharmacological approaches to the treatment of youth suicidality are correct *except*

    A. The Treatment of Adolescent Depression Study (TADS) showed a twofold increase in suicide-related adverse events among youth receiving medication compared with placebo groups.
    B. The U.S. Food and Drug Administration's (FDA's) meta-analysis of short-term placebo-controlled trials of selective serotonin reuptake inhibitors (SSRIs) and other antidepressants in youth indicated an increased risk of suicidality in patients taking antidepressants.
    C. The mechanism by which SSRIs might increase risk for suicidal behavior is not known.
    D. The recent decrease in SSRI prescriptions was associated with a marked decrease in youth suicide in the United States.
    E. Recent analysis supports the assertion that many more youth will show a good clinical response to SSRIs than will become suicidal.

The correct response is option D.

Although causation has not been demonstrated, there is a significant correlation in time between an increase in SSRI prescriptions and sales and a decline in both the overall suicide rate and the suicide rate among adolescents (Ludwig and Marcotte 2005). Additionally, the decrease in SSRI prescriptions following the public health warning of a possible association between SSRIs and suicide in youth was associated with a marked increase in youth suicide in the United States (Gibbons et al. 2007).

There is concern regarding a possible association between SSRI treatment and emergent suicidality in children and adolescents. The TADS documented a twofold increase in suicide-related adverse events among youth receiving active medication as compared with those taking placebo. Similarly, the FDA's meta-analysis of short-term placebo-controlled trials of SSRIs and other antidepressants in youth also indicated an increased risk of suicidal ideation or attempt in patients taking antidepressants.

The mechanism by which SSRIs might increase risk for suicidal behavior is not known. However, a recent meta-analysis supports the assertion that many more youth will show a good clinical response to SSRIs than will become suicidal (Bridge et al. 2007). **(p. 538)**

Bridge J, Iyengar S, Salary CB, et al: Clinical response and risk for reported suicidal ideation and suicide attempts in pediatric antidepressant treatment: a meta-analysis of randomized controlled trials. JAMA 297:1683–1696, 2007

Gibbons RD, Brown CH, Hur K, et al: Early evidence on the effects of regulators' suicidality warnings on SSRI prescriptions and suicide in children and adolescents. Am J Psychiatry 164:1356–1363, 2007

Ludwig J, Marcotte DE: Anti-depressants, suicide, and drug regulation. J Policy Anal Manage 24:249–272, 2005

Chapter 36

Gender Identity and Sexual Orientation

Select the single best response for each question.

36.1 By which age have most children established their gender identity?

    A. By the age of 2.
    B. By the age of 3.
    C. By the age of 5.
    D. By the age of 8.
    E. By the age of 12.

The correct response is option B.

Gender identity refers to a person's basic sense of self as a male, a female, or some other "third" type of gendered subjectivity. By the age of 3 years, most children demonstrate the rudimentary capacity to self-label their gender identity. **(p. 543)**

36.2 All of the following statements regarding epidemiology and comorbidity of gender identity disorder (GID) in children and adolescents are correct *except*

    A. GID in youth is relatively uncommon.
    B. People are less tolerant of cross-gender behavior in boys than in girls.
    C. The number of annual adolescent referrals for GID tripled between 2004 and 2007.
    D. In boys with GID, externalizing comorbid disorders predominate, whereas in girls with GID, there is a mixture of comorbid internalizing and externalizing disorders.
    E. Children and adolescents with GID should be evaluated systematically for comorbid conditions.

The correct response is option D.

In boys with GID, internalizing disorders predominate, whereas in girls with GID, there is a mixture of internalizing and externalizing disorders.

Epidemiological studies have not examined GID in youth. There is consensus that GID is relatively uncommon.

There is considerable evidence that parents, teachers, and peers are less tolerant of cross-gender behavior in boys than in girls; however, in adolescence, social pressures may be equally salient for boys and girls with pervasive cross-gender behavior. In Zucker's clinic, the number of child referrals per year has remained quite stable over the past 20 years; in contrast, the number of adolescent referrals per year tripled between the years 2004 and 2007 (Zucker et al. 2008).

Children and youth with GID should be evaluated systematically for the presence of other behavior problems and/or psychiatric disorders. **(p. 544)**

Zucker KJ, Bradley SJ, Owen-Anderson A, et al: Is gender identity disorder in adolescents coming out of the closet? (letter to the editor). J Sex Marital Ther 34:287–290, 2008

36.3 Based on up-to-date research, all of the following statements regarding the etiology of gender identity disorder (GID) are correct *except*

 A. The vast majority of children with GID do not have a disorder of sex development (DSD).
 B. Within-sex variation in sex-dimorphic behavior has a heritable component.
 C. Boys with GID have an elevated rate of right-handedness.
 D. A greater-than-average proportion of boys with GID have older male siblings.
 E. There is no evidence that parents of children with GID disproportionately wished for a child of the opposite sex during the pregnancy.

The correct response is option C.

Boys with GID have an elevated rate of left-handedness (Zucker et al. 2001), which may be a sign of prenatal developmental perturbations, and they are later in birth order relative to their brothers (Blanchard et al. 1995), which may be a marker of a progressive maternal immune response to male-specific antigens that results in a demasculinization of the male fetal brain (Blanchard and Klassen 1997).

Regarding biological factors, the vast majority of children with GID do not have a DSD (formerly known as physical intersex conditions).

There is some evidence that within-sex variation in sex-dimorphic behavior has a heritable component, but studies of identical twins discordant for GID suggest that genetic factors do not tell the whole story (Segal 2006).

There is no evidence that parents of children with GID disproportionately wished for a child of the opposite sex during the pregnancy. **(pp. 544–545)**

> Blanchard R, Klassen P: H-Y antigen and homosexuality in men. J Theor Biol 185:373–378, 1997
> Blanchard R, Zucker KJ, Bradley SJ, et al: Birth order and sibling sex ratio in homosexual male adolescents and probably prehomosexual feminine boys. Dev Psychol 31:22–30, 1995
> Segal NL: Two monozygotic twin pairs discordant for female-to-male transsexualism. Arch Sex Behav 35:347–358, 2006
> Zucker KJ, Beaulieu N, Bradley SJ, et al: Handedness in boys with gender identity disorder. J Child Psychol Psychiatry 42:767–776, 2001

36.4 Based on up-to-date follow-up studies of both boys and girls with gender identity disorder (GID), which of the following psychosexual outcomes is found?

 A. Persistence of GID with a co-occurring homosexual/bisexual sexual orientation.
 B. Desistence of GID with a co-occurring homosexual/bisexual sexual orientation.
 C. Desistence of GID with a co-occurring heterosexual orientation.
 D. All of the above.
 E. None of the above.

The correct response is option D.

Follow-up studies of both boys and girls with GID have provided data on at least three types of psychosexual outcomes: 1) persistence of GID with a co-occurring homosexual/bisexual sexual orientation, 2) desistence of GID with a co-occurring homosexual/bisexual sexual orientation, and 3) desistence of GID with a co-occurring heterosexual orientation. **(p. 545)**

36.5 Homosexuality was delisted from DSM as a mental disorder more than 30 years ago. Mental health professionals should remain current about what is known of people with a minority sexual orientation because

 A. It represents a form of cultural competence in delivering clinical care.
 B. It requires sensitivity in training clinicians.
 C. There may be heightened mental health challenges associated with a minority sexual orientation.

D. Many youth struggle with their emerging minority sexual orientation.

E. All of the above.

The correct response is option E.

In 1973, the American Psychiatric Association delisted homosexuality from DSM as a mental disorder. There are, however, reasons why mental health professionals need to remain current about what is known about people with a minority sexual orientation. First, it represents a form of cultural competence in delivering clinical care. Second, it requires sensitivity in training clinicians (Townsend et al. 1997). Third, there may be unique (or heightened) mental health challenges associated with a minority sexual orientation. Fourth, there remain many youth who struggle with their emerging minority sexual orientation, and the practitioner needs to know how best to help them in the consolidation of their sexual identity. **(p. 549)**

Townsend MH, Wallick MM, Pleak RR, et al: Gay and lesbian issues in child and adolescent psychiatry training as reported by training directors. J Am Acad Child Adolesc Psychiatry 36:764–768, 1997

Chapter 37

Aggression and Violence

Select the single best response for each question.

37.1 Which of the following medical conditions may carry risk for transient or permanent aggressive behavior?

A. Encephalitis.
B. Endocrine abnormalities.
C. Seizure disorders.
D. Traumatic brain injury (TBI).
E. All of the above.

The correct response is option E.

Several medical conditions carry risk for transient or more permanent aggressive behavior—because of inhibitory dyscontrol, impaired insight and judgment, and/or disorientation; these include delirious states secondary to infections (e.g., meningitis, encephalitis) or endocrine abnormalities and seizure disorders (occurring during either ictal or postictal periods). These conditions may present with acute onset of aggression, even if there is no preexisting pattern of antisocial acts; however, if treated properly, the aggression is generally time limited. In contrast, individuals who develop aggressive behavior following TBI often have a more chronic course. **(p. 554)**

37.2 Which of the following statements regarding the neurochemical and hormonal mechanisms and risk factors of aggression and violence is *false*?

A. An inverse relationship between central serotonin (5-hydroxytryptophan [5-HT]) function and impulsive aggression has been established in children.
B. Blunted prolactin response to fenfluramine at ages 7–11 years predicts aggressive outcome in adolescence.
C. Higher 5-HT responsivity in childhood might be a protective factor.
D. Aggression has been linked with both elevated peripheral cortisol and reduced cortisol.
E. Testosterone concentration and aggressive behavior are correlated in boys only after puberty.

The correct response is option A.

Convergent data from studies in animals and human adults have found an inverse relationship between central 5-HT function and impulsive aggression, but this has not been established in children.

Blunted prolactin response to fenfluramine at ages 7–11 years (indicative of low 5-HT activity) predicted aggressive outcome in adolescence, above and beyond the effect of early childhood aggression (Halperin et al. 2006).

Low 5-HT responsivity in childhood was necessary but not sufficient for aggressive outcome at follow-up; concomitant psychosocial risk was also required. However, psychosocial risk was not associated with aggression at follow-up in youth with higher 5-HT responsivity in childhood, suggesting that this may be a protective factor (Marks et al. 2007).

Aggression is associated with hormonal changes that occur in response to stress. Aggression has been linked with both elevated peripheral cortisol, which is characteristic of acute stress or anxiety states, and reduced cortisol, which may accompany posttraumatic stress.

Testosterone concentration and aggressive behavior are correlated in boys only after puberty, suggesting the importance of developmental mechanisms. Moreover, testosterone is primarily associated with aggression following provocation, very likely through interactions with a variety of neurotransmitters. (p. 555)

> Halperin JM, Kalmar JH, Schulz KP, et al: Elevated childhood serotonergic function protects against adolescent aggression in disruptive boys. J Am Acad Child Adolesc Psychiatry 45:833–840, 2006
> Marks DJ, Miller SR, Schulz KP, et al: The interaction of psychosocial adversity and biological risk in childhood aggression. Psychiatry Res 151:221–230, 2007

37.3 All of the following statements regarding genetic factors in aggression and violence are correct *except*

    A. The variability in heritability across studies indicates that genes account for only a portion of the variance.

    B. The candidate genes most consistently linked to aggression are the monoamine oxidase A (MAOA) and serotonin (5-hydroxytryptophan [5-HT]) transporter (5-HTT) genes.

    C. A rare mutation in the MAOA gene has been associated with impulsively violent behavior.

    D. Youth with one or more 5-HTT long variants show high levels of externalizing behavior.

    E. Two polymorphisms of the tryptophan hydroxylase gene are associated with increased irritability and assaultiveness.

The correct response is option D.

Youth with one or more 5-HTT short variants had high levels of externalizing behavior but in conjunction with genetic risk for alcoholism (Miczek et al. 2007).

Considerable data indicate that aggression runs in families. Twin studies consistently report higher concordance rates for aggression among monozygotic compared with dizygotic twins (Button et al. 2004). However, the variability in heritability across studies indicates that genes account for only a portion of the variance.

The candidate genes most consistently linked to aggression are the MAOA and 5-HTT genes. In humans, a rare mutation in the MAOA gene was found to be associated with impulsively violent behavior over multiple generations.

Two polymorphisms of the tryptophan hydroxylase gene have been associated with increased scores on the total and irritability/assaultiveness scales of the Buss-Durkee Hostility Inventory and with impulsive-aggressive suicidal behavior. (p. 556)

> Button TM, Scourfield J, Martin N, et al: Do aggressive and non-aggressive antisocial behaviors in adolescents result from the same genetic and environmental effects? Am J Med Genet B Neuropsychiatr Genet 129B:59–63, 2004
> Miczek KA, de Almeida RM, Kravitz EA, et al: Neurobiology of escalated aggression and violence. J Neurosci 27:11803–11806, 2007

37.4 Which of the following are characteristics of successful intervention programs for aggression and violence?

    A. Multimodal intervention.

    B. Consistently delivered interventions on a daily to weekly basis.

    C. School/family collaboration.

    D. Application of individual management techniques.

    E. All of the above.

The correct response is option E.

Characteristics of successful intervention programs include 1) multimodal intervention for children and parents, parent support, teacher involvement, and early childhood education; 2) delivery of interventions consistently on a daily to weekly basis; 3) duration of 2 years or longer; 4) specific interventions to remediate coercive family process and harsh and inconsistent parenting techniques through skill building, and development of problem-solving and coping skills; 5) interventions that begin in early childhood; 6) application of individual management techniques; and 7) collaboration among community, school, family, and mental health professionals. **(p. 558)**

37.5   Which of the following medications is the best studied, and has been approved by the U.S. Food and Drug Administration (FDA) for treating aggression in children with posttraumatic stress disorder?

    A. Lithium.
    B. Risperidone.
    C. Fluoxetine.
    D. Clonidine.
    E. Divalproex sodium.

The correct response is option B.

Second-generation "atypical" antipsychotics have shown significant efficacy in decreasing aggression and regulating mood in youth. Risperidone is the best studied of these agents; positive findings from controlled trials of risperidone efficacy in the treatment of aggression in children with pervasive developmental disorders (Aman et al. 2002; McDougle et al. 2005) led to approval by the FDA for this indication. (**Note:** This is the only medication approved for the treatment of aggression in any diagnostic group.) In addition to improvement in aggressive behavior, risperidone produces robust improvement in impulsivity, social interactions, explosivity, self-injury, sleep, and hygiene. **(p. 562)**

Aman MG, De Smedt G, Derivan A, et al: Double-blind, placebo-controlled study of risperidone for the treatment of disruptive behaviors in children with subaverage intelligence. Am J Psychiatry 159:1337–1346, 2002

McDougle CJ, Scahill L, Aman MG, et al: Risperidone for the core symptom domains of autism: results from the study by the autism network of the research units on pediatric psychopharmacology. Am J Psychiatry 162:1142–1148, 2005

Chapter 38

Genetics

Fundamentals Relevant to Child and Adolescent Psychiatry

Select the single best response for each question.

38.1   How frequently do DNA mutations occur in every replication cycle?

    A. 1 per each 100,000 base pairs (bp).
    B. 1 per each 10,000 bp.
    C. 1 per each 1,000 bp.
    D. 1 per each 500 bp.
    E. 1 per each 100 bp.

The correct response is option C.

Mutations occur normally at a rate of 1 per each 1,000 bp in every replication cycle but can increase following exposure to environmental stressors such as radiation, chemical toxins, or viruses. **(p. 568)**

38.2   Nonharmful changes in DNA can be passed on to subsequent generations. Mutations may or may not have effects on functioning. Which of the following describes a mutation that occurs in more than 1% of the population?

    A. Genetic drift.
    B. Polymorphism.
    C. Hardy-Weinberg equilibrium.
    D. Single nucleotide polymorphisms (SNPs).
    E. None of the above.

The correct response is option B.

Most mutations randomly disappear over time. However, the frequency of some mutations within populations can increase, solely by chance. When a given mutation occurs in more than 1% of a population it is called a *polymorphism*.

Nonharmful changes in DNA can be passed on to subsequent generations. Unless a DNA change causes an advantage or disadvantage in a particular environment, the mutation's frequency will vary randomly in the population from generation to generation in a phenomenon known as *genetic drift*.

Over time, the frequencies of different alleles within the same gene exhibit relative stability, called *Hardy-Weinberg equilibrium*. Polymorphisms can be defined as major or minor alleles according to their population frequency.

SNPs are found in both coding and noncoding genomic regions, and each reflects a mutation that probably occurred once during human evolution. Consequently, SNPs usually have two variants, and the degree to which two individuals share common SNPs provides a measure of relatedness. SNPs have been particularly useful in mapping genes and locating genes that contribute susceptibility to disease. **(p. 568)**

38.3 Which of the following statements regarding chromosomes is *false?*

    A. They are in the nucleus.
    B. The human genome consists of 22 pairs of autosomal chromosomes and a pair of sex chromosomes—XY in males or XX in females.
    C. The autosomal chromosomes are numbered 1 through 22 in order of increasing size.
    D. The shorter arms are designated "p," whereas the longer arms are designated "q."
    E. An ordered list of loci within a particular genome provides a genetic map.

The correct response is option C.

Chromosomes comprise large molecules of DNA and associated proteins that package genomic material within the nucleus. DNA makes up less than one-third of chromosomal mass, with the remainder comprised of histone proteins that package DNA and facilitate RNA synthesis. The human genome consists of 22 pairs of autosomal chromosomes, numbered 1 through 22 in order of decreasing size, and a pair of sex chromosomes: XY in males or XX in females. The shorter arms of each chromosome are designated "p" (for petit), and the longer arms are designated "q" (for the next letter in the alphabet). An ordered list of loci within a particular genome provides a genetic map. **(p. 568)**

38.4 All of the following statements regarding the regulation of gene expression are correct *except*

    A. Each of an individual's nucleated cells (other than eggs or sperm) contains the same DNA and associated genes.
    B. Gene transcription can be induced or silenced by transcription factors.
    C. Genes can be induced by exposure to exogenous compounds.
    D. Histone acetylation can enhance DNA transcription.
    E. DNA methylation can promote DNA transcription.

The correct response is option E.

DNA methylation prevents the interaction of genomic regions with transcriptional factors and subsequently silences transcription.

    Each of an individual's nucleated cells (other than eggs or sperm) contains the same DNA and associated genes. Mechanisms that regulate gene expression enable this finite set of genes to control all the body's diverse functions. Gene transcription can be induced or silenced by transcription factors. Genes can by induced by other products synthesized within the cell or by exposure to exogenous compounds such as hormones or bacterial antigens. Changes in chromatin structure control the accessibility of genomic regions for DNA transcription. Histone acetylation facilitates the interaction of genomic sequences with gene regulator proteins and RNA polymerase, leading to enhanced DNA transcription. **(p. 573)**

38.5 According to up-to-date research, which of the following statements regarding the Mendelian patterns of inheritance of medical and psychiatric disorders is *false?*

    A. Most psychiatric disorders follow Mendelian patterns of inheritance.
    B. Huntington disease is inherited as an autosomal dominant disorder.
    C. Both dominant and recessive patterns of inheritance have been associated with Alzheimer's disease.
    D. X-linked dominant inheritance has been suggested in Rett syndrome.
    E. Recessive pattern of inheritance is associated with cystic fibrosis.

The correct response is option A.

Simple traits arise from changes in single genes and usually follow Mendelian patterns of inheritance. *Complex traits* arise from the interplay of multiple genes, usually with varying small degrees of effect, and the environment. Almost all psychiatric disorders represent complex traits and are not explained by Mendelian patterns of inheritance.

Huntington's disease is inherited as an autosomal dominant disorder stemming from an abnormal triplet repeat CAG within a gene on chromosome 4 (Roses 1996).

Polymorphisms in genes coding for the amyloid precursor protein, presenilin 1, and presenilin 2 have been associated with Alzheimer's disease (Liddell et al. 2002), although both dominant and recessive patterns of inheritance have been proposed.

Most cases of Rett syndrome arise from sporadic mutations, but patterns in family pedigrees suggest X-linked dominant inheritance in females and lethality in males (Schanen et al. 1997).

Cystic fibrosis results from recessive mutations in the CF gene located on chromosome 7 (Riordan et al. 1989). **(p. 574)**

Liddell MB, Williams J, Owen MJ: The dementias, in Psychiatric Genetics and Genomics. Edited by McGuffin P, Owen MJ, Gottesman II. New York, Oxford University Press, 2002, pp 341–397

Riordan JR, Rommens JM, Kerem B, et al: Identification of the cystic fibrosis gene: cloning and characterization of complementary DNA. Science 245:1066–1073, 1989

Roses AD: From genes to mechanisms to therapies: lessons to be learned from neurological disorders. Nature Med 2:267–269, 1996

Schanen NC, Dahle EJ, Capozzoli F, et al: A new Rett syndrome family consistent with X-linked inheritance expands the X chromosome map. Am J Hum Genet 61:634–641, 1997

38.6   Linkage studies examine the relationship between a phenotype and a genetic locus. The degree of linkage is expressed by a lod score. Which of the following lod scores is considered evidence of linkage?

   A. >0.5.
   B. >1.
   C. >2.
   D. >3.
   E. >4.

The correct response is option D.

The degree of linkage is expressed by a *lod score*, which is a log ratio reflecting the frequency of recombination between two markers divided by the expected frequency with independent assortment. In order to provide a common point of discussion between researchers, lod scores >2 are suggestive of linkage, lod scores >3 are considered evidence of linkage, and lod scores >4 are evidence of strong linkage with a gene of major effect (Lander and Kruglyak 1995). **(pp. 574–575)**

Lander E, Kruglyak L: Genetic dissection of complex traits: guidelines for interpreting and reporting linkage results. Nat Genet 11:241–247, 1995

Chapter 39

Psychiatric Emergencies

Select the single best response for each question.

39.1 All of the following statements regarding assessing suicidal youth in an emergency room are correct *except*

    A. Parental consent should be obtained prior to assessment.
    B. Safety is a primary concern.
    C. Assessment includes a careful physical examination and mental status examination.
    D. Lethality and intent are two important aspects for assessment.
    E. Precipitants and predisposing factors need to be addressed.

The correct response is option A.

The mental health clinician in the emergency room can evaluate the suicidal adolescent (under age 18 years in all but four states) without parental consent.

Safety is a primary concern in the emergency room assessment that begins at the time of admission. The psychiatric assessment includes a careful physical examination, including mental status. The assessment of the suicidal patient focuses on two aspects of the behavior: lethality and intent. The clinician should realize that there are precipitants of the suicide attempt and that a primary purpose of the assessment is to uncover and address those issues as well as predisposing factors. **(pp. 584–585)**

39.2 Which of the following statements regarding youth evaluated in emergency settings for suicidal behavior is *false?*

    A. About 14% of patients evaluated in the emergency room for suicidality never attend an outpatient mental health appointment.
    B. Patients with higher levels of suicidal behavior and depression are more likely to attend outpatient appointments.
    C. Patients who actively express suicidal ideation and intent should be hospitalized.
    D. Patients who have low levels of suicidality and who agree to participate in outpatient sessions with family support may require outpatient treatment only.
    E. A no-suicide contract is an important and valid indicator of future risk.

The correct response is option E.

Studies do not support the validity of "no-suicide contracts" created as part of the assessment as an indicator of future dangerousness.

For the clinician trying to determine relative risk, the likelihood of successful follow-up is critically important. Approximately 14% of patients evaluated in an emergency setting for suicidal behavior never attend an outpatient mental health appointment. Patients with higher levels of suicidal behavior and depression are more likely to attend outpatient appointments (Spirito et al. 1992, 2002).

A recommendation for psychiatric hospitalization is made when the patient actively voices suicidal ideation with intent.

Outpatient treatment is appropriate for patients who exhibit low levels of suicidal behavior and who are prepared to participate in outpatient sessions with the support of their caregivers. **(pp. 585–586)**

Spirito A, Plummer B, Gispert M, et al: Adolescent suicide attempters: outcomes at follow-up. Am J Orthopsychiatry 62:464–468, 1992

Spirito A, Boergers J, Donaldson D, et al: An intervention trial to improve adherence to community treatment by adolescents following a suicide attempt. J Am Acad Child Adolesc Psychiatry 41:435–442, 2002

39.3   An intervention is defined as *seclusion* if the patient is placed alone in a room under which of the following circumstances?

   A. The patient is behind a locked door.
   B. The door is either held by staff or locked with a spring-loaded latch.
   C. Free movement of the patient is inhibited.
   D. The patient is actively separated and taken to a specific location away from the group.
   E. All of the above.

The correct response is option E.

Interventions are defined as *seclusion* when the patient is placed alone in a room under the following circumstances: 1) the patient is behind a locked door, 2) the door is either held by staff members or locked with a spring-loaded latch, 3) free movement of the patient is inhibited, and 4) the patient is actively separated and taken to a specific location away from the group. **(pp. 590–591)**

39.4   All of the following statements regarding chemical restraints in an emergency department setting are correct *except*

   A. *Chemical restraint* is defined as the use of medication for behavioral control.
   B. To avoid chemical restraint, medications should be prescribed in a manner consistent with the diagnosis.
   C. Pharmacological management of aggression is preferable to the use of restraints.
   D. There is a clear consensus on the most appropriate medication strategy for the pediatric emergency psychiatry patient.
   E. Some atypical antipsychotics are effective for the treatment of aggression and self-injurious behavior in children with pervasive developmental disorder (PDD).

The correct response is option D.

There is no consensus on the most appropriate medication strategy for the pediatric emergency psychiatry patient. However, some simple recommendations can improve the quality of the patient's care: 1) administer repeated low-dose medications rather than a single high dose when titrating the drug, 2) apply combined treatments with caution and care, and 3) use low-dose benzodiazepines carefully because of concerns about paradoxical reactions.

Chemical restraint is loosely defined as the use of medications for the sole purpose of behavioral control rather than as part of a plan of care for a diagnosable condition.

In order to avoid chemical restraint, the patient should be appropriately assessed and medications prescribed in a manner consistent with the diagnosis.

Pharmacological management of aggression is preferable to the use of restraints, particularly when considering the time and potential complications.

Atypical antipsychotics present a lower risk of extrapyramidal side effects than high-potency medications and are effective for the treatment of aggression and self-injurious behavior in mentally retarded and developmentally delayed patients, as well as children with pervasive developmental disorder. **(p. 592)**

39.5   Which of the following recommendations for restraint of children and adolescents is *correct*?

   A. Makeshift restraints are preferable to those prescribed for adults.
   B. In certain circumstances, it is appropriate to tie down only one limb.

C. There are no randomized trials on the most appropriate method or position for restraint.

D. The prone restraint position is better for the clinician but not for the patient.

E. Patients with medical conditions should never be restrained supine.

The correct response is option C.

There are no randomized trials on the most appropriate method or position for restraint. No clinical trials demonstrate the most effective way to release a patient from restraints either. The process is best approached as an ongoing negotiation, with the clinician constantly communicating and reassuring the patient. Restraint devices should only be those that are designed specifically for this purpose. These devices include limb holders, abdominal belts, and vests. Makeshift restraints are always contraindicated because the devices are typically difficult to apply, are frequently tied too tightly but ineffectively, and are often uncomfortable and dangerous for the patient. Restraints are gradually released one step at a time, but the patient should never be left with one limb tied down. When applying a restraint, the prone position is initially safer for both patient and clinician because there is a lower risk of asphyxiation and of biting injury. Patients with medical considerations are restrained supine with their arms at their sides. **(pp. 592–593)**

Chapter 40

Family Transitions

Challenges and Resilience

Select the single best response for each question.

40.1   In which decade did a white, middle-class, intact nuclear household headed by a breadwinner father and a homemaker mother represent the model family?

  A. 1920s.
  B. 1930s.
  C. 1950s.
  D. 1980s.
  E. None of the above.

The correct response is option C.

In the midst of social, economic, and political upheavals over recent decades, families have become more diverse and complex (Walsh 2003). The 1950s model family—white, middle-class, intact nuclear household, headed by a breadwinner father and a homemaker mother—is now only a narrow band on the wide spectrum of families (Coontz 1997). **(p. 595)**

> Coontz S: The Way We Really Are: Coming to Terms With America's Changing Families. New York, Basic Books, 1997
> Walsh F (ed): Normal Family Processes: Growing Diversity and Complexity, 3rd Edition. New York, Guilford, 2003

40.2   Which of the following statements regarding changing family structures and gender roles in the United States is *false*?

  A. More than 70% of all mothers were in the workforce by 2001.
  B. The assumption that mothers' work outside the home harms children has not been supported by research.
  C. Divorce rates continue to climb up, especially for first marriages.
  D. Research shows children raised by gay and lesbian couples fare as well as those who are raised by hetero-sexual ones.
  E. Most adoptions are now open.

The correct response is option C.

Divorce rates, after rising in recent decades, have leveled off at around 45% for first marriages. Most children in divorced families undergo further transition with parental remarriage and stepfamily formation.

Economic pressures, career aspirations, and divorce have brought over 70% of all mothers into the workforce (Barnett and Hyde 2001).

The assumption that mothers' work outside the home harms children has fueled maternal guilt and blame but has not been supported in research. What matters most is stable, quality care.

Increasing numbers of gay and lesbian single parents and couples are raising children. Research clearly shows that their children fare as well as those with heterosexual parents, although they are challenged by social stigma (Green 2004; Stacey and Biblarz 2001).

Most adoptions are now open, based on findings that children benefit developmentally if they know who their birth families are, have the option for contact, and in biracial and international adoption are encouraged to develop bicultural identities and connections. **(pp. 595–596)**

Barnett RC, Hyde J: Women, men, work, and family. An expansionist theory. Am Psychol 56:781–796, 2001

Green RJ: Risk and resilience in lesbian and gay couples: comment on Solomon, Rothblum, and Balsam (2004). J Fam Psychol 18:290–292, 2004

Stacey J, Biblarz TJ: How does the sexual orientation of parents matter? American Sociological Review 66:159–183, 2001

40.3   Family systems–oriented practice is guided by a developmental, multisystemic perspective on human problems and processes of change. All of the following statements regarding family systems practice approaches are accurate *except*

   A. Tools such as the genogram and timeline are of only limited value in elucidating key elements of family systems.
   B. The family is viewed as a transactional system evolving over the life course and across the generations.
   C. Family processes can heighten risk or foster positive adaptation.
   D. Key members in the family system must be identified.
   E. It is important to identify processes that promote resilience.

The correct response is option A.

The *genogram* and timeline (McGoldrick et al. 2008) are essential tools for mapping the family system, noting relationship information, and tracking system patterns to guide intervention planning.

Family systems practice approaches address the complex interplay of individual, family, and social influences, including school, workplace, court, and health care systems. The family is viewed as a transactional system evolving over the life course and across the generations (Carter and McGoldrick 1999). Individual and family development are intertwined, with each phase posing new challenges.

Stressful transitions affect the family as a functional unit, with reverberations for all members and their relationships. In turn, family processes can heighten risk or foster positive adaptation (Walsh 2003). Thus, the family is an essential partner in assessment and treatment.

A systemic lens is required to identify key members in the family system, including all household members, nonresidential parents and steprelations, the extended kin network, and other significant relationships (e.g., intimate partner, informal kin, and caregivers).

Family strain increases exponentially if a current crisis, such as a threatened separation, reactivates past trauma or loss (Carter and McGoldrick 1999). It is important to identify processes that promote resilience, such as active coping and perseverance, and to draw out stories of positive adaptation in facing other life challenges. **(p. 597)**

Carter B, McGoldrick M (eds): The Expanded Life Cycle: Individual, Family, and Social Perspectives, 3rd Edition. Needham Heights, MA, Allyn & Bacon, 1999

McGoldrick M, Gerson R, Petry S: Genograms: Assessment and Intervention, 3rd Edition. New York, WW Norton, 2008

Walsh F (ed): Normal Family Processes: Growing Diversity and Complexity, 3rd Edition. New York, Guilford, 2003

40.4   Which of the following situations can increase the risk for child and family dysfunction?

    A. Sudden death.
    B. Lingering death.
    C. Ambiguous loss.
    D. Disenfranchised losses.
    E. All of the above.

The correct response is option E.

The nature and circumstances of loss can increase risk for child and family dysfunction. Such situations include 1) *sudden death* without time to prepare for the loss, to say goodbyes, or to deal with unfinished business; 2) *lingering death* after a long illness, depleting family resources and generating relief and guilt that a prolonged ordeal is over; 3) *ambiguous loss* when there is unclarity about the fate of a loved one who is missing, or when, as in dementia, there is psychological and relational loss of a loved one who is still alive (Boss 1999); 4) *disenfranchised losses*, with socially unacknowledged losses (such as miscarriage or pet loss) or stigmatized deaths (as with HIV/AIDS or suicide) producing secrecy, guilt, and estrangement; 5) *violent deaths* such as a fatal accident, homicide, or suicide, generating lingering anger, guilt, or remorse and forgiveness issues. **(pp. 598–599)**

> Boss P: Ambiguous Loss. Cambridge, MA, Harvard University Press, 1999

40.5   Which of the following are tasks that may facilitate adaptation for children and strengthen the family as a functional unit, according to Walsh and McGoldrick (2004)?

    A. Share acknowledgment of reality of death.
    B. Share experiences of loss.
    C. Reorganize family system.
    D. Transform bonds with deceased.
    E. All of the above.

The correct response is option E.

Family adaptation to loss involves sharing grief, gaining meaning and perspective, and moving ahead with life. Four core family tasks facilitate immediate and long-term adaptation for children and strengthen the family as a functional unit (Walsh and McGoldrick 2004): 1) *share acknowledgment* of reality of death/loss through information and communication; 2) *share experience of loss* through memorial rituals or empathic sharing of feelings and meaning-making; 3) *reorganize family system* by realigning relationships and role functions to provide continuity, cohesion, and adaptive flexibility; and 4) *reinvest in relationships and life pursuits and transform bonds with deceased* from living presence to spiritual connections, memories, and legacies. **(p. 600)**

> Walsh F, McGoldrick M (eds): Living Beyond Loss: Death in the Family, 2nd Edition. New York, WW Norton, 2004

Chapter 41

Psychiatric Aspects of Chronic Physical Disorders

Select the single best response for each question.

41.1 All of the following statements regarding the psychological adjustment of children with chronic health problems are correct *except*

    A. Suffering from chronic illnesses increases risks for emotional adjustment problems.

    B. Patients with chronic illnesses are more likely to suffer from externalizing syndrome.

    C. Disease-related factors are relatively less significant than family/child-related factors.

    D. Disease involving the central nervous system (CNS) has a significant impact on adjustment.

    E. Patients with multiple chronic physical conditions are at higher risk for psychiatric disorders.

The correct response is option B.

Patients with chronic illnesses are more likely to suffer from internalizing syndromes, including depressive and anxiety disorders that appear early and persist over time (Breslau and Marshall 1985; Stuber 1996; Thompson et al. 1990).

There is evidence that children and adolescents suffering from chronic illnesses are at increased risk for emotional adjustment problems (Wallander et al. 2003).

In general, disease-related factors seem to play a relatively small part in affecting the child's psychological adjustment. Although illness severity might be expected to affect psychological adjustment to a chronic condition, in fact its significance is relatively minor and much less than family factors such as parental mental health (Lavigne and Faier-Routman 1993).

Of greater significance than severity of the disorder in affecting the child's adjustment is the degree to which the CNS is involved in the disease process. Disorders affecting CNS functioning (e.g., epilepsy, cerebral palsy, hydrocephalus) show higher rates of psychological problems than other disorders (DeMaso et al. 1990; Lavigne and Faier-Routman 1992; Noeker et al. 2005).

Numerous studies have found that, among conditions not involving the brain (e.g., cystic fibrosis, diabetes mellitus, or asthma), there is no relationship between disease severity and psychosocial adjustment (Campis et al. 1995; DeMaso et al. 1991, 1995; Shaw and DeMaso 2006). Exceptions may be found in cases where adolescents must cope with multiple chronic physical conditions (Newacheck et al. 1991) and/or long-term physical disability (Holmbeck et al. 2003). These patients are at greater risk for psychiatric disorder. **(pp. 607–608)**

Breslau N, Marshall IA: Psychological disturbance in children with physical disabilities: continuity and change in a 5-year follow-up. J Abnorm Child Psychol 12:199–216, 1985

Campis LB, DeMaso DR, Twente AW: The role of maternal factors in the adaptation of children with craniofacial disfigurement. Cleft Palate Craniofac J 32:55–61, 1995

DeMaso DR, Beardslee WR, Silbert AR, et al: Psychological functioning in children with cyanotic heart defects. J Dev Behav Pediatr 11:289–294, 1990

DeMaso DR, Campis LK, Wypij D, et al: The impact of maternal perceptions and medical severity on the adjustment of children with congenital heart disease. J Pediatr Psychol 16:137–149, 1991

DeMaso DR, Twente AW, Spratt EG, et al: The impact of psychological functioning, medical severity, and family functioning in pediatric heart transplantation. J Heart Lung Transplant 14:1102–1108, 1995

Holmbeck GN, Westhoven VC, Phillips WS, et al: A multimethod, multi-informant, multidimensional perspective on psychosocial adjustment in preadolescents with spina bifida. J Consult Clin Psychol 71:782–796, 2003

Lavigne JV, Faier-Routman J: Psychological adjustment to pediatric physical disorders: a meta-analytic review. J Pediatr Psychol 17:133–157, 1992

Lavigne JV, Faier-Routman J: Correlates of psychological adjustment to pediatric physical disorders: a meta-analytic review and comparison to existing models. J Dev Behav Pediatr 14:117–123, 1993

Newacheck PW, McManus MA, Fox HB: Prevalence and impact of chronic illness among adolescents. Am J Dis Child 145:1367–1373, 1991

Noeker M, Haverkamp-Krois A, Haverkamp F: Development of mental health dysfunction in childhood epilepsy. Brain Dev 27:5–16, 2005

Shaw RJ, DeMaso DR: Clinical Manual of Pediatric Psychosomatic Medicine: Mental Health Consultation With Physically Ill Children and Adolescents. Washington, DC, American Psychiatric Publishing, 2006

Stuber ML: Psychiatric sequelae in seriously ill children and their families. Psychiatr Clin North Am 19:481–493, 1996

Thompson RJ, Hodges K, Hamlett KW: A matched comparison of adjustment in children with cystic fibrosis and psychiatrically. J Pediatr Psychol 15:745–759, 1990

Wallander JL, Thompson RJ, Alriksson-Schmidt A: Psychosocial adjustment of children with chronic physical conditions, in Handbook of Pediatric Psychology, 3rd Edition. Edited by Roberts MC. New York, Guilford, 2003, pp 141–158

41.2 Which of the following statements regarding models of adaptation to the effects of chronic illness is *true*?

A. Wright's model posited a central role for the effect of chronic illness.
B. According to Wright, an individual with chronic illness highly values a physical status "like everyone else."
C. More recent models that emphasize the interplay between child and parent have been developed.
D. The transactional model emphasizes the interplay between chronic illness and exposure to negative life events.
E. All of the above.

The correct response is option E.

One of the earliest models of adaptation was proposed by Beatrice Wright (1960). Wright's model posited a central role for the effects of chronic illness on the self-system, including body image, and on the individual's values.

More recently, better articulated and integrative models of adaptation to pediatric illnesses (Thompson and Gustafson 1996; Wallander and Varni 1992) have been developed that emphasize the interplay between child and parent adaptation in adjustment.

The ecological-systems theory relies on a transactional model of stress and coping. Successful adaptation to the chronic illness by the patient and family is dependent upon an interaction between the disease and a variety of biomedical, developmental, and psychosocial factors (Wallander et al. 2003). The transactional model emphasizes the interplay between chronic illness and exposure to negative life events in the etiology of adjustment disorders. **(p. 608)**

Thompson RJ, Gustafson KE: Adaptation to Chronic Childhood Illness. Washington, DC, American Psychological Association, 1996

Wallander JL, Varni JW: Adjustment in children with chronic physical disorders: programmatic research on a disability-stress-coping model, in Stress and Coping in Child Health. Edited by La Greca AM, Siegel LJL, Wallander JL, et al. New York, Guilford, 1992, pp 279–299

Wallander JL, Thompson RJ, Alriksson-Schmidt A: Psychosocial adjustment of children with chronic physical conditions, in Handbook of Pediatric Psychology, 3rd Edition. Edited by Roberts MC. New York, Guilford, 2003, pp 141–158

Wright B: Physical Disability: A Psychosocial Approach. New York, Harper & Row, 1960

41.3 All of the following statements concerning the impact on families of a child's chronic illness are correct *except*

    A. High levels of parental attention, reassurance, and empathy are essential for strengthening the child's ability to cope with his or her illness.

    B. Most families with a medically ill child are well adjusted and productive.

    C. Parents must deal with their feelings of loss of control over their child's life.

    D. Overconcern with medical information can cause parents to neglect both their child's and their family's psychosocial needs.

    E. Siblings may sometimes withdraw from engagement in activities with the affected child.

The correct response is option A.

Overresponding to the child (via excessive parental attention, reassurance, empathy, and apologies) can interfere with the child's ability to cope with his or her illness (Frank et al. 1995; Logan and Scharff 2005).

Most families with a medically ill child are well adjusted and productive. Individual members, however, are more likely to experience symptoms of irritability, anxiety, depression, and somatic complaints than the general population (Jacobs 2000).

Along with providing the instrumental care and emotional support their child needs, parents must also deal with their own feelings about being unable to protect their child from disease and their loss of control over their child's life. Parents can become overly concerned with medical information and neglect both their child's and family's psychosocial needs. The demands of caring for an ill child may affect the parents' marital relationship (Kazak et al. 2003). Parents may be highly supportive of one another and even be drawn closer to one another, but there is a risk that the marital relationship may be weakened, particularly if marital problems existed before the child's illness developed.

Siblings may occasionally become emotionally disengaged from busy parents, less able to engage in activities with the affected child, jealous of the attention directed toward the ill child, and feel guilt about not being affected. **(p. 611)**

Frank NC, Blount RL, Smith AJ, et al: Parent and staff behavior, previous child medical experience, and maternal anxiety as they relate to child procedural distress and coping. J Pediatr Psychol 20:277–289, 1995

Jacobs J: Family therapy in chronic medical illness, in Psychiatric Care of the Medical Patient, 2nd Edition. Edited by Stoudemire A, Fogel BS, Greenberg DB. Oxford, England, Oxford University Press, 2000, pp 31–39

Kazak AE, Rourke MT, Crump TA: Families and other systems in pediatric psychology, in Handbook of Pediatric Psychology, 3rd Edition. Edited by Roberts MC. New York, Guilford, 2003, pp 159–175

Logan DE, Scharff L: Relationships between family and parent characteristics and functional abilities in children with recurrent pain syndromes: an investigation of moderating effects on the pathway from pain to disability. J Pediatr Psychol 30:698–707, 2005

41.4 Which of the following statements regarding psychopharmacological management of youth with chronic physical disorders is *false?*

    A. Medically ill children represent the exception to the axiom "start low, go slow" when initiating treatment with psychotropic medication.

    B. Drug levels for psychotropic medications are not reliable indicators of efficacy or toxicity.

    C. It is best to use one medication at a time and to choose a drug with a short half-life.

    D. Most psychotropic drugs are highly protein bound.

    E. Drug metabolism and drug-drug interactions may be altered in medically ill patients.

The correct response is option A.

Young patients are affected by illnesses that impair organ systems and change drug metabolism—particularly those patients with hepatic, gastrointestinal, renal, and cardiac diseases. It is, therefore, wise to follow the axiom "start low, go slow" when initiating medication.

Drug levels for psychotropic medications are not reliable indicators of efficacy or toxicity. In medically ill children, it is best to use one medication at a time and to choose a drug with a short half-life that can be administered in single doses and that quickly reaches a therapeutic level.

Most psychotropic medications, with the exception of lithium, venlafaxine, divalproex sodium, methylphenidate, gabapentin, and topiramate, are bound to protein at an 80%–90% rate.

Clinicians should be aware of medications that either potentiate or inhibit the hepatic cytochrome P450 (CYP450) system, particularly in medically ill patients on multiple-drug regimens. In these situations, drug metabolism is altered and drug-drug interactions are more likely (Shaw and DeMaso 2006). **(pp. 611–612)**

Shaw RJ, DeMaso DR: Clinical Manual of Pediatric Psychosomatic Medicine: Mental Health Consultation With Physically Ill Children and Adolescents. Washington, DC, American Psychiatric Publishing, 2006

41.5   Which of the following is the most common cause of delirium in pediatric patients?

    A. Cancer.
    B. Trauma.
    C. Central nervous system (CNS) infections.
    D. Diabetes.
    E. All of the above.

The correct response is option C.

Pediatric patients seem to be especially vulnerable to delirium following toxic, metabolic, or traumatic CNS insults and fever regardless of the etiology. The most common causes of delirium are infections of the CNS (meningitis) or medication toxicity.

Delirium is characterized by impairments in attention and orientation, deficits in language and visual spatial skills, and deterioration in cognition not explained by an underlying dementia (Murphy 2000). Patients should be evaluated several times over an extended period before making the diagnosis. **(p. 617)**

Murphy BA: Delirium. Emerg Med Clin North Am 18:243–252, 2000

Chapter 42

Children of Parents With Psychiatric and Substance Abuse Disorders

Select the single best response for each question.

42.1 Which of the following interventions for families at high risk because of parental mental illness is supported by the Institute of Medicine Committee on Prevention?

A. Indicated prevention programs.
B. Selective prevention programs.
C. Universal prevention programs.
D. All of the above.
E. None of the above.

The correct response is option D.

Research on preventive interventions for families at high risk due to parental mental illness and associated factors has shown considerable positive effects. The Institute of Medicine Committee on Prevention supports the following system of classification of prevention programs (Mrazek and Haggerty 1994; Munoz et al. 1996): 1) *indicated prevention programs*, which target at-risk individuals who already have symptoms or a biological marker but do not meet full diagnostic criteria; 2) *selective prevention programs*, which target individuals presumed to be at high risk for the development of a disorder; prevention programs that target children of parents with mental illness are selective preventions, whereas those that target children who themselves have symptoms are a combination of selective and indicated programs; 3) *universal prevention programs*, which target entire populations, regardless of risk factors. **(p. 624)**

> Mrazek PJ, Haggerty RJ: Reducing Risks for Mental Disorders. Washington, DC, Institute of Medicine, National Academy Press, 1994
> Munoz RF, Mrazek PJ, Haggerty RJ: Institute of Medicine report on prevention of mental disorders: summary and commentary. Am Psychol 51:1116–1122, 1996

42.2 There are several well-established risk factors for depression and other disorders. Some of them are specific for depression. All of the following are specific risks for depression *except*

A. Social isolation.
B. Extensive family history of depression.
C. Prior history of depression.
D. Depressogenic cognitive style.
E. Bereavement.

The correct response is option A.

There are several well-established risk factors for depression and other disorders for which there is empirical justification. Risk factors specific for depression include extensive family history of depression, especially in parents; prior history of depression; depressogenic cognitive style, and bereavement. **(p. 625; see also Table 42–1)**

42.3 Children growing up with parents with a psychiatric disorder are at significantly higher risk of developing a mental disorder during their life span. All of the following statements regarding risks and outcomes are correct *except*

   A. The risk increases significantly when both parents are ill.
   B. Parent-child interaction with parents with certain psychiatric disorders can be a risk factor for children.
   C. The relationship between risk factors and later outcome for children is deterministic.
   D. The risk and protective factors can be additive, interactive, and accumulative in nature.
   E. It is not the diagnosis of the parent but the chronicity, severity, and amount of impairment that is associated with effects on the child.

The correct response is option C.

The relationship between risk factors and later outcome for children is probabilistic, not deterministic (Beardslee et al. 2005).

The risk increases substantially when both parents are ill (Bijl et al. 2002). Numerous studies have documented that the children of depressed parents are at two to four times higher risk for developing depression in adolescence. They are also at risk for interpersonal difficulties, school dropout, and a variety of other psychiatric difficulties (Beardslee et al. 1998).

Parent-child interaction patterns characteristic of parents with certain psychiatric disorders can also be a risk factor for children. Depressed mothers have been shown to have greater negative feelings toward their children and exhibit less warmth and greater use of psychological control (Cornish et al. 2006; Cummings et al. 2005).

An equally important conceptual framework that operates for risk and protective factors is the additive, interactive, and cumulative nature of such factors (Cicchetti and Cohen 1995; Sameroff et al. 1998).

It is not the diagnostic category of the parent but the chronicity, severity, and amount of impairment that is associated with effects on the child. **(pp. 625–626)**

Beardslee WR, Versage E, Gladstone TR: Children of affectively ill parents: a review of the past ten years. J Am Acad Child Adolesc Psychiatry 37:1134–1141, 1998

Beardslee WR, Boris N, Compton W, et al: The Prevention of Mental Disorders in General Psychiatric Practice: Implications for Assessment, Intervention and Research. A Report Submitted by the Task Force on Prevention to the Council on Research. Washington, DC, American Psychiatric Association, 2005

Bijl RV, Cuijpers P, Smit F: Psychiatric disorders in adult children of parents with a history of psychopathology. Soc Psychiatry Psychiatr Epidemiol 37:7–12, 2002

Cicchetti D, Cohen DJ (eds): Perspectives on developmental psychopathology, in Developmental Psychopathology, Vol 2: Risk, Disorder, and Adaptation. New York, Wiley, 1995

Cornish AM, McMahon CA, Ungerer J, et al: Maternal depression and the experience of parenting in the second postnatal year. Journal of Reproductive and Infant Psychology 24:121–132, 2006

Cummings EM, Keller PS, Davies PT: Towards a family process model of maternal and paternal depressive symptoms: exploring multiple relations with child and family functioning. J Child Psychol Psychiatry 46:479–489, 2005

Sameroff A, Bartko WT, Baldwin A, et al: Family and social influences on the development of child competence, in Families, Risk, and Competence. Edited by Feiring C, Lewis M, Mahwah, NJ, Lawrence Erlbaum, 1998, pp 161–185

42.4 According to a study by Beardslee and Podorefsky (1988), which of the following characteristics do children with good functioning exhibit?

   A. They are active in pursuing and accomplishing age-appropriate developmental tasks.
   B. They are committed to relationships.
   C. They understand they are not to blame for their parent's illness.
   D. All of the above.
   E. None of the above.

The correct response is option D.

In one study of children of parents with mood disorders, investigators examined a subset of resilient children from a larger group of children at risk (Beardslee and Podorefsky 1988). Using a combination of structured and semistructured interviews, 18 children (from 14 families) who exhibited good functioning were interviewed. Three domains robustly characterized these youngsters. First, they were active in pursuing and accomplishing age-appropriate developmental tasks (e.g., going to school, excelling academically, being committed to outside activities, dedicated to religious and community activities). Second, they were deeply committed to relationships and had strong friendships and good relationships within families and often with teachers and mentors. Third, they reported that understanding that their parents had an illness and that they were not to blame was crucial in their being able to move on with their own lives. **(pp. 626–627)**

> Beardslee WR, Podorefsky D: Resilient adolescents whose parents have serious affective and other psychiatric disorders: the importance of self-understanding and relationships. Am J Psychiatry 145:63–69, 1988

42.5 Which of the following programs is *not* ordinarily used as a prevention program for children of parents with substance abuse disorders?

    A. FRIENDS.
    B. Nurse-Family Partnership.
    C. Strengthening Families Program (SFP).
    D. Family Check-up Preventive Intervention (FCU).
    E. All of the above.

The correct response is A.

FRIENDS, a school-based cognitive-behavioral therapy program developed in Australia (www.friendsinfo.net), has shown promising effects in children at risk for anxiety disorders.

In general, family-centered care and psychoeducation are important components of prevention programs in the domain of substance abuse (e.g., Nurse-Family Partnership; Olds 2002).

The SFP is a 14-session family skills training program with multiple components that was originally developed for children of parents with alcohol or drug addiction (Kumpfer et al. 2003). There are three components to the intervention: parent skills training, child skill training, and family life-skills training.

The FCU (Dishion and Kavanagh 2003) targets early starter pathways to antisocial behavior and substance abuse through inclusion of families with environmental adversity (low socioeconomic status), maternal depression and/or substance abuse, and child conduct problems. **(pp. 629–630)**

> Dishion TJ, Kavanagh K: Intervening in Adolescent Problem Behavior: A Family Centered Approach. New York, Guilford, 2003
>
> Kumpfer KL, Alvarado R, Whiteside HO: Family based interventions for substance use and misuse prevention. Subst Use Misuse 38:1759–1787, 2003
>
> Olds DL: Prenatal and infancy home visiting by nurses: from randomized trials to community replication. Prev Sci 3:153–172, 2002

Chapter 43

Legal and Ethical Issues

Select the single best response for each question.

43.1 Which of the following statements regarding the concept of *parens patriae* is *true?*

A. It is related to child privacy.
B. It is related to state taking over guardianship.
C. It is related to involuntary hospitalization.
D. It is related to children being charged as adults.
E. It is related to mandatory warning process.

The correct response is option B.

If a child is orphaned or abandoned, the child might come under the authority of the state under the concept of parens patriae, derived from the notion that the crown or the state had guardianship over individuals unable to legally act for themselves. Our contemporary society's perception and treatment of minors continues to fluctuate between the legal doctrines of *parens patriae* and "the best interests of the child." Parens patriae traditionally has empowered state initiatives to protect persons who are unable to care for or protect themselves and also has allowed state agencies to interfere with parental prerogatives when there is evidence of neglect, inability to perform parental responsibilities, or evidence of abuse of minors. **(pp. 637–638)**

43.2 According to a consensus developed at a White House Conference on Children in 1970, which of the following rights is specific to a child's well-being?

A. The right to grow in a society with respect.
B. The right to grow up nurtured by affectionate parents.
C. The right to be a child during childhood.
D. The right to have social mechanisms to enforce the foregoing rights.
E. All of the above.

The correct response is option E.

A consensus regarding children's rights and needs was developed at the White House Conference on Children convened in 1970, asserting specific rights essential to a child's well-being (U.S. Government Printing Office 1971): 1) the right to grow in a society that respects the dignity of life and is free of poverty, discrimination, and other forms of degradation; 2) the right to be born and to be healthy and wanted through childhood; 3) The right to grow up nurtured by affectionate parents; 4) the right to be a child during childhood, to have meaningful choices in the process of maturation and development, and to have a meaningful voice in the community; 5) the right to be educated to the limits of one's capacity and through processes designed to elicit one's full potential; and 6) the right to have social mechanisms to enforce the foregoing rights. **(p. 638)**

> U.S. Government Printing Office: Report to the President: White House Conference on Children. Washington, DC, U.S. Government Printing Office, 1971

43.3   Informed consent in treatment and research and maintaining appropriate professional boundaries and confidences are related to which of the following concepts?

    A. Confidentiality.
    B. Autonomy.
    C. Beneficence.
    D. Justice.
    E. None of the above.

The correct response is option B.

Ethics can be defined as the study of moral principles and values that guide and determine the conduct of individuals in particular, usually professional circumstances and relationships. Ethical guidelines are evolving to highlight several principal issues: respect for the patient's autonomy, beneficence, and justice.

The ethical principle of *confidentiality* is considered the cornerstone for building trust and honest communication in the physician-patient relationship.

The concept of respect for the person's *autonomy* includes informed consent in treatment and research, including maintaining appropriate professional boundaries and confidences, as well as factual honesty and avoidance of misrepresentations.

The concept of *beneficence* expands the "do no harm" concept to include acting in the patient's best interests and minimizing risks and maximizing benefits in professional judgments and relationships.

The concept of *justice* has more recently come into ethical consideration in the biomedical arena, having to do with social justice in the allocation of resources and fair and equitable distribution of risks and benefits. **(pp. 639–640)**

43.4   According to American Academy of Child and Adolescent Psychiatry guidelines, important factors to consider in evaluating the need for involuntary hospitalization of young patients include all of the following *except*

    A. A qualified psychiatrist's evaluation.
    B. Diagnosis by DSM criteria.
    C. Severity of impairment in one area of daily functioning.
    D. Likelihood of benefit from the proposed treatment.
    E. Prior consideration of less restrictive treatment procedures.

The correct response is option C.

Parents, legal guardians, and state agencies may occasionally need to hospitalize a seriously disturbed child or adolescent, and this necessity may conflict with the child's or adolescent's desire for autonomy and self-determination. The American Academy of Child and Adolescent Psychiatry (1989) has published guidelines regarding this issue and listed the following factors to consider: 1) a qualified psychiatrist's evaluation; 2) diagnosis by DSM criteria; 3) severity of impairment in two or more areas of daily functioning; 4) likelihood of benefit from the proposed treatment; 5) prior consideration of less restrictive treatment procedures and the judgment that they are inappropriate or inadequate to meet the patient's needs; 6) encouragement of the child to voluntarily participate in the admission, treatment planning, and discharge process; and 7) parent's full information about and participation in the hospitalization and treatment planning decisions. **(p. 641)**

American Academy of Child and Adolescent Psychiatry: Policy Statement: Inpatient Hospital Treatment of Children and Adolescents. Washington, DC, American Academy of Child and Adolescent Psychiatry, 1989

43.5 All of the following elements must be presented by the plaintiff to the court during a professional negligence lawsuit against a child psychiatrist *except*

    A. Intentionality.
    B. Duty.
    C. Dereliction.
    D. Damage.
    E. Direct causation.

The correct response is option A.

Malpractice lawsuits are based on principles of tort law or civil wrongful behavior, in which the practitioner may be liable for the unintended consequences of alleged harm or injury to the patient or to a third party that could have or should have been prevented by the practitioner's action. The four elements of a claim of professional negligence include: 1) *duty:* a duty of care was owed to the patient by the physician; 2) *dereliction:* the duty of care was breached; 3) *damages:* the patient experienced actual damage due to the breach of duty; and 4) *direct causation:* the dereliction was the direct cause of the damages. The plaintiff must demonstrate to the court the existence of these elements according to the standard of care in the community at the time. In civil cases, the standard of proof is preponderance of evidence (i.e., more likely than not). **(pp. 641–642)**

Chapter 44

Telepsychiatry

Select the single best response for each question.

44.1 Which of the following terms is correctly described by the definition "use of interactive televideo communication (ITV) to deliver medical care that is usually delivered in person"?

    A. E-health.
    B. Telemedicine.
    C. Telepsychiatry.
    D. Bandwidth.
    E. Telecommunication connectivity.

The correct response is option B.

Telemedicine is the use of interactive televideo communication to deliver medical care that is usually delivered in person. Telepsychiatry is the application of telemedicine to psychiatry.

E-health describes health services provided from a clinician to a patient or the lay public through any electronic medium, in real time or store-and-forward modality, including the Internet, telephone, or facsimile.

Bandwith is the theoretical maximum rate that data can travel through a network in a fixed period of time. Bandwidth is often expressed in units of kilobits per second (kb/sec). The higher the bandwidth, the greater the amount of data that can be transmitted. Standard telephones that transmit audio signals are low-bandwidth devices, whereas cable television and telecommunications lines that transmit audio and video signals simultaneously are high-bandwidth devices. Most health care applications use bandwidths at or above 384 kb/sec, often referred to as "virtually live" or "80% television quality."

Telecommunication connectivity describes the technical methods or protocols used to establish an ITV connection. **(p. 650 [Table 44–1])**

44.2 Based on current data, child and adolescent telepsychiatry programs have been sited in all of the following settings *except*

    A. Inpatient psychiatric hospitals.
    B. Community medical and mental health centers.
    C. Urban daycare and rural schools.
    D. Corrections and residential settings.
    E. Private practice.

The correct response is option A.

Telepsychiatry has not been sited in inpatient psychiatric hospitals.

Child and adolescent telepsychiatry programs are now sited in diverse settings such as community medical centers (Alicata et al. 2008; Myers et al. 2004), community mental health centers (Cain and Spaulding 2006), urban day care (Cain and Spaulding 2006), rural schools (Adelsheim and Mattison 2008; Alicata et al. 2006; Harper 2006), corrections facilities (Myers et al. 2006), residential settings (Storck 2007), and private practice (Cassidy and Glueck 2008; George 2007; Glueck 2007). **(p. 652)**

Adelsheim S, Mattison R: Telepsychiatry with rural school-based health centers in New Mexico. Clinical perspectives presentation at the 55th Annual Meeting of the American Academy of Child and Adolescent Psychiatry, Chicago, IL, October 28–November 2, 2008

Alicata D, Saltman D, Ulrich D: Child and adolescent telepsychiatry in rural Hawaii. Presented at the 53rd Annual Meeting of the American Academy of Child and Adolescent Psychiatry, San Diego, CA, October 2006

Alicata D, Koyanagi C, Guerrero A, et al: Telepsychiatry in rural Hawaii: The Big Island Telepsychiatry Initiative. Clinical perspectives presentation at the 55th Annual Meeting of the American Academy of Child and Adolescent Psychiatry, Chicago, IL, October 28–November 2, 2008

Cain S, Spaulding R: Telepsychiatry: lessons from two models of care. Presented at the 53rd Annual Meeting of the American Academy of Child and Adolescent Psychiatry, San Diego, CA, October 2006

Cassidy L, Glueck D: Private practice telepsychiatry. Workshop presentation at the 55th Annual Meeting of the American Academy of Child and Adolescent Psychiatry, Chicago, IL, October 28–November 2, 2008

George R: A private practice model of telepsychiatry for residential treatment. Presented at the 54th Annual Meeting of the American Academy of Child and Adolescent Psychiatry, Boston, MA, October 2007

Glueck D: Telepsychiatry and the Adolescent Treatment Outcomes Module. Presented at the 54th Annual Meeting of the American Academy of Child and Adolescent Psychiatry, Boston, MA, October 2007

Harper RA: Telepsychiatry consultation to schools and mobile clinics in rural Texas. Presented at the 53rd Annual Meeting of the American Academy of Child and Adolescent Psychiatry, San Diego, CA, October 2006

Myers KM, Sulzbacher S, Melzer SM: Telepsychiatry with children and adolescents: are patients comparable to those evaluated in usual outpatient care? Telemed J E Health 10:278–285, 2004

Myers K, Valentine J, Morganthaler R, et al: Telepsychiatry with incarcerated youth. J Adolesc Health 38:643–648, 2006

Storck M: Bringing the community to the state hospital through teleconferencing. Presented at the 54th Annual Meeting of the American Academy of Child and Adolescent Psychiatry, Boston, MA, October 2007

44.3   A growing literature has examined telepsychiatry with children and adolescents. Based on up-to-date research data on this issue, which of the following statements is *false?*

    A. Telepsychiatry with children and adolescents has shown to be feasible, acceptable, and sustainable in consultation to primary care clinicians.

    B. Studies measuring satisfaction showed that providers, families, and youth are very satisfied with their care.

    C. Scientific evidence of its efficacy has been well supported.

    D. Cost effectiveness remains to be demonstrated.

    E. All of the above.

The correct response is option C.

Despite the successes of and the increasing demand for telepsychiatry services, there is little scientific evidence of its efficacy. A reasonable conclusion from the limited evidence is that telepsychiatry is a viable option when usual in-person psychiatric care is not available. Cost effectiveness also remains to be demonstrated.

Telepsychiatry with children and adolescents has been shown to be feasible, acceptable, and sustainable in consultation to primary care clinicians (Myers et al. 2007). Most studies have measured satisfaction (Elford et al. 2000, 2001; Kopel et al. 2001; Myers et al. 2004, 2006; Pesamaa et al. 2004) and have found that providers (Myers et al. 2007), families (Myers et al. 2008), and youth (Myers et al. 2006) are very satisfied with their care. **(p. 652)**

Elford R, White H, Bowering R, et al: A randomized, controlled trial of child psychiatric assessments conducted using videoconferencing. J Telemed Telecare 6:73–82, 2000

Elford R, White H, St John K, et al: A prospective satisfaction study and cost analysis of a pilot child telepsychiatry service in Newfoundland. J Telemed Telecare 7:73–81, 2001

Kopel H, Nunn K, Dossetor D: Evaluating satisfaction with a child and adolescent psychological telemedicine outreach service. J Telemed Telecare 7 (suppl):35–40, 2001

Myers KM, Sulzbacher S, Melzer SM: Telepsychiatry with children and adolescents: are patients comparable to those evaluated in usual outpatient care? Telemed J E Health 10:278–285, 2004

Myers K, Valentine J, Melzer SM, et al: Telepsychiatry with incarcerated youth. J Adolesc Health 38:643–648, 2006

Myers KM, Valentine JM, Melzer SM: Feasibility, acceptability, and sustainability of telepsychiatry with children and adolescents. Psychiatr Serv 58:1493–1496, 2007

Myers KM, Valentine JM, Melzer SM: Child and adolescent telepsychiatry: utilization and satisfaction. Telemed J E Health 14:131–137, 2008

Pesamaa L, Ebeling H, Kuusimaki ML, et al: Videoconferencing in child and adolescent telepsychiatry: a systematic review of the literature. J Telemed Telecare 10:187–192, 2004

44.4 All of the following statements regarding regulatory and ethical issues in telemedicine are correct *except*

    A. The Joint Commission for the Accreditation of Healthcare Organizations (JCAHO; now known as the Joint Commission) has regulations applicable to telemedicine at the national level.

    B. Most states require telepsychiatrists to be licensed only in the state in which they practice.

    C. Familiarity with laws regarding involuntary commitment and reporting child maltreatment across states is essential.

    D. Televideo transmission needs to be compliant with the Health Insurance Portability and Accountability Act (HIPAA).

    E. Until nationally accepted telepsychiatry care guidelines are available, telepsychiatrists should adhere to existing procedures for in-person care.

The correct response is option B.

Most states require telepsychiatrists to be licensed both in the state in which they practice and in the state where the patient receives care.

At the national level, Medicare and the Joint Commission have regulations applicable to telemedicine. More extensive regulations are determined by state laws. Laws regarding involuntary commitment and reporting child maltreatment may vary across jurisdictions. Other factors to consider include the patient's privacy and compliance of the televideo transmission with HIPAA. Until nationally accepted telepsychiatry care guidelines are available, telepsychiatrists should adhere to existing procedures for in-person care (American Academy of Child and Adolescent Psychiatry 2008). **(pp. 658, 661)**

American Academy of Child and Adolescent Psychiatry: Practice parameter for telepsychiatry with children and adolescents. J Am Acad Child Adolesc Psychiatry 47:1468–1483, 2008

C h a p t e r   4 5

Principles of Psychopharmacology

Select the single best response for each question.

45.1 Which of the following goals needs to be reached during a psychiatric assessment of youth before considering psychopharmacological treatment?

    A. Psychiatric symptoms that reflect possible underlying psychiatric disorders must be identified.

    B. Determine which elements of the disorder need to be addressed by psychopharmacological treatments.

    C. Decide which elements of the disorder may need a combination of psychosocial intervention with medications.

    D. Determine which modalities might be most suitable for the particular patient.

    E. All of the above.

The correct response is option E.

The first step in the psychiatric treatment of a child or adolescent is the completion of a thorough assessment. This initial assessment has several goals, one of which is for the clinician to identify psychiatric symptoms that may indicate one or more underlying psychiatric disorders. The clinician can then decide which elements of these disorders might be best addressed by psychopharmacological treatments, which might be best treated with psychosocial treatments and/or environmental interventions, and which elements might deserve a combination therapy approach. Another goal of the psychiatric assessment is to uncover relevant patient and family historical information that may determine which modalities of psychiatric treatment or which psychotropic medications might be most suitable for this patient. **(pp. 668–669)**

45.2 Which of the following medications is least likely to affect electrocardiogram (ECG) at therapeutic doses?

    A. Alpha-2-adrenergic agonists (clonidine or guanfacine).

    B. Thioridazine or pimozide.

    C. Escitalopram or citalopram.

    D. Clozapine or ziprasidone.

    E. Lithium or tricyclic antidepressants.

The correct response is option C.

Escitalopram and citalopram are the medications least likely to affect ECG.

In patients with a history or symptoms of cardiovascular illness or a family history of heart disease, clinicians may elect to obtain a baseline ECG to assess the presence of cardiac illness before initiating psychotropic medication. Certain medications may either prolong the QTc interval or substantively affect cardiovascular functioning at therapeutic doses. These psychotropic medications include (McNally et al. 2007) alpha-2-adrenergic agonists such as clonidine or guanfacine; first-generation antipsychotics (neuroleptics) such as thioridazine and pimozide; atypical (second-generation) antipsychotics such as clozapine and ziprasidone; tricyclic antidepressants; and lithium. **(p. 672)**

McNally P, McNichols F, Oslizlok P: The QT interval and psychotropic medications in children: recommendations for clinicians. Eur Child Adolesc Psychiatry 16:33–47, 2007

45.3 All of the following statements regarding the principles of diagnosing and treating youth with psychiatric disorders are correct *except*

    A. Primary psychiatric diagnosis and possible comorbid conditions need to be identified.

    B. Treatment planning should be based on a biopsychosocial formulation.

    C. Treating target symptoms is more important than treating the psychiatric disorders.

    D. In many treatment settings, an authoritative approach is advisable for clinicians.

    E. The efficacy and safety of a medication is only one of the factors to consider when selecting psychopharmacological agents.

The correct response is option C.

Clinical guidelines do not recommend psychiatric pharmacotherapy solely to address specific target psychiatric symptoms. Rather, clinicians generally treat psychiatric syndromes with medications and then measure treatment response by tracking specified target symptoms.

After the psychiatric assessment, the clinician is next faced with the task of identifying the primary psychiatric diagnosis (if one exists), as well as recognizing any comorbid disorders.

Factors other than a DSM-IV-TR (American Psychiatric Association 2000) diagnosis can affect a youth's emotions and behaviors and include comorbid medical conditions, level of development, psychological distress, family relationships, social relationships, environmental stressors, and educational functioning. A biopsychosocial formulation supplements the diagnosis by describing the predisposing, precipitating, perpetuating, and protective factors that have shaped the patient's clinical presentation.

In many treatment settings, it is advisable for clinicians to take an authoritative approach to the family. This approach may be necessary when the patient's parents are either having difficulty making treatment choices or are requesting treatment approaches that may result in harm to the patient or others.

Clinicians typically rely on several principles when selecting and dosing psychotropic medications for children and adolescents. These considerations include the differences in drug metabolism between children and adults, data on the efficacy and safety of psychotropic medication in children, regulatory issues associated with the off-label use of psychotropic medications, and ethical issues surrounding the psychopharmacological treatment of children and adolescents. **(pp. 672, 673, 674)**

American Psychiatric Association: Diagnostic and Statistical Manual of Mental Disorders, 4th Edition, Text Revision. Washington, DC, American Psychiatric Association, 2000

45.4 Which of the following statements regarding the differences in pharmacokinetics between children and adults is *false?*

    A. Youth have proportionally more liver tissue than adults when adjusted for body weight.

    B. Children may have higher glomerular filtration rates than adults when adjusted for body weight.

    C. Children may have higher weight-based dosing for hydrophilic drugs.

    D. Children may have higher weight-based dosing for lipophilic drugs.

    E. There is greater variability of oral drug absorption in youth compared to adults.

The correct response is option D.

Children have proportionally more extracellular and total-body water than adults, which may lead to lower plasma concentrations of hydrophilic drugs. As a result, some drugs (e.g., lithium) may require higher weight-based dosing in youth.

Youth have proportionally more liver tissue than adults, when adjusted for body weight. As a result, youth may have more rapid hepatic drug metabolism than adults, possibly resulting in more rapid elimination of drugs that use hepatic pathways (Kearns et al. 2003).

When adjusted for body weight, children may have higher glomerular filtration rates than adults, possibly resulting in more rapid excretion of drugs that use renal pathways (Chen et al. 2006).

Drugs may also be absorbed and distributed differently in children's bodies. As a result, some drugs may require further dosing adjustments when compared to dosing for adults.

Children have proportionally less fat tissue than adults, so higher plasma concentrations of some lipophilic drugs (e.g., paroxetine) may be expected in children. The functioning of the gastrointestinal tract does not fully mature until 10–12 years of age. This phenomenon may lead to greater variability of oral drug absorption in the young when compared with adults. **(pp. 674–675)**

Chen N, Aleksa K, Woodland C, et al: Ontogeny of drug elimination by the human kidney. Pediatr Nephrol 21:160–168, 2006

Kearns GL, Abdel-Rahman SM, Alander SW, et al: Developmental pharmacology: drug disposition, action, and therapy in infants and children. N Engl J Med 349:1157–1167, 2003

45.5   Which of the following elements should be considered during the informed consent and assent processes?

    A. The process needs to be completed prior to the initiation of the psychopharmacological treatment.

    B. Parents or legal guardians should be competent and able to make decisions freely without coercion.

    C. Parents or legal guardians should have an understanding of the nature of the patient's illness and the potential risks, benefits, and side effects of the proposed treatment.

    D. The expected prognosis with and without the proposed treatment should be discussed.

    E. All of the above.

The correct response is option E.

As treatment options are presented to the patient and parents, the clinician should provide education to help the family understand the purpose of the therapeutic interventions and the potential risks and benefits associated with each treatment option. This initiates both an informed consent process with the parents and an assent process with the patient that generally occur before beginning psychopharmacological treatment. Informed consent to initiate or continue a psychotropic medication generally requires the patient's parents to be competent, to demonstrate adequate knowledge about the proposed medication, and to make the treatment decision freely, without coercion. "Adequate knowledge" about a psychotropic medication usually includes an understanding of the nature of the patient's psychiatric disorder; the potential risks, benefits, and side effects of the proposed psychopharmacological treatment; the possible alternatives to the proposed treatment; and the patient's expected prognosis both with and without the proposed treatment. **(p. 676)**

Chapter 46

Medications Used for Attention-Deficit/Hyperactivity Disorder

Select the single best response for each question.

46.1 Emerging neuropsychological and neuroimaging literature suggests that the underlying neural substrate of attention-deficit/hyperactivity disorder (ADHD) is a dysfunction of which of the following?

  A. The parietal-temporal region.
  B. The limbic lobe.
  C. The frontostriatal region.
  D. The parietal lobe.
  E. The hippocampus.

The correct response is option C.

ADHD is a heterogeneous disorder of unknown etiology. An emerging neuropsychological and neuroimaging literature suggests that abnormalities in frontal networks or frontostriatal dysfunction is the disorder's underlying neural substrate, and catecholamine dysregulation is its underlying pathophysiology. The pattern of neuropsychological deficits found in children with ADHD implicates executive functions and working memory. This pattern is similar to what has been found among adults with frontal lobe damage, which suggests that the frontal cortex or regions projecting to the frontal cortex are dysfunctional in at least some subjects with ADHD. **(p. 681)**

46.2 The most commonly abused substance in adolescents and adults with attention-deficit/hyperactivity disorder (ADHD) is

  A. Alcohol.
  B. Marijuana.
  C. Stimulants.
  D. Benzodiazepines.
  E. Barbiturates.

The correct response is option B.

The most commonly abused substance in adolescents and adults with ADHD is marijuana (Biederman et al. 1995).
  The U.S. Food and Drug Administration (FDA) recently reviewed the prescribing information on stimulants in an effort to clarify risks and benefits. After this careful review, the only black box warning for stimulants concerns their abuse potential. Although misuse for treating fatigue can be accomplished by oral administration, abuse for euphoria typically requires insufflation, and thus there is greater risk in immediate-release formulations that can be crushed. Despite the concern that ADHD may increase the risk of drug abuse in adolescents and young adults (or their associates), to date there is no clear evidence that stimulant-treated youth with ADHD abuse prescribed medication when they are appropriately diagnosed and carefully monitored. **(p. 683)**

Biederman J, Wilens T, Mick E, et al: Psychoactive substance use disorder in adults with attention deficit hyperactivity disorder: effects of ADHD and psychiatric comorbidity. Am J Psychiatry 152:1652–1658, 1995

46.3   Which of the following medications (brand names) is a long-acting preparation of amphetamine?

    A. Concerta.
    B. Metadate-CD.
    C. Focalin XR.
    D. Adderall XR.
    E. Daytrana.

The correct response is option D.

Adderall XR is a combination of mixed salts of levo- and dextroamphetamines. It has a half-life of 10–12 hours and can be administered once or twice a day.

A new generation of highly sophisticated, well-developed, safe, and effective long-acting preparations of stimulant drugs has reached the market and revolutionized the treatment of ADHD. These compounds employ novel delivery systems to overcome acute tolerance termed *tachyphylaxis* and allow a reduced number of doses per day.

Concerta uses an osmotic pump mechanism to create an ascending level of methylphenidate in the blood. This provides effective extended treatment that approximates three-times-per-day dosing of methylphenidate immediate release (MPH-IR).

Metadate-CD is a capsule with a mixture of immediate- and delayed-release beads containing methylphenidate, 30% of which are immediate release and 70% of which are delayed. It is designed to provide effective treatment for 6–8 hours.

A new extended-release dosage form of Focalin (Focalin XR) has been developed to provide effective methylphenidate treatment for 10–12 hours. Focalin XR uses the same bimodal release system as Ritalin LA, producing pharmacokinetic characteristics that in single-dose administration resemble those of two doses of Focalin tablets administered 4–5 hours apart.

A transdermal delivery system for methylphenidate has been developed (methylphenidate transdermal system—MTS). Methylphenidate is contained within a multipolymeric adhesive layer attached to a transparent backing. Patches are applied once daily and deliver a consistent amount of methylphenidate during the time the patch is worn. **(pp. 685–688; see also Table 46–2)**

46.4   Which of the following medications has *not* been shown to be effective in the treatment of attention-deficit/hyperactivity disorder (ADHD)?

    A. Desipramine.
    B. Nortriptyline.
    C. Bupropion.
    D. Modafinil.
    E. Venlafaxine.

The correct response is option E.

The usefulness of the mixed serotonergic/noradrenergic atypical antidepressant venlafaxine in the treatment of ADHD is uncertain. Although a 77% response rate was reported in completers in four open studies of ADHD adults ($N = 61$ combined), 21% dropped out because of side effects (Adler et al. 1995; Findling et al. 1996; Hornig-Rohan and Amsterdam 1995; Reimherr et al. 1995). Additionally, a single open study of venlafaxine in 16 ADHD children reported a 50% response rate in completers with a 25% rate of dropout because of side effects, most prominently increased hyperactivity.

In the largest controlled study of tricyclic antidepressants in children, Biederman et al. (1989) reported favorable results with desipramine in 62 clinically referred ADHD children, most of whom had previously failed to respond to psychostimulant treatment. The study was a randomized, placebo-controlled, parallel-design, 6-week clinical trial. Clinically and statistically significant differences in behavioral improvement were found for desipramine over placebo, at an average daily dosage of 5 mg/kg.

In a prospective placebo-controlled discontinuation trial, nortriptyline in dosages of up to 2 mg/kg daily in 35 school-age youth with ADHD (Prince et al. 2000) was deemed efficacious. ADHD youth receiving nortriptyline also were found to have more modest but statistically significant reductions in oppositionality and anxiety. Nortriptyline was well tolerated, with some weight gain. Weight gain is frequently considered to be a desirable side effect in this population.

Bupropion hydrochloride is a novel-structured antidepressant of the aminoketone class related to the phenylisopropylamines but pharmacologically distinct from known antidepressants. Although its specific site or mechanism of action remains unknown, bupropion seems to have an indirect mixed agonist effect on dopamine and norepinephrine neurotransmission. Bupropion has been shown to be effective for ADHD in children in a controlled multisite study ($N=72$) (Casat et al. 1987, 1989; Conners et al. 1996) and in a comparison with methylphenidate ($N=15$) (Barrickman et al. 1995). A double-blind, controlled clinical trial of bupropion in adults with ADHD documented superiority over a placebo (Wilens et al. 1999, 2005), with an effect size highly consistent with the pediatric trials.

Modafinil is an antinarcoleptic agent that is structurally and pharmacologically different from other agents approved to treat ADHD. Although the mechanism of action is unknown, it may improve symptoms of ADHD via the same mechanism by which it improves wakefulness. While initial studies demonstrated significant improvement in ADHD symptoms, recent studies reported increased efficacy with higher dosages (340–425 mg/day) in children and adolescents (Swanson et al. 2006). A concentrated form of modafinil was developed to produce a small tablet that would ease administration of these doses in the pediatric population. A 9-week randomized, double-blind, placebo-controlled, flexible-dosage trial evaluated the efficacy and tolerability of this new formulation of modafinil in once-daily dosing (Biederman et al. 2005). Medication was titrated to an optimal dose based on efficacy and tolerability (range: 170–425 mg once daily). Patients ($N=246$) were treated with modafinil ($n=164$) or placebo ($n=82$). Significant improvements were observed with modafinil treatment on the ADHD-RS-IV School Version at week 1, with an effect size of 0.69 by the final visit. (pp. 690–694)

Adler L, Resnick S, Kunz M, et al: Open-Label Trial of Venlafaxine in Attention Deficit Disorder. Orlando, FL, New Clinical Drug Evaluation Unit Program, 1995

Barrickman L, Perry P, Allen AJ, et al: Bupropion versus methylphenidate in the treatment of attention-deficit hyperactivity disorder. J Am Acad Child Adolesc Psychiatry 34:649–657, 1995

Biederman J, Baldessarini RJ, Wright V, et al: A double-blind placebo controlled study of desipramine in the treatment of ADD, I: efficacy. J Am Acad Child Adolesc Psychiatry 28:777–784, 1989

Biederman J, Swanson J, Wigal SB, et al: Efficacy and safety of modafinil film-coated tablets in children and adolescents with attention-deficit/hyperactivity disorder: results of a randomized, double-blind, placebo-controlled, flexible-dose study. Pediatrics 116:e777–e784, 2005

Casat CD, Pleasants DZ, Van Wyck Fleet J: A double-blind trial of bupropion in children with attention deficit disorder. Psychopharmacol Bull 23:120–122, 1987

Casat CD, Pleasants DZ, Schroeder DH, et al: Bupropion in children with attention deficit disorder. Psychopharmacol Bull 25:198–201, 1989

Conners CK, Casat CD, Gualtieri CT, et al: Bupropion hydrochloride in attention deficit disorder with hyperactivity. J Am Acad Child Adolesc Psychiatry 35:1314–1321, 1996

Findling R, Schwartz M, Flannery DJ, et al: Venlafaxine in adults with ADHD: An open trial. J Clin Psychiatry 57:184–189, 1996

Hornig-Rohan M, Amsterdam J: Venlafaxine vs. Stimulant Therapy in Patients With Dual Diagnoses of ADHD and Depression. Orlando, FL, New Clinical Drug Evaluation Unit Program, 1995

Prince JB, Wilens TE, Biederman J: A controlled study of nortriptyline in children and adolescents with attention deficit hyperactivity disorder. J Child Adolesc Psychopharmacol 10:193–204, 2000

Reimherr F, Hedges D, Strong R, et al: An Open Trial of Venlafaxine in Adult Patients With Attention Deficit Hyperactivity Disorder. Orlando, FL, New Clinical Drug Evaluation Unit Program, 1995

Swanson JM, Greenhill LL, Lopez FA, et al: Modafinil film-coated tablets in children and adolescents with attention-deficit/hyperactivity disorder: results of a randomized, double-blind, placebo-controlled, fixed-dose study followed by abrupt discontinuation. J Clin Psychiatry 67:137–147, 2006

Wilens T, Spencer T, Biederman J, et al: A Controlled Trial of Bupropion SR for Attention Deficit Hyperactivity Disorder in Adults. Boca Raton, FL, New Clinical Drug Evaluation Unit Program, 1999

Wilens T, Haight BR, Horrigan JP, et al: Bupropion XL in adults with ADHD: a randomized, placebo-controlled study. Biol Psychiatry 57:793–801, 2005

Chapter 47

Antidepressants

Select the single best response for each question.

47.1 All of the following statements regarding antidepressant use in youth are correct *except*

A. Half-lives of antidepressants are generally longer in children because of their lower weight.
B. Randomized controlled trials (RCTs) are the gold standard for assessing both efficacy and safety of drugs.
C. It is wrong to assume that antidepressants adverse effects are the same in children and in adults.
D. The increased rates of suicidality in clinical trials using antidepressants occur not only in children but also in young adults.
E. The difference in suicidality between active treatment and placebo is approximately 4% vs. 2%.

The correct response is option A.

Because antidepressants are metabolized primarily in the liver and children have a proportionately large liver mass, half-lives of antidepressants are generally shorter in children.

RCTs are the gold standard for assessing not only efficacy but also safety. Without a placebo control it is very difficult to identify whether adverse events are related to the medication, especially if they occur relatively frequently (e.g., headaches).

To assume that antidepressant adverse events are the same in children and adolescents as adults would be erroneous. It appears, for example, that increased rates of suicidality reported in children and adolescents treated with antidepressants relative to placebo (Hammad et al. 2006) extend only to age 25 (Friedman and Leon 2007).

The controversy around increases in suicidality in children and adolescents treated with antidepressants also highlighted problems in assessing adverse effects in clinical trials. This resulted in the U.S. Food and Drug Administration (FDA) requesting an independent reanalysis of the adverse event data. Even with the reanalysis and the findings that suicidality (not suicide) occurred in 4% of children on antidepressants compared with 2% on placebo based on spontaneous report, the prospectively collected rating scales from those studies did not demonstrate any difference in suicidality between active treatment and placebo (Bridge et al. 2007; Hammad et al. 2006). **(pp. 702–703)**

> Bridge JA, Iyengar S, Salary CB, et al: Clinical response and risk for reported suicidal ideation and suicide attempts in pediatric antidepressant treatment: a meta-analysis of randomized controlled trials. JAMA 297:1683–1696, 2007
> Friedman RA, Leon AC: Expanding the black box: depression, antidepressants, and the risk of suicide. N Engl J Med 356:2343–2346, 2007
> Hammad TA, Laughren T, Racoosin J: Suicidality in pediatric patients treated with antidepressant drugs. Arch Gen Psychiatry 63:332–339, 2006

47.2 Which of the following antidepressants has not received any U.S. Food and Drug Administration (FDA)–approved pediatric indications?

A. Citalopram (Celexa).
B. Fluoxetine (Prozac).
C. Fluvoxamine (Luvox).

D. Sertraline (Zoloft).

E. Imipramine.

The correct response is option A.

Citalopram and escitalopram are not FDA approved for use with children.

Fluoxetine is approved for depression in children 8 years and older and for obsessive-compulsive disorder (OCD) in children 7 years and older.

Fluvoxamine is approved for OCD in children 8 years and older.

Zoloft is approved for OCD in children 6 years and older.

The FDA has approved imipramine for nocturnal enuresis for children age 6 years and older. **(p. 705 [Table 47–2])**

47.3   Which of the following statements regarding fluoxetine is *false?*

A. To date, there have been only two large randomized controlled trials (RCTs) in pediatric major depressive disorder (MDD) demonstrating superiority of fluoxetine over placebo.

B. In contrast to other selective serotonin reuptake inhibitors (SSRIs), fluoxetine seems to be equally effective in children younger than 12 years.

C. There are three positive RCTs in children and adolescents with obsessive-compulsive disorder (OCD).

D. Fluoxetine is the only antidepressant to have more than one positive RCT for MDD, OCD, and anxiety disorders.

E. Fluoxetine is the only antidepressant FDA-approved for treatment of pediatric MDD.

The correct response is option A.

To date, three large RCTs in pediatric MDD have been conducted with fluoxetine, with all three demonstrating superiority over placebo (Emslie et al. 1997, 2002; March et al. 2004).

Unlike some of the other SSRIs, fluoxetine appears to be equally effective in the younger age group (<12 years).

Fluoxetine has also been studied in three RCTs of children and adolescents with OCD, totaling 160 subjects (Geller et al. 2001; Liebowitz et al. 2002; Riddle et al. 1992).

Fluoxetine is the only antidepressant to have more than one positive RCT for MDD, OCD, and anxiety disorders. It is the only antidepressant FDA-approved for treatment of pediatric depression, and is one of three antidepressants indicated for treatment of pediatric OCD. **(p. 709)**

Emslie GJ, Rush AJ, Weinberg WA, et al: A double-blind, randomized, placebo-controlled trial of fluoxetine in children and adolescents with depression. Arch Gen Psychiatry 54:1031–1037, 1997

Emslie GJ, Heiligenstein JH, Wagner KD, et al: Fluoxetine for acute treatment of depression in children and adolescents: a placebo-controlled, randomized clinical trial. J Am Acad Child Adolesc Psychiatry 41:1205–1215, 2002

Geller DA, Hoog SL, Heiligenstein JH, et al: Fluoxetine treatment for obsessive-compulsive disorder in children and adolescents: a placebo-controlled clinical trial. J Am Acad Child Adolesc Psychiatry 40:773–779, 2001

Liebowitz MR, Turner SM, Piacentini J, et al: Fluoxetine in children and adolescents with OCD: a placebo-controlled trial. J Am Acad Child Adolesc Psychiatry 41:1431–1438, 2002

March J, Silva S, Petrycki S, et al: Fluoxetine, cognitive-behavioral therapy, and their combination for adolescents with depression: Treatment for Adolescents With Depression Study (TADS) randomized controlled trial. JAMA 292:807–820, 2004

Riddle MA, Scahill L, King RA, et al: Double-blind, crossover trial of fluoxetine and placebo in children and adolescents with obsessive-compulsive disorder. J Am Acad Child Adolesc Psychiatry 31:1062–1069, 1992

47.4 Which of the following atypical antidepressants is a norepinephrine and dopamine reuptake inhibitor?

    A. Duloxetine.
    B. Bupropion.
    C. Trazodone.
    D. Mirtazapine.
    E. Venlafaxine.

The correct response is option B.

Bupropion is a structurally novel antidepressant that resembles diethylpropion and is related to phenylethylamine. Bupropion is a norepinephrine and dopamine reuptake inhibitor. Its effects on serotonin are negligible. It does not have cholinergic activity and is not sympathomimetic (DeVane 1998). **(p. 714)**

DeVane CL: Differential pharmacology of newer antidepressants. J Clin Psychiatry 59 (suppl):85–93, 1998

47.5 Which of the following antidepressants is currently a third-line treatment option for youth with treatment-resistant major depressive disorder (MDD) because of the increased risk of emergent suicidal thinking?

    A. Bupropion.
    B. Duloxetine.
    C. Mirtazapine.
    D. Venlafaxine.
    E. Trazodone.

The correct response is option D.

Three double-blind, controlled trials of venlafaxine have been conducted in children and adolescents with MDD, none of which demonstrated efficacy of venlafaxine over placebo (Emslie et al. 2007; Mandoki et al. 1997). As a result of limited acute efficacy support and the increased risk of emergent suicidal thinking, venlafaxine is currently a third-line treatment option for youth with treatment-resistant MDD. **(p. 718)**

Emslie GJ, Findling RL, Yeung PP, et al: Venlafaxine ER for the treatment of pediatric subjects with depression: results of two placebo-controlled trials. J Am Acad Child Adolesc Psychiatry 46:479–488, 2007

Mandoki MW, Tapia MR, Tapia MA, et al: Venlafaxine in the treatment of children and adolescents with major depression. Psychopharmacol Bull 33:149–154, 1997

C h a p t e r   4 8

Mood Stabilizers

Select the single best response for each question.

48.1   You decide to start a 16-year-old girl on lithium for treatment of hypomania associated with her bipolar II disorder. Which of the following tests does *not* need to be ordered?

    A. Serum electrolytes.
    B. Lipid panel.
    C. Thyroid function tests.
    D. Complete blood count with differential.
    E. Electrocardiogram (ECG).

The correct response is option B.

A lipid panel is not required.

Baseline studies prior to initiating treatment with lithium should include a general medical history and physical examination; serum electrolytes; creatinine, serum urea nitrogen, and serum calcium levels; thyroid function tests; ECG; complete blood count with differential; and a pregnancy test for sexually active females (Danielyan and Kowatch 2005). Renal function should be tested every 2–3 months during the first 6 months of treatment, and thyroid function should be tested during the first 6 months of treatment (McClellan et al. 2007). Thereafter, renal and thyroid functions should be checked every 6 months or when clinically indicated. Chronic treatment with lithium can cause hyperparathyroidism; therefore, serum calcium levels should be checked once a year (Bendz et al. 1996a, 1996b). **(p. 727)**

> Bendz H, Sjodin I, Aurell M: Renal function on and off lithium in patients treated with lithium for 15 years or more: a controlled, prospective lithium-withdrawal study. Nephrol Dial Transplant 11:457–460, 1996a
> Bendz H, Sjodin I, Toss G, et al: Hyperparathyroidism and long-term lithium therapy: a cross-sectional study and the effect of lithium withdrawal. J Intern Med 240:357–365, 1996b
> Danielyan A, Kowatch RA: Management options for bipolar disorder in children and adolescents. Paediatr Drugs 7:277–294, 2005
> McClellan J, Kowatch R, Findling RL: Practice parameter for the assessment and treatment of children and adolescents with bipolar disorder. J Am Acad Child Adolesc Psychiatry 46:107–125, 2007

48.2   With the adolescent girl in the last question, you change the formulation of lithium from lithium carbonate to a slower-release preparation. For which of the following common side effects would this change have a beneficial effect?

    A. Acne.
    B. Weight gain.
    C. Hypothyroidism.
    D. Polyuria.
    E. Nausea and diarrhea.

The correct response is option E.

Common side effects of lithium in children and adolescents include nausea, diarrhea, abdominal distress, sedation, tremor, polyuria, weight gain, enuresis, and acne. A slow-release preparation is an effective treatment of tremor, sedation, headache, nausea, and diarrhea. It would not have an effect on any of the other side effects listed above. **(p. 727; see also Table 48–1)**

48.3   Which of the following baseline studies should be ordered in children and adolescents for whom valproate is to be initiated?

      A. Complete blood count with differential.
      B. Serum electrolytes.
      C. Thyroid function tests.
      D. ECG.
      E. Urinalysis.

The correct response is option A.

Baseline studies prior to initiating treatment with valproate in children and adolescents should include: general medical history and physical examination with height and weight, liver function tests, complete blood count with differential and platelets, and a pregnancy test for sexually active females. A complete blood count with differential, platelet count, and liver functions should be checked every 6 months or when clinically indicated as divalproex can cause liver dysfunction and lower platelet counts. **(p. 730)**

48.4   You start a 17-year-old girl on valproate. You order all the necessary baseline tests, which are within normal limits. Three months later, she develops irregular menstruation, weight gain, hirsutism, and acne. Which clinical condition should you be concerned about?

      A. Pregnancy.
      B. Hyperammonemia.
      C. Polycystic ovarian syndrome (PCOS).
      D. Pancreatitis.
      E. Liver failure.

The correct response is option C.

There are increasing concerns about the possible association between valproate and PCOS. PCOS is an endocrine disorder characterized by ovulatory dysfunction and hyperandrogenism, affecting between 3% and 5% of women who are not taking psychotropic medications (Rasgon 2004). Common symptoms of PCOS include irregular or absent menstruation, lack of ovulation, weight gain, hirsutism, and/or acne. The initial reports of the association between PCOS and divalproex exposure were in women with epilepsy. The association was particularly strong if their exposure was during adolescence (Isojarvi et al. 1993). In a report on adults with bipolar disorder, there was a sevenfold increased risk of new-onset amenorrhea/oligomenorrhea with hyperandrogenism in women who were treated with valproate (Joffe et al. 2006). All females who are treated with valproate should have a baseline assessment of menstrual cycle patterns and continued monitoring for menstrual irregularities, weight gain, hirsutism, and/or acne that may develop during valproate treatment. If symptoms of PCOS develop, referral to an endocrinologist should be considered.

    Valproate-induced hyperammonemia has been observed in children and adolescents treated with valproate for psychiatric disorders (Carr and Shrewsbury 2007; Raskind and El-Chaar 2000). It can present as lethargy, disorientation, and reversible cognitive deficits, which may progress to marked sedation, coma, and even death. It is a transient and asymptomatic phenomenon but can become chronic if undetected. **(p. 730)**

Carr RB, Shrewsbury K: Hyperammonemia due to valproic acid in the psychiatric setting. Am J Psychiatry 164:1020–1027, 2007

Isojarvi JI, Laatikainen TJ, Pakarinen AJ, et al: Polycystic ovaries and hyperandrogenism in women taking valproate for epilepsy. N Engl J Med 329:1383–1388, 1993

Joffe H, Cohen LS, Suppes T, et al: Valproate is associated with new-onset oligoamenorrhea with hyperandrogenism in women with bipolar disorder. Biol Psychiatry 59:1078–1086, 2006

Rasgon N: The relationship between polycystic ovary syndrome and antiepileptic drugs: a review of the evidence. J Clin Psychopharmacol 24:322–334, 2004

Raskind JY, El-Chaar GM: The role of carnitine supplementation during valproic acid therapy. Ann Pharmacother 34:630–638, 2000

48.5   You begin carbamazepine in a 15-year-old boy who is also on atypical antipsychotic medication. Which of the following potential drug-drug interactions should you be concerned about?

   A. A decrease in carbamazepine serum levels.
   B. An increase in carbamazepine serum levels.
   C. A decrease in serum levels of the atypical antipsychotic.
   D. An increase in serum levels of the atypical antipsychotic.
   E. None.

The correct response is option C.

Carbamazepine decreases the serum levels of many of the atypical antipsychotics (Besag and Berry 2006), leading to symptomatic relapses in some patients.

Because of its stimulation of the hepatic cytochrome P450 (CYP) isoenzyme system, carbamazepine has many clinically significant drug interactions. Carbamazepine decreases lithium clearance and increases the risk of lithium toxicity. Medications that will increase carbamazepine levels include erythromycin, cimetidine, fluoxetine, verapamil, and valproate. Carbamazepine may increase the levels of the following medications: oral contraceptives, phenobarbital, primidone, phenytoin, tricyclics, and lamotrigine (Ciraulo et al. 1995). **(p. 732)**

Besag FM, Berry D: Interactions between antiepileptic and antipsychotic drugs. Drug Saf 29:95–118, 2006

Ciraulo DA, Shader RJ, Greenblatt DJ, et al (eds): Drug Interactions in Psychiatry. Baltimore, MD, Williams & Wilkins, 1995

48.6   The U.S. Food and Drug Administration (FDA) has issued the following black box warning for lamotrigine: "Lamictal is not indicated for use in patients below the age of 16." Which of the following serious medical conditions was the FDA concerned about in this patient population?

   A. Leukopenia.
   B. Lupus.
   C. Agranulocytosis.
   D. Serious rash.
   E. Hepatic failure.

The correct response is option D.

Benign rashes develop in 12% of adult patients, typically within the first 8 weeks of lamotrigine therapy (Calabrese et al. 2002). The risk of developing a serious rash is approximately three times greater in children and adolescents younger than 16 years old compared with adults. The FDA has issued a black box warning that states, "Lamictal is not indicated for use in patients below the age of 16 years." The frequency of serious rash associated with lamotrigine (defined as rashes requiring hospitalization and discontinuation of treatment), including Stevens-Johnson syndrome, is approximately 1/100 (1%) in children younger than 16 years and 3/1,000 (0.3%) in adults (GlaxoSmithKline 2001).

Cases of lupus, leukopenia, agranulocytosis, hepatic failure, and multiorgan failure associated with lamotrigine treatment have been reported (reviewed in Sabers and Gram 2000). However, lamotrigine has been well tolerated as long-term treatment in pediatric patients with epilepsy. **(p. 734)**

Calabrese JR, Sullivan JR, Bowden CL, et al: Rash in multicenter trials of lamotrigine in mood disorders: clinical relevance and management. J Clin Psychiatry 63:1012–1019, 2002

GlaxoSmithKline: Lamictal (lamotrigine) product information, in Physicians Desk Reference, 56th Edition. Research Triangle Park, NC, Thomson Healthcare, 2001

Sabers A, Gram L: Newer anticonvulsants: comparative review of drug interactions and adverse effects. Drugs 60:23–33, 2000

Chapter 49

Antipsychotic Medications

Select the single best response for each question.

49.1 Cytochrome P450 (CYP) enzymes metabolize antipsychotics. The CYP2C19 and 2C9 enzymes are relevant for which of the following antipsychotic medications?

   A. Aripiprazole.
   B. Clozapine.
   C. Molindone.
   D. Perphenazine.
   E. Risperidone.

The correct response is option B.

Knowledge about specific CYP enzymes that metabolize antipsychotics is important in predicting and managing potential drug-drug interactions. Medications that can induce CYP enzyme production may lower antipsychotic serum levels. CYP2C19 and 2C9 are relevant only for clozapine clearance.

   Aripiprazole, molindone, perphenazine, and risperidone are predominantly cleared by CYP2D6. **(pp. 743–746)**

49.2 Which of the following antipsychotic medications has the shortest half-life when administered orally?

   A. Aripiprazole.
   B. Olanzapine.
   C. Quetiapine.
   D. Risperidone.
   E. Ziprasidone.

The correct response is option D.

Knowledge about the half-life of antipsychotics can help predict how quickly steady state is achieved and how fast the body eliminates the drug. In general, it takes about five times the half-life of a drug for both steady state and elimination. The half-life of antipsychotics differs considerably. Risperidone has the shortest half-life (3 hours) of all the antipsychotics listed above. **(p. 746; see also Table 49–1)**

49.3 The degree of receptor occupancy is one of the determinants of an antipsychotic's therapeutic and adverse effects. With a full antagonist, what percentage of dopamine receptor occupancy is needed for antipsychotic efficacy?

   A. 40%–50%.
   B. 50%–60%.
   C. 60%–70%.
   D. 70%–80%.
   E. 80%–90%.

The correct response is option C.

The dosage, degree of receptor occupancy, and intrinsic activity at the receptor to which the antipsychotic binds are all important determinants of therapeutic and adverse effects. With a full antagonist, approximately 60%–70% dopamine receptor occupancy is needed for antipsychotic efficacy.

With a partial agonist (e.g., aripiprazole), receptor occupancy is not equivalent to blockade, and a higher degree of occupancy (at least 80%–85%) is required to achieve the same level of blockade (Burris et al. 2002). **(p. 747)**

Burris KD, Molski TF, Xu C, et al: Aripiprazole, a novel antipsychotic, is a high-affinity partial agonist at human dopamine D2 receptors. J Pharmacol Exp Ther 302:381–389, 2002

49.4 All of the following statements regarding neuromotor adverse effects of antipsychotic medications in children and adolescents are accurate *except*

A. Youth are more sensitive than adults to extrapyramidal side effects (EPS).
B. In studies of youth with psychotic disorders, risperidone and olanzapine have been associated with substantial EPS.
C. Withdrawal dyskinesias experienced by youth are usually irreversible.
D. Meta-analytic studies have shown relatively low rates of tardive dyskinesia (TD) in youth.
E. Even though neuroleptic malignant syndrome (NMS) appears to be rare in youth, vigilance is still needed.

The correct response is option C.

During first-generation antipsychotic (FGA) treatment, youth are at risk of developing withdrawal dyskinesias, yet unlike in adults, the dyskinesias are frequently reversible (Campbell et al. 1997).

In general, children and adolescents are more sensitive than adults to EPS associated with FGAs and second-generation antipsychotics (SGAs) (Correll et al. 2006). A randomized controlled trial of 40 youth with psychotic disorders comparing haloperidol (mean dosage: 5 mg/day), risperidone (mean dosage: 4 mg/day), and olanzapine (mean dosage: 12 mg/day) found substantial EPS not only with haloperidol (67%) but also with olanzapine (56%) and risperidone (53%), although haloperidol-treated patients reported more severe EPS (Sikich et al. 2004). Clozapine and quetiapine appear to be associated with relatively low rates of EPS in pediatric patients (as in adults). For aripiprazole and ziprasidone, rates of EPS appear to increase with increasing dose.

A meta-analysis of 10 studies lasting at least 11 months reported on TD rates in 783 patients ages 4–18 years (weighted mean: 10 years). Across these studies, only three cases of TD were reported, resulting in an annualized incidence rate of 0.4% (Correll and Kane 2007). Although this pediatric rate is approximately half the rate found in a meta-analysis including 1,964 nonelderly adults (Correll et al. 2004), firm conclusions are precluded by the fact that none of the pediatric studies was designed specifically to detect TD, antipsychotic doses were low, and lifetime exposure was relatively short.

NMS is a rare but potentially fatal complication of antipsychotic treatment. In children and adolescents, several cases of NMS have been reported even with SGAs. Thus, clinicians should be vigilant and rule out NMS in antipsychotic-treated youth presenting with fever, tachycardia, and marked motor rigidity, by measuring white cell count and creatine kinase levels, which would both be elevated—with creatine kinase levels typically found to be 1,000 or higher in cases of true NMS. **(pp. 753–755)**

Campbell M, Armenteros JL, Malone RP, et al: Neuroleptic-related dyskinesias in autistic children: a prospective, longitudinal study. J Am Acad Child Adolesc Psychiatry 36:835–843, 1997
Correll CU, Kane JM: One-year tardive dyskinesia rates in children and adolescents treated with second-generation antipsychotics: a systematic review. J Child Adolesc Psychopharmacol 17:647–655, 2007
Correll CU, Leucht S, Kane JM: Lower risk for tardive dyskinesia associated with second-generation antipsychotics: a systematic review of 1-year studies. Am J Psychiatry 161:414–425, 2004
Correll CU, Penzner JB, Parikh UH, et al: Recognizing and monitoring adverse events of second-generation antipsychotics in children and adolescents. Child Adolesc Psychiatr Clin N Am 15:177–206, 2006
Sikich L, Hamer RM, Bashford RA, et al: A pilot study of risperidone, olanzapine, and haloperidol in psychotic youth: a double-blind, randomized, 8-week trial. Neuropsychopharmacology 29:133–145, 2004

49.5   Which of the following antipsychotics is *least* likely to cause prolactin-related side effects, such as hyperpro-
lactinemia?

    A. Risperidone.
    B. Olanzapine.
    C. Ziprasidone.
    D. Quetiapine.
    E. Aripiprazole.

The correct response is option E.

First-generation antipsychotics and second-generation antipsychotics can elevate prolactin levels. Hyperpro-
lactinemia can result in sexual side effects, such as amenorrhea or oligomenorrhea, erectile dysfunction, decreased libido, hirsutism, and breast symptoms including enlargement, engorgement, pain, or galactorrhea, although prolactin levels are not tightly correlated with these symptoms (Correll and Carlson 2006). Data also
suggest that hyperprolactinemia is dose-dependent, reduces over time, and resolves after antipsychotic discontinuation. The relative potency of antipsychotic drugs in increasing prolactin levels is higher in adolescents than
in adults but follows roughly the same pattern: paliperidone ≥ risperidone > haloperidol > olanzapine > ziprasidone > quetiapine ≥ clozapine > aripiprazole. **(p. 760)**

Correll CU, Carlson HE: Endocrine and metabolic adverse effects of psychotropic medications in children and
    adolescents. J Am Acad Child Adolesc Psychiatry 45:771–791, 2006

Chapter 50

Alpha-Adrenergics, Beta-Blockers, Benzodiazepines, Buspirone, and Desmopressin

Select the single best response for each question.

50.1 Research suggests that guanfacine may be useful for treatment of the hyperactivity, impulsiveness, and distractibility associated with which of the following disorders?

    A. Panic disorder.
    B. Pervasive developmental disorder (PDD).
    C. Impulse control disorder.
    D. Generalized anxiety disorder.
    E. None of the above.

The correct response is option B.

Guanfacine entered clinical practice in the early 1990s. Accumulated evidence to date suggests that it appears to be useful as a nonstimulant alternative for the treatment of attention-deficit/hyperactivity disorder (ADHD) and the target symptoms of hyperactivity, impulsiveness, and distractibility in children with PDD. **(pp. 775–776)**

50.2 Clonidine may be an effective treatment for which of the following disorders?

    A. Major depressive disorder.
    B. Bipolar disorder.
    C. Attention-deficit/hyperactivity disorder (ADHD).
    D. Social phobia.
    E. None of the above.

The correct response is option C.

Two large-scale, 16-week trials with clonidine have targeted ADHD (Palumbo et al. 2008; Tourette's Syndrome Study Group 2002). In both trials, clonidine was compared with placebo, methylphenidate only, and combined treatment (clonidine plus methylphenidate). After subtracting out the placebo effect in the trial with children with ADHD and a tic disorder, the clonidine group showed a 21% improvement on a teacher rating compared with 16% for the methylphenidate group and 37% for combined treatment group (calculated from graphic display of results). All three active treatments were superior to placebo. **(p. 776)**

Palumbo DR, Sallee FR, Pelham WE, et al: Clonidine for attention-deficit/hyperactivity disorder, I: efficacy and tolerability outcomes. J Am Acad Adolesc Psychiatry 47:180–188, 2008
Tourette's Syndrome Study Group: Treatment of ADHD in children with tics: a randomized controlled trial. Neurology 58:527–536, 2002

50.3 Prior to beginning an alpha-2 agonist and during treatment, which of the following clinical areas should be evaluated or tests obtained?

    A. Blood pressure.
    B. Kidney function.
    C. Liver function.
    D. Electrocardiogram (ECG).
    E. All of the above.

The correct response is option A.

Several areas of concern are specific to the alpha-2 agonists. Although blood pressure is rarely a clinically significant problem in healthy children treated with usual doses, blood pressure and pulse should be measured at baseline and during the dose adjustment phase. The placebo-controlled trial with guanfacine showed a slight drop in the average diastolic blood pressure and pulse at week 4 that resolved by week 8 (Scahill et al. 2001). In young children, it may be useful to enlist help from the school nurse to monitor blood pressure in the early weeks of treatment. Once the dose is established and it is clear that the child is tolerating the medication, only periodic monitoring of pulse and blood pressure is warranted.

In a recent review, the Medical Advisory Board of the Tourette Syndrome Association noted the lack of consensus on the need for ECGs before and after treatment with the alpha-2 agonists (Scahill et al. 2006). A companion report from the Palumbo et al. (2008) trial supports the view that ECG monitoring is not required in clinical practice for healthy children (Daviss et al. 2008). **(pp. 777–778)**

Daviss WB, Patel NC, Robb AS, et al: Clonidine for attention-deficit/hyperactivity disorder, II: ECG changes and adverse events analysis. J Am Acad Adolesc Psychiatry 47:189–198, 2008

Palumbo DR, Sallee FR, Pelham WE, et al: Clonidine for attention-deficit/hyperactivity disorder, I: efficacy and tolerability outcomes. J Am Acad Adolesc Psychiatry 47:180–188, 2008

Scahill L, Chappell PB, Kim YS, et al: A placebo-controlled study of guanfacine in the treatment of children with tic disorders and attention deficit hyperactivity disorder. Am J Psychiatry 158:1067–1074, 2001

Scahill L, Erenberg G, Berlin CM, et al: Contemporary assessment and pharmacotherapy of Tourette syndrome. NeuroRx 3:192–206, 2006

50.4 Beta-blockers have been reported to be effective, either alone or in combination with other medications, in treating which of the following disorders in children?

    A. Aggression.
    B. Panic disorder.
    C. Social phobia.
    D. Specific phobias.
    E. Posttraumatic stress disorder (PTSD).

The correct response is option A.

Aggression may occur in the context of multiple disorders, including intermittent explosive disorder, psychotic disorders, traumatic brain injury, autism, attention-deficit/hyperactivity disorder, and Tourette's syndrome. Beta-blockers have been used in adults and children with intellectual disabilities for the treatment of aggression or self-injurious behaviors. Pediatric trials include case studies and small controlled trials (see Schur et al. 2003 for a review).

Anxiety disorders such as panic disorder, social phobia, and specific phobias have not shown a positive response to beta-blockers (Hidalgo et al. 2007). Although studies in adults with PTSD provide some support for beta-blockers (Pitman et al. 2002), this strategy has not been attempted in children. There are no placebo-controlled studies of a beta-blocker in children for the treatment of anxiety. **(p. 779)**

Hidalgo RB, Tupler LA, Davidson JR: An effect-size analysis of pharmacologic treatments for generalized anxiety disorder. J Psychopharmacol 21:864–872, 2007

Pitman RK, Sanders KM, Zusman RM, et al: Pilot study of secondary prevention of posttraumatic stress disorder with propranolol. Biol Psychiatry 51:189–192, 2002

Schur SB, Sikich L, Findling RL, et al: Treatment recommendations for the use of antipsychotics for aggressive youth (TRAAY), part I: a review. J Am Acad Child Adolesc Psychiatry 42:132–144, 2003

50.5 There is considerable evidence to support the use of benzodiazepines to treat which of the following disorders in children?

    A. Panic disorder.
    B. Generalized anxiety disorder.
    C. Posttraumatic stress disorder (PTSD).
    D. Social phobia.
    E. None of the above.

The correct response is option E.

Although there is considerable research support for the use of benzodiazepines in adults with anxiety disorders, the evidence in children is limited and often negative (Rynn and Ryan 2008). Despite the positive findings in open trials with alprazolam and clonazepam, small controlled trials have failed to demonstrate efficacy for several benzodiazepines for anxiety (Graae et al. 1994; Simeon et al. 1992). One trial (Graae et al. 1994) was stopped early because of a high frequency of disinhibition and irritability. Other drawbacks include the possibility of dependence and loss of motor coordination. **(p. 780)**

Graae F, Milner J, Rizzotto L, et al: Clonazepam in childhood anxiety disorders. J Am Acad Child Adolesc Psychiatry 33:372–376, 1994

Rynn MA, Ryan J: Anxiety disorders, in Clinical Manual of Child and Adolescent Psychopharmacology. Edited by Findling RL. Washington, DC, American Psychiatric Publishing, 2008, pp 143–196

Simeon JG, Ferguson HB, Knott V, et al: Clinical, cognitive, and neurophysiological effects of alprazolam in children and adolescents with overanxious and avoidant disorders. J Am Acad Child Adolesc Psychiatry 31:29–33, 1992

Chapter 51

Medications Used for Sleep

Select the single best response for each question.

51.1   Which of the following neurotransmitters is responsible for the regulation of sleep?

    A. Gamma-aminobutyric acid (GABA).
    B. Melatonin.
    C. Histamine.
    D. Norepinephrine.
    E. All of the above.

The correct response is option E.

The regulation of sleep is related to neurotransmitters, including GABA, melatonin, histamine, and norepinephrine. Medications used to treat insomnia act at the receptors of these neurotransmitters. **(p. 787)**

51.2   Medications exert their sedative effect through different mechanisms, affecting different receptors. All of the following medications are correctly paired with their receptors/mechanisms *except*

    A. Benzodiazepines—benzodiazepine receptor.
    B. Trazodone—anticholinergic mechanism.
    C. Diphenhydramine—antihistamine mechanism.
    D. Mirtazapine—gamma-aminobutyric acid (GABA) receptor and chloride channels.
    E. Clonidine—alpha-adrenergic agonist.

The correct response is option D.

Mirtazapine exerts its sedative effect through anticholinergic mechanisms.

    Benzodiazepines and benzodiazepine receptor agonists bind to the benzodiazepine receptor site, leading to modulation of the GABA receptor and its chloride ion channels. Antidepressants such as trazodone, mirtazapine, and amitriptyline exert this sedative effect through anticholinergic mechanisms. Antihistamines, available in a wide variety of compounds such as diphenhydramine, are sedating and often used to treat pediatric insomnia. Alpha-adrenergic agonists such as clonidine and guanfacine, although antihypertensives, are also prescribed for their sedative qualities. **(pp. 787–788)**

51.3   Which of the following statements regarding melatonin is *false*?

    A. In the United States, melatonin is a widely sold licensed, over-the-counter drug.
    B. There are a number of placebo-controlled trials of melatonin in the treatment of pediatric insomnia.
    C. Melatonin has been used to treat insomnia in a number of pediatric populations.
    D. Melatonin has been used in the treatment of adolescents with delayed sleep phase syndrome.
    E. Melatonin is relatively short acting, with a short half-life that makes it more effective in treating initial insomnia.

The correct response is option A.

In the United States, melatonin is a widely sold nutritional supplement, not a licensed drug.

To date, there have been more placebo-controlled trials of melatonin in the treatment of pediatric insomnia than other licensed drugs (Smits et al. 2001, 2003; Weiss et al. 2006).

Melatonin has been used to treat insomnia in a number of pediatric populations, including normally developing children with initial insomnia, children with attention-deficit/hyperactivity disorder (ADHD) and comorbid insomnia, children with neurodevelopmental disabilities, and children with autism spectrum disorder (Garstang and Wallis 2006; Jan and Freeman 2004; Smits et al. 2003; Weiss et al. 2006). Additionally, melatonin has been used in the treatment of adolescents with delayed sleep phase syndrome, a circadian rhythm sleep disorder (Szeinberg et al. 2006).

Melatonin is relatively short acting, with a half-life of approximately 1 hour; therefore, it is much more effective in treating initial insomnia rather than sleep maintenance insomnia or terminal insomnia. **(p. 788)**

Garstang J, Wallis M: Randomized controlled trial of melatonin for children with autistic spectrum disorders and sleep problems. Child Care Health Dev 32:585–589, 2006

Jan JE, Freeman RD: Melatonin therapy for circadian rhythm sleep disorders in children with multiple disabilities: what have we learned in the last decade? Dev Med Child Neurol 46:776–782, 2004

Smits MG, Nagtegaal EE, van der Heijden J, et al: Melatonin for chronic sleep onset insomnia in children: a randomized placebo-controlled trial. J Child Neurol 16:86–92, 2001

Smits MG, van Stel HF, van der Heijden K, et al: Melatonin improves health status and sleep in children with idiopathic chronic sleep-onset insomnia: a randomized placebo-controlled trial. J Am Acad Child Adolesc Psychiatry 42:1286–1293, 2003

Szeinberg A, Borodkin K, Dagan Y: Melatonin treatment in adolescents with delayed sleep phase syndrome. Clin Pediatr 45:809–818, 2006

Weiss MD, Wasdell MB, Bomben MM, et al: Sleep hygiene and melatonin treatment for children and adolescents with ADHD and initial insomnia. J Am Acad Child Adolesc Psychiatry 45:512–519, 2006

51.4   Among the following sedative-hypnotic medications, which has the shortest half-life?

   A. Eszopiclone.
   B. Zaleplon.
   C. Zolpidem.
   D. Temazepam.
   E. Estazolam.

The correct response is option B.

Zaleplon has a half-life of 1 hour, eszopiclone 6 hours, zolpidem 2.5 hours, temazepam 8–22 hours, and estazolam 10–24 hours. **(p. 790 [Tables 51–1 and 51–2])**

51.5   Which of the following medications has been reported to likely be associated with Stevens-Johnson syndrome?

   A. Mirtazapine.
   B. Chloral hydrate.
   C. Modafinil.
   D. Sodium oxybate.
   E. Pramipexole.

The correct response is option C.

Modafinil (brand name Provigil) is an alerting oral agent approved by the U.S. Food and Drug Administration for the treatment of adults with excessive daytime sleepiness associated with narcolepsy, shift work sleep disorder, and residual sleepiness despite the use of nasal continuous positive airway pressure in patients with obstructive sleep apnea. Modafinil has a Schedule IV designation by the U.S. Drug Enforcement Administration (DEA) and is not approved for any indication in the pediatric population.

In 2007, a new warning was added to the labeling related to pediatric clinical trials data. In these clinical trials, a rash developed in 0.8% of patients treated with modafinil and in 0% of patients treated with placebo. These dermatological reactions included Stevens-Johnson syndrome and multiorgan hypersensitivity. **(pp. 791–792)**

Chapter 52

Electroconvulsive Therapy, Transcranial Magnetic Stimulation, and Deep Brain Stimulation

Select the single best response for each question.

52.1 Rates of response to electroconvulsive therapy (ECT) in adolescents are similar to those reported in adults, with the exception of one disorder. For which disorder are ECT response rates in adolescents lower than those in adults?

    A. Bipolar mania.
    B. Bipolar depression.
    C. Schizophrenia.
    D. Major depressive disorder.
    E. Major depressive disorder with psychosis.

The correct response is option C.

With the exception of schizophrenia (i.e., higher ECT response rates are reported for adults), the improvement rates in adolescents are very similar to ECT improvement rates in adults, suggesting that teenagers may respond to ECT in a fashion similar to adults.

    Retrospective open case studies over the past 60 years suggest that ECT is an effective treatment for adolescents with treatment-resistant affective disorders and possibly for some adolescents with schizophrenia. Response rates range between 50% and 100%, with higher response rates generally reported for mood disorders as compared with psychotic disorders (Ghaziuddin et al. 2004). There appear to be no gender differences in response rates. **(p. 796)**

> Ghaziuddin N, Kutcher SP, Knapp P, et al: Practice parameter for use of electroconvulsive therapy with adolescents. J Am Acad Child Adolesc Psychiatry 43:1521–1539, 2004

52.2 The American Academy of Child and Adolescent Psychiatry (AACAP) has established consensus eligibility criteria for electroconvulsive therapy (ECT) in adolescents. Which of the following are ECT indications?

    A. Adolescents unable to achieve a therapeutic medication dose because they are not able to tolerate an adequate psychopharmacological trial.
    B. Adolescents with treatment-resistant depression who have failed at least two adequate antidepressant drug trials of at least 8 weeks' duration at a therapeutic dose and serum level without even mild improvement.
    C. Adolescents with bipolar disorder who have failed at least one antipsychotic-mood stabilizer/antidepressant combination treatment trial of at least 6 weeks' duration without even mild improvement.
    D. Adolescents with schizophrenia with mood symptoms.
    E. All of the above.

The correct response is option E.

For severely ill patients with life-threatening neuropsychiatric symptoms, waiting for a response to a psychopharmacological treatment trial may endanger the life of the adolescent. For example, some adolescents are unable to achieve a therapeutic medication dose because they are not able to tolerate an adequate psychopharmacology trial. In such cases, earlier consideration of ECT may be necessary (Ghaziuddin et al. 2004).

Before the clinician recommends ECT, treatment refractoriness and the adequacy of previous psychological and pharmacological interventions must be documented. *Treatment-resistant depression* is defined as failure of at least two adequate antidepressant drug trials of at least 8–10 weeks' duration, each at a therapeutic dose and serum level (if available) without even mild improvement (Ghaziuddin et al. 1996, 2004; Kutcher and Robertson 1995; Walter and Rey 1997).

For bipolar disorder, failure of at least one antipsychotic–mood stabilizer/antidepressant combination treatment trial of at least 6 weeks' duration without even mild improvement is considered evidence for treatment refractoriness (Ghaziuddin et al. 2004; Kutcher and Robertson 1995; Walter et al. 1999).

By extension from data on adults, some schizophrenic episodes in youth may respond to ECT, especially when mood symptoms are prominent. ECT may also be used to treat catatonia and neuroleptic malignant syndrome (Ghaziuddin et al. 2004). **(pp. 796–798)**

Ghaziuddin N, King CA, Naylor MW, et al: Electroconvulsive treatment in adolescents with pharmacotherapy-refractory depression. J Child Adolesc Psychopharmacol 6:259–271, 1996

Ghaziuddin N, Kutcher SP, Knapp P, et al: Practice parameter for use of electroconvulsive therapy with adolescents. J Am Acad Child Adolesc Psychiatry 43:1521–1539, 2004

Kutcher S, Robertson HA: Electroconvulsive therapy in treatment resistant bipolar youth. J Child Adolesc Psychopharmacol 5:167–175, 1995

Walter G, Rey JM: An epidemiological study of the use of ECT in adolescents. J Am Acad Child Adolesc Psychiatry 36:809–815, 1997

Walter G, Rey JM, Mitchell PB: Practitioner review: electroconvulsive therapy in adolescents. J Child Psychol Psychiatry 40:325–334, 1999

52.3 In which of the following child or adolescent populations would use of electroconvulsive therapy (ECT) be contraindicated?

    A. Adolescents who are pregnant.
    B. Adolescents with mental retardation.
    C. Adolescents with a seizure disorder.
    D. Adolescents with a space-occupying central nervous system (CNS) lesion.
    E. Prepubertal children.

The correct response is option E.

Prepubertal children should not receive ECT because scientific data on ECT use in this age group are lacking.

There is insufficient information at present to draw firm conclusions about absolute contraindications to use of ECT in adolescents, but suggestions may be extrapolated from the adult literature. In adults, there are no absolute contraindications to ECT. ECT has been successfully given to adults with comorbid psychiatric disorders, mental retardation, CNS space-occupying lesions, seizures, a history of myocardial infarction, and active chest infection. ECT has been successfully given to pregnant women, especially if they have a history of previous ECT response. Although these conditions remain relative contraindications, ECT may be safely administered after a prospective assessment of risk versus benefit from the procedure (Ghaziuddin et al. 2004). **(p. 798)**

Ghaziuddin N, Kutcher SP, Knapp P, et al: Practice parameter for use of electroconvulsive therapy with adolescents. J Am Acad Child Adolesc Psychiatry 43:1521–1539, 2004

52.4   Prior to beginning electroconvulsive therapy (ECT) in an adolescent, which of the following clinical or medical assessments should be completed?

    A. Age-appropriate cognitive assessment.
    B. Consultation with a second child and adolescent psychiatrist who is knowledgeable about ECT but not involved in the current treatment of the patient.
    C. Complete physical examination.
    D. Laboratory evaluations of physiological parameters that may influence the administration of anesthesia.
    E. All of the above.

The correct response is option E.

Because ECT may affect memory, an age-appropriate cognitive assessment is required before treatment, after treatment, and 3–6 months posttreatment (Ghaziuddin et al. 2004). Cognitive testing should emphasize short-term memory and new knowledge acquisition.

Consultation with a second child and adolescent psychiatrist who is knowledgeable about and experienced in the use of ECT and not involved in the current treatment of the patient is recommended by ECT guidelines (Ghaziuddin et al. 2004; Walter et al. 1999, 2003).

Every patient considered for ECT should receive 1) a complete physical examination, 2) laboratory investigations appropriate for the findings from the medical history and physical examination, and 3) laboratory evaluation of physiological parameters that may influence the administration or tolerability of anesthesia (Ghaziuddin et al. 2004). **(pp. 798–799)**

Ghaziuddin N, Kutcher SP, Knapp P, et al: Practice parameter for use of electroconvulsive therapy with adolescents. J Am Acad Child Adolesc Psychiatry 43:1521–1539, 2004

Walter G, Rey JM, Mitchell PB: Practitioner review: electroconvulsive therapy in adolescents. J Child Psychol Psychiatry 40:325–334, 1999

Walter G, Rey JM, Ghaziuddin N: Electroconvulsive therapy and transcranial magnetic stimulation, in Pediatric Psychopharmacology Principles and Practice. Edited by Martin A, Scahill L, Charney DS, et al. New York, Oxford University Press, 2003, pp 377–386

52.5   Modern electroconvulsive therapy (ECT) is generally well tolerated by patients, and side effects are usually mild and transient. In a study of more than 800 ECT treatments in patients younger than 19 years, the most frequently reported adverse event was

    A. Prolonged seizures.
    B. Nausea/vomiting.
    C. Subjective memory problems.
    D. Headaches.
    E. Tardive seizures.

The correct response is option D.

In a study that identified all persons younger than age 19 years who received ECT in the Australian state of New South Wales between 1990 and 1999 (Walter and Rey 2003), the most common adverse events reported in 826 ECT treatments were headache (61%), confusion (20%), subjective memory problems (19%), nausea/vomiting (15%), and muscle aches/pains (4%). Instances of prolonged seizure (>180 seconds) were very rare (0.4%). No tardive seizures or fatalities were reported. **(p. 801 [Table 52–4])**

Walter G, Rey JM: Has the practice and outcome of ECT in adolescents changed? Findings from a whole-population study. J ECT 19:84–87, 2003

52.6   Which type of transcranial magnetic stimulation (TMS) is used clinically to treat depression and other conditions?

     A. Single-pulse TMS.
     B. Paired-pulse TMS.
     C. Repetitive TMS.
     D. Nonrepetitive TMS.
     E. All of the above.

The correct response is option C.

There are three types of TMS. Single-pulse TMS is best suited to diagnostic and research applications. Paired-pulse TMS is used to evaluate cortical excitability. Repetitive TMS (rTMS) has been used in therapeutic applications because it is capable of producing rapid bursts of pulses lasting approximately 60 seconds using an oscillatory magnetic field output (Curra et al. 2002; Quintana 2005).

To date, only two small case series (totaling nine subjects) have reported on the use of rTMS in adolescent depression (Loo et al. 2006; Walter et al. 2001). In the first case series, seven patients (ages 16–18 years) were treated with rTMS. Three patients had unipolar depression, three had schizophrenia, and one had bipolar disorder. Five of the seven patients improved. Tension headaches reported in one patient were the only adverse effects noted from the rTMS procedure (Walter et al. 2001). Another report included two new adolescent patients with depression. Both improved after a course of rTMS and reported no adverse effects of the procedure. **(p. 802)**

Curra A, Modugno N, Inghilleri M, et al: Transcranial magnetic stimulation techniques in clinical investigation. Neurology 59:1851–1859, 2002
Loo C, McFarquhar T, Walter G: Transcranial magnetic stimulation in adolescent depression. Australas Psychiatry 14:81–85, 2006
Quintana H: Transcranial magnetic stimulation in persons younger than the age of 18. J ECT 21:88–95, 2005
Walter G, Tormos JM, Israel JA, et al: Transcranial magnetic stimulation in young persons: a review of known cases. J Child Adolesc Psychopharmacol 11:69–75, 2001

Chapter 53

Individual Psychotherapy

Select the single best response for each question.

53.1 Child psychiatry incorporates both uncovering and support in its general approach to psychotherapy. Which of the following techniques would a child therapist be *less* likely to employ in supportive therapy?

  A. Clarification.
  B. Education.
  C. Suggestion.
  D. Modeling.
  E. Reinforcement.

The correct response is option A.

Child psychotherapy followed adult psychiatry in separating the idea of *uncovering* (Freudian-minded psychotherapy) from *support* (ego building, conscience building, community-related helps, and education). But child psychiatry eventually came to incorporate both forms—uncovering and support—into its general approach to psychotherapy. To uncover with an adult, the therapist needed interpretation and *clarification*. The therapist also needed to maintain a neutral and relatively passive stance. This rather distant approach was intended to encourage *transference*, the displacement of old attitudes, especially those about the patient's family of origin, to the therapist. To support a child, on the other hand, the therapist was taught to employ more *education, suggestion, modeling*, and positive or negative *reinforcement* (largely in the therapist's attitude toward the patient). **(p. 809)**

53.2 If a therapist treats a child through the parent (who takes the doctor's ideas home and tries them out on the young person), the therapy is called

  A. Uncovering psychotherapy.
  B. Supportive psychotherapy.
  C. Family therapy.
  D. Filial therapy.
  E. Collaborative therapy.

The correct response is option D.

The "Little Hans" means of child treatment—by working only with a parent and then having the parent make the suggested therapeutic interventions and commentaries—has been elaborated by Erna Furman into what is known as *filial therapy*. This treatment can be especially useful in preschoolers or with crisis management situations, such as coping with a seriously ill adolescent or a health emergency in a latency-age child (Furman 1957). **(p. 814; see also Table 53–1)**

Furman E: Treatment of under-fives by way of parents. Psychoanal Study Child 12:250–262, 1957

53.3 All of the following statements regarding individual psychotherapy are correct *except*

A. Establishing a therapeutic alliance with the child is essential to performing effective therapy.
B. The therapist should be calm, unhurried, willing to listen, and nonjudgmental.
C. The child therapist should be a passive listener and occasional communicator to allow the child free expression.
D. A thorough acquaintance with the concepts of transference and countertransference is important.
E. Individual child psychotherapy requires a room where appropriate toys and games are available.

The correct response is option C.

Although for adult patients, the classic psychodynamic psychotherapeutic persona is that of passive listener and occasional commentator, the child and adolescent psychotherapeutic persona is often more activist, serving as "tutor" or "coach."

Forming a therapeutic alliance with a child is essential to performing effective individual psychotherapy. The clinician must be professional; this includes being calm, unhurried, willing to listen, nonjudgmental, relatively objective, focused on the patient, and committed to the basic principle behind the Hippocratic oath (actually enunciated by Florence Nightingale as "First, do no harm").

Countertransference (the therapist's feelings, often based on old unresolved conflicts that the patient's attitudes may bring to the surface) occasionally must be dealt with in order to save the therapeutic alliance with the child (Marshall 1979; Tsiantis et al. 1996). A thorough acquaintance with the concepts of transference and countertransference is important in doing psychotherapy with children (see Winnicott 1958). It is also important to be able to talk with a supervisor or with colleagues about these types of very personal responses to children.

Individual child and adolescent psychotherapy requires a room in which to be alone with the young patient that is as appealing as possible. A youngster's conflicts and concerns are often expressed in terms of animals (hence, animal puppets and small dinosaurs are important office equipment); vehicles (thus, a set of cars, fire and rescue equipment, pickup and tow trucks, and police cars—and even a bus to the local prison—are helpful); a baby doll; older girl dolls, and if possible, a boy doll; a deck of cards; checkers; a doll house with miniature furniture and a small doll family; an army including men (and women) and their equipment; and some pop-culture items (e.g., a Little Mermaid, Star Wars figures, Hello Kitty, Power Rangers). Other kinds of objects, including some larger dolls and some movable ones—such as circus figures—and some simple games for two— such as cards or checkers—are also useful. **(pp. 814–817)**

Marshall R: Countertransference in the psychotherapy of children and adolescents. Contemp Psychoanal 15:599–629, 1979

Tsiantis J, Sandler A-M, Anastasopoulos D, et al: Countertransference in Psychoanalytic Psychotherapy With Children and Adolescents. London, England, Karnac, 1996

Winnicott DW: Clinical varieties of transference, in Collected Papers: Through Pediatrics to Psychoanalysis. New York, Basic, 1958, pp 295–299

53.4 Which of the following concepts is relevant when a therapist makes interpretations during the individual therapy with a child?

A. Ego ideal.
B. Defense and coping.
C. Secret unattainable desires.
D. Transference.
E. Countertransference.

The correct response is option A.

Therapeutic statements to children cover a wide range of issues. Present realities—trouble at school, problems with classmates, joblessness at home, bullies in the neighborhood—are given far more room for exploration and discussion than they were in the past. What a child wishes for in the future and whom a child might wish to emulate as an *ego ideal* are also important (Terr 2003) as the clinician makes contemporary interpretations. How does the youngster envision what will happen next? Later in adulthood? How will he or she die? When? What about marriage, children, career? Discussing the future in terms of the youngster's present coping skills or behaviors often offers a new perspective to the child and thus, a new way to combat old conflicts. These issues are taken into account right along with the classic issues—defenses and coping, secret unattainable desires, transference, and countertransference. **(p. 820; see also Table 53–1)**

Terr L: Wild child: how three principles of healing organized 12 years of psychotherapy. J Am Acad Child Adolesc Psychiatry 42:1401–1409, 2003

Chapter 54

Parent Counseling, Psychoeducation, and Parent Support Groups

Select the single best response for each question.

54.1   Which of the following is a basic principle of parent counseling interventions?

  A. Education and therapy are provided directly to the child.
  B. Parents' expertise in caring for their children is not used, since parental shortcomings are frequently the source of their children's problems.
  C. It is assumed that parent-child conflicts are due to parental problems.
  D. Parents are helped to understand normal child development, their own child, and his or her needs and problems.
  E. None of the above.

The correct response is option D.

Underlying parent counseling is a sincere valuing of parents for their experience in caring for their children and their expertise in understanding their children and their needs (Arnold 1978). Parents are essential to treatment because they spend the most time with their child. Parent counseling interventions help parents modify their own attitudes, behaviors, and parenting that may be unwittingly contributing to the problem. Education and therapy are provided to the parents rather than directly to the child. The experience and expertise parents have from caring for their children are valued and utilized in treatment. The assumption is made that parent-child conflicts are two-way vicious cycles. Parents are helped to understand normal child development, their own child, and his or her needs and problems. The professional acts as a consultant to help parents identify problems and learn skills needed to manage the child's illness successfully on their own. Efficiency, effectiveness, and practicality to the exclusion of moral judgment or blame are emphasized. Finally, appropriate choice of intervention depends on the problem, the circumstances, and the family. **(p. 827 [Table 54–2])**

Arnold LE (ed): Helping Parents Help Their Children. New York, Brunner/Mazel, 1978

54.2   What is an advantage of multifamily psychoeducation groups over individual family psychoeducation?

  A. Increased privacy.
  B. Flexibility to tailor to individual needs.
  C. Development of a support network.
  D. Ease of scheduling.
  E. All of the above.

The correct response is option C.

As described by Fristad (2006), individual family psychoeducation and multifamily psychoeducation groups have different strengths. Multifamily psychoeducation groups are a cost-effective way to deliver services within a large clinic. They offer families the opportunity to talk and share with both professionals and other families, to develop a support network, and to identify with and learn from other families' successes.

By contrast, individual family psychoeducation is easy for private practice clinicians to implement. It offers privacy, flexibility in scheduling, and flexibility to tailor topics to individualized needs. **(p. 828; see also Table 54–4)**

> Fristad MA: Psychoeducational treatment for school-aged children with bipolar disorder. Dev Psychopathol 18:1289–1306, 2006

54.3 Which of the following are age adjustments needed for psychoeducation with children and adolescents with mental illness?

    A. Less emphasis on social skills training.
    B. Less intensive treatment.
    C. Emphasis on the home environment.
    D. Shorter follow-up.
    E. Little attention given to environmental circumstances.

The correct response is option C.

Adaptation of psychoeducation for children and adolescents requires several changes in the content and format of the intervention (Fristad et al. 1996). When treating children and adolescents, it is important to place emphasis on the home environment.

Children may not have had an opportunity to develop a healthy identity separate from their symptoms, so it is important to clarify what is the disorder and what are the child's traits. Emphasis should be placed on social skills training and assistance should be given to help children adjust to their environment to be able to succeed despite their symptoms. Treatment needs to focus on the appropriate developmental level and is of longer duration and greater intensity than required by adults. **(p. 829; see also Table 54–5)**

> Fristad MA, Gavazzi SM, Centolella DM, et al: Psychoeducation: a promising intervention strategy for families of children and adolescents with mood disorders. Contemporary Family Therapy: An International Journal 18:371–384, 1996

54.4 Family or parent psychoeducation interventions have been designed for all the following disorders *except*

    A. Attention-deficit/hyperactivity disorder (ADHD).
    B. Obsessive-compulsive disorder (OCD).
    C. Bipolar disorder.
    D. Eating disorder.
    E. Depressive disorders.

The correct response is option B.

No family interventions have been developed for OCD.

Family or parent psychoeducation interventions have been designed for anxiety disorders, ADHD, depressive disorders, bipolar disorder, disruptive behavior disorders, and eating disorders. Programs have also been designed for general emotional and behavioral disturbances rather than for specific disorders. Across diagnoses, the active treatment components of these family psychoeducation interventions were all very similar and included medications, other forms of treatment, symptom management, parenting, and coping and communication skills. **(p. 830; see also Table 54–6)**

54.5   A variety of techniques are used in psychoeducation. The technique whereby a child develops a variety of pleasant or relaxing activities to use in affect regulation is called

A. Toolkit.
B. Thinking, feeling, doing.
C. Naming the enemy.
D. Mood chart.
E. Daily routine tracking.

The correct response is option A.

Techniques commonly used in family psychoeducation groups include bibliotherapy, daily routine tracking, mood charting, "naming the enemy," "thinking–feeling–doing," and "toolkit" (see Table 54–1). **(p. 838 [Table 54–10])**

Table 54–1.   Examples of techniques used in psychoeducation

Psychoeducational techniques	Description of technique
Bibliotherapy	Using written materials, video, or Web sites to further educate families about mental illness.
Daily routine tracking	Tracking daily routines such as sleep-wake cycles, eating, and other daily activities to determine their effect on mood and behavior.
Mood chart	Tracking changes in mood, when they occur, and the circumstances that happen around the time of the changes.
Naming the enemy[a]	Helping the child and parents determine the difference between the child's symptoms and his or her own personality.
Thinking, feeling, doing[a]	Increasing insight of parents and child into the connections among their thoughts, feelings, and behavior.
Tool kit[a]	Develop a variety of pleasant or relaxing activities for the child to use in affect regulation.

[a]Techniques used in multifamily psychoeducational psychotherapy.

Chapter 55

Behavioral Parent Training

Select the single best response for each question.

55.1 Which of the following is *not* one of the four key concepts of contingency-based behavioral interventions?

    A. Shaping.
    B. Positive reinforcement.
    C. Negative reinforcement.
    D. Punishment.
    E. Extinction.

The correct response is option A.

Shaping is not a key concept of contingency-based behavioral interventions.

    Behavior therapy has a long history of success in treating childhood problems. Behavior therapy approaches emphasize the importance of environmental and social contingencies in fostering and maintaining problem behavior—i.e., *contingency theory* (Patterson 1982). Contingency-based behavioral interventions involve one or more of four key concepts. Behavior is increased either by following it with something desirable *(positive reinforcement)* or by removing something desirable *(negative reinforcement)*; behavior is decreased either by following it with something undesirable *(punishment)* or by removing something desirable *(extinction)*. **(p. 845)**

    Patterson GR: Coercive Family Process. Eugene, OR, Castalia Publishing, 1982

55.2 Which of the following is a key component of functional behavior analysis?

    A. Specifying behaviors (either positive or negative behaviors).
    B. Identifying each behavior's antecedents.
    C. Identifying each behavior's consequences.
    D. All of the above.
    E. None of the above.

The correct response is option D.

Behavioral interventions usually begin with a *functional behavior analysis*, which involves specifying behaviors (positive behaviors to increase or negative behaviors to decrease) and then identifying each behavior's antecedents (variables setting the stage for or preceding the behavior) and consequences (variables maintaining the behavior). Based on this analysis, specific strategies for modifying antecedents and consequences are selected for a behavioral intervention plan with the goal of reducing problem behavior and promoting desired behavior. **(pp. 845–846)**

55.3 Which of the following is considered a supplemental topic—rather than a core session topic—of parent training programs?

    A. Psychoeducation/background information.
    B. Praise and positive reinforcement.
    C. Parent stress/emotion management.

D. Time-out.

E. Home-school report card.

The correct response is option C.

Parent stress management is a supplemental topic of behavioral parent training. Parents usually are receptive to the idea that their own stress levels affect their child's behavior and that higher levels of parental stress are related to increased behavior problems on the part of the child (as well as relational stress between the child and the parent). Likewise, parents usually agree that when they are able to manage their own stress levels, they also are better able to meet their children's needs.

Although a number of different approaches to parent training exist, all approaches generally involve some combination of the following core topics:

- *Psychoeducation/background information:* The first session of behavioral parent training generally involves providing parents with background information and psychoeducation regarding childhood behavior problems, family interactions, and behavior therapy.
- *Praise and positive reinforcement:* Because negative behavior generally is much more salient to parents than is positive behavior, parents often unintentionally ignore positive behaviors when these behaviors do occur. Session content consequently focuses on reinforcing and rewarding positive behavior with praise and tangible reinforcers such as activities or token prizes.
- *Time-out:* "Time-out," or time away from positive reinforcement (e.g., parental attention, another enjoyable activity), can be a powerful consequence of negative behavior. This session involves reviewing parents' past experiences with time-out as well as discussion of mechanical and logistical issues of the time-out procedure.
- *Home-school report cards:* Many parent training intervention programs include a session teaching families to develop a daily behavior report card targeting between one and four problem behaviors that the teacher fills out and sends home with the child each day (Kelley 1990).

(pp. 848–853; see also Appendix 55–1)

Kelley ML: School-Home Notes: Promoting Children's Classroom Success. New York, Guilford, 1990

55.4 In regard to potential adverse effects resulting from behavioral parent training, those complications likely to be most serious relate to which of the following topics?

A. Positive reinforcement.

B. Attending.

C. Token economy.

D. Punishment.

E. Developing a plan for homework.

The correct response is option D.

Unwanted effects in behavioral parent training usually are mild and transient results of parents using skills taught in an inappropriate manner and can be addressed by making modifications to the program. The most serious complications may occur around the topic of punishment, because overly critical or potentially violent parents may overuse these approaches to the exclusion of the more positive ones. In these cases, an errorless learning approach may be particularly helpful (Ducharme et al. 2000). *Errorless learning* is a success-based noncoercive intervention that involves the gradual introduction of more demanding requests so that child noncompliance and associated consequences for noncompliance are minimized throughout treatment. Likewise, children presenting with aggressive behavior may become aggressive toward parents or other authority figures when punishment is used. In these cases, reward-only programs may be best, or there may be a need for additional interventions, such as collaborative family problem-solving (Greene 2004) or medication. **(p. 856)**

> Ducharme JM, Atkinson L, Poulton L: Success-based, noncoercive treatment of oppositional behavior in children from violent homes. J Am Acad Child Adolesc Psychiatry 39:995–1004, 2000
> Greene RW: Effectiveness of collaborative problem solving in affectively dysregulated children with oppositional defiant disorder: initial findings. J Consult Clin Psychol 72:1157–1164, 2004

55.5   Based on recent studies, all of the following statements regarding the outcomes of behavioral parent training (BPT) are accurate *except*

- A. Evidence shows that low socioeconomic status (SES) predicts higher dropout rates for behavioral parent training versus other psychosocial treatments.
- B. Having both parents attending the training may not affect posttreatment outcome.
- C. Severe marital discord can reduce efficacy of parent training.
- D. Children with conduct disorder, who are high on callous-unemotional traits, show poorer response.
- E. Therapist warmth, likeability, and communication skills are likely to contribute to more positive outcomes.

The correct response is option A.

For families facing financial disadvantage, an individual approach to parent training that allows for more tailoring of treatment to individual family circumstances may be significantly more effective than group-based approaches (Harwood and Eyberg 2004; Lundahl et al. 2005). There is no evidence that low SES increases dropout differentially for behavior therapy versus other psychosocial treatments.

There has been some question as to whether fathers need to attend parent training; outcome studies tend to show that having both parents attend may not affect posttreatment outcome but may improve maintenance of treatment gains (Miller and Prinz 1990).

Severe marital discord, parent psychopathology (e.g., depression, attention-deficit/hyperactivity disorder, antisocial behavior), and parental drug abuse or dependence can all reduce efficacy of parent training (Chronis et al. 2004).

A number of child factors also predict response to parent training. The severity and nature of symptoms and problems likely are the strongest predictors of whether or not (or to what degree) treatment produces desired change. Children with conduct disorder who are high on callous-unemotional traits show a poorer response to parent training in general than do children low on these traits, and these children show an especially poor response to time-out as compared with reward programs (Hawes and Dadds 2005).

As with any intervention, the therapist-client relationship influences outcome in behavior therapy (Webster-Stratton and Herbert 1993). Therapist warmth, knowledge of social learning principles and disruptive behavior disorders, likeability, and communication skills all are likely to contribute to more positive outcomes. **(pp. 859–860)**

> Chronis A, Chacko A, Fabiano G, et al: Enhancements to the behavioral parent training paradigm for families of children with ADHD: review and future directions. Clin Child Fam Psychol Rev 7:1–27, 2004
> Harwood MD, Eyberg SM: Therapist verbal behavior early in treatment: relation to successful completion of parent-child interaction therapy. J Clin Child Adolesc Psychol 33:601–612, 2004
> Hawes DJ, Dadds MR: The treatment of conduct problems in children with callous-unemotional traits. J Consult Clin Psychol 73:737–741, 2005
> Lundahl B, Risser HJ, Lovejoy MC: A meta-analysis of parent training: moderators and follow-up effects. Clin Psychol Rev 26:86–104, 2005
> Miller GE, Prinz RJ: Enhancement of social learning family intervention for childhood conduct disorder. Psychol Bull 108:291–307, 1990
> Webster-Stratton C, Herbert M: "What really happens in parent training?" Behav Modif 17:407–456, 1993

Chapter 56

Family Therapy

Select the single best response for each question.

56.1 Which form of family therapy uses the emotional reactions of family members to guide assessment and intervention?

    A. Structural family therapy.
    B. Experiential family therapy.
    C. Family systems therapy.
    D. Strategic family therapy.
    E. None of the above.

The correct response is option B.

Experiential family therapies, represented by Carl Whitaker and Virginia Satir, demonstrate that a keen awareness of the here-and-now experience of family members is beneficial to treatment. This attunement to the emotional reactions of family members guides assessment and intervention. These models brought to the field an appropriate emphasis on in-session interaction. An example would be asking a conflicted parent-child dyad to talk about a problem in session. This allows the clinician to see firsthand the strengths and weaknesses of the relationship.

Structural family therapy, represented by Salvador Minuchin of the Philadelphia Child Guidance Clinic, emphasizes aspects of family structure. Family boundaries that are too rigid, disengaged, diffuse, or enmeshed are areas of intervention (Cuffe et al. 2005). Triangles, coalitions, and over- and underinvolvement are also concerns. Often, we see one parent overtly or covertly aligned with a child against the other parent, thus weakening overall parental effectiveness. A triangle exists when the emotionality between two persons spills over to a third.

Historically, Bowen family systems therapy is noteworthy for its equal regard for both the individual and familial dimensions contributing to human problems. This model assesses and intervenes through seven interlocking concepts: differentiation of the self, emotional triangles, nuclear family emotional process, multigenerational transmission, family projections, sibling positions, and emotional cutoffs. The centerpiece of this approach is a self that is sufficiently secure to be both less reactive to others and able to form viable relationships with other family members.

Strategic family therapy, a historically important model that is now rarely used, views problem formation in terms of failed solutions and interventions in terms of paradoxical injunctions. For example, parents become concerned that their child's school performance is declining and so increase their surveillance of the child's homework and studies. The child becomes anxious and resents what she or he sees as parental pressure and continues to fail. A strategic intervention would encourage the parents to do more of the same (paradoxical injunction) until they become frustrated and open to different solutions. **(pp. 870–871)**

Cuffe SP, McKeown RE, Addy CL, et al: Family and psychosocial risk factors in a longitudinal epidemiological study of adolescents. J Am Acad Child Adolesc Psychiatry 44:121–129, 2005

56.2 Who is viewed as the originator of structural family therapy?

    A. James Alexander.
    B. Carl Whitaker.
    C. Virginia Satir.

D. Salvador Minuchin.

E. D. W. Winnicott.

The correct response is option D.

Structural family therapy, represented by Salvador Minuchin of the Philadelphia Child Guidance Clinic, emphasizes aspects of family structure.

Functional family therapy is most often associated with James Alexander (Alexander and Parsons 1982). Functional family therapists observe how symptoms and behaviors function and then seek to remedy the manifesting problems.

Experiential family therapies, represented by Carl Whitaker and Virginia Satir, demonstrate that a keen awareness of the here-and-now experience of family members is beneficial to treatment.

D. W. Winnicott, an early major figure in child psychiatry, emphasized the significance of the social environment for the child in terms of two interlocking processes: 1) the developmental process from absolute dependence through relative dependence to independence (Winnicott 1960/1965, 1963/1965), and 2) the profoundly beneficial influence of an emotionally facilitating environment. **(pp. 870–871, 872–873, 874)**

Alexander JF, Parsons BV: Functional Family Therapy: Principles and Procedures. Carmel, CA, Brooks and Cole, 1982

Winnicott DW: The theory of the parent-infant relationship (1960), in The Maturational Processes and the Facilitating Environment: Studies in the Theory of Emotional Development. New York, International Universities Press, 1965, pp 37–55

Winnicott DW: From dependence towards independence in the development of the individual (1963), in The Maturational Processes and the Facilitating Environment: Studies in the Theory of Emotional Development. New York, International Universities Press, 1965, pp 83–92

56.3 A number of frameworks and models have been developed for use in assessing and conceptualizing family issues and problems. Which of the following models asks the questions "Why can't people solve their own problems? What is constraining a person or family from overcoming the difficulty?"

A. Linear causality.

B. Emotion regulation.

C. Clinical constraints.

D. Developmental trajectories.

E. Circular causality.

The correct response is option C.

The notion of *clinical constraints* was developed by Breunlin et al. (1992). It asks the questions, "Why can't people solve their own problems? What is constraining a person or a family from overcoming the difficulty?" By thinking in terms of constraints, the clinician is guided to potential sources of the patient's problems and can readily develop a workable intervention focus.

Linear causality seeks to identify, in a sequential fashion, when and how a certain problem began. For instance, the child's behavior problems increased when a parent moved out of the household.

Emotion (or *affect*) *regulation* deals with how well-functioning individuals downregulate negative emotion and upregulate positive emotions (related to mastery and achievement, which builds emotional security and self-esteem).

From the beginning, family therapy has thought in terms of several parallel and sometimes intertwined *developmental trajectories*. Besides the developmental needs of the identified patient, family therapists consider the developmental processes of couple and family formation and how parent-child interactions are affected by them and how interactional styles must change with maturation.

The interlocking nature of family interactions is, perhaps, best captured in the term *circular causality*. Many human difficulties arise within a social or interactional context, and a specific moment of change when the problem emerged cannot be identified. Employing circular causality frees the clinician from evaluating "Who (what) started it?" Seeing the circular causality prevents the useless search for a first cause or perpetrator and allows for interventions that address how both individuals may be a little right and a little wrong—but can change the cycle if they choose. **(pp. 871–872)**

Breunlin DC, Schwartz RC, MacKune-Karrer B: Metaframeworks: Transcending the Models of Family Therapy. San Francisco, CA, Jossey-Bass, 1992

56.4   Which newer form of family therapy encourages therapists to observe how symptoms and behavior function and then seek to remedy the presenting problem?

     A. Functional family therapy.
     B. Solution-focused family therapy.
     C. Narrative family therapy.
     D. Emotionally focused therapy.
     E. Strategic family therapy.

The correct response is option A.

Functional family therapy is most often associated with James Alexander (Alexander and Parsons 1982). Functional family therapists observe how symptoms and behaviors function and then seek to remedy the manifesting problems.

The 1990s saw *solution-focused family therapy* grow in popularity. This model deemphasizes problems and instead focuses on solutions. When families want to talk about problems, solution-focused clinicians explore exceptions to the problem (i.e., identify times or circumstances in which the problem does not exist).

Narrative family therapy (Freeman et al. 1997) focuses on the stories families tell and how these narratives both define roles of family members and constrain the family from seeking alternative narratives (leading to more adaptive behaviors).

Emotionally focused therapy (EFT) has received empirical support for the treatment of couples and depression in adults (Bradley and Johnson 2005; Dessaulles et al. 2003; Greenberg and Johnson 1988; Johnson and Greenberg 1985) and is growing in influence. EFT draws from the experiential family therapy tradition and focuses on how both individual members and dyads in families regulate affects.

Strategic family therapy, a historically important model that is now rarely used, views problem formation in terms of failed solutions and interventions in terms of paradoxical injunctions. For example, parents become concerned that their child's school performance is declining and so increase their surveillance of the child's homework and studies. The child becomes anxious and resents what she or he sees as parental pressure and continues to fail. A strategic intervention would encourage the parents to do more of the same (paradoxical injunction) until they become frustrated and open to different solutions. **(pp. 871, 874)**

Alexander JF, Parsons BV: Functional Family Therapy: Principles and Procedures. Carmel, CA, Brooks and Cole, 1982

Bradley B, Johnson SM: EFT: an integrative contemporary approach, in Handbook of Couples Therapy. Edited by Harway M. Hoboken, NJ, John Wiley & Sons, 2005, pp 179–193

Dessaulles A, Johnson SM, Denton WH: Emotion-focused therapy for couples in the treatment of depression: a pilot study. American Journal of Family Therapy 31:345–353, 2003

Freeman J, Epston D, Lobovits D: Playful Approaches to Serious Problems: Narrative Therapy With Children and Their Families. New York, WW Norton, 1997

Greenberg LS, Johnson SM: Emotionally Focused Therapy for Couples. New York, Guilford, 1988

Johnson SM, Greenberg LS: Emotionally focused couples therapy: an outcome study. J Marital Fam Ther 11:313–317, 1985

56.5   D. W. Winnicott emphasized the significance of the social environment for normal human development and psychological growth. A critical component to this theory is

   A. The identified patient.
   B. Nuclear family emotional process.
   C. Multigeneration transmission process.
   D. Family projection process.
   E. The holding environment.

The correct response is option E.

Winnicott posited that the adequacy of the social environment is essential for normal human development and psychological growth. Perhaps more than anything else, it is the dependence of infants, children, and adolescents and the sensitivity and reactivity of young people to their environment that distinguish working with children and adolescents from the treatment of adults. Winnicott's theory is now firmly established in the literature. There are a variety of regulatory processes, biologically based and environmentally shaped, that influence emotional outcomes from health and vitality to the manifestation of behavioral disorders. A critical component of Winnicott's theory is the *holding environment:* that is, the provision of a safe and need-fulfilling social context within which the infant and young child can develop. The creation of this holding environment requires an early and primary parental preoccupation in order to facilitate the growth of children, which gradually recedes as the child matures. This is one reason why the family is so important to child and adolescent mental health practice. Adults may be able to be treated without reference to their family (although many rightly question this), but the dependency of children requires the assessment and involvement of the family.

   The *identified patient* is the person (the child or adolescent) originally presenting for treatment. Family therapy uses this term to remind clinicians that other family members and the family as a whole, in some sense, are "patients" requiring assessment and intervention. **(pp. 871, 872–873)**

Chapter 57

Interpersonal Psychotherapy for Depressed Adolescents

Select the single best response for each question.

57.1 Which of the following statements regarding interpersonal psychotherapy for depressed adolescents (IPT-A) is *false?*

    A. IPT-A is a time-limited, manualized, psychotherapeutic intervention adapted from IPT for adults.

    B. It is based on the principle that depression occurs within an interpersonal context.

    C. Its goal is to decrease depressive symptoms.

    D. It can be used for the treatment of adolescents who have either psychotic or nonpsychotic depression.

    E. It is not recommended for adolescents who are mentally retarded, actively suicidal or homicidal, or have bipolar disorders.

The correct response is option D.

IPT-A is designed to treat adolescents (ages 12–18 years) with nonpsychotic, unipolar depression. IPT-A is not recommended for adolescents who are mentally retarded, actively suicidal or homicidal, psychotic, bipolar, or are actively abusing substances.

    IPT-A (Mufson et al. 2004) is a time-limited, manualized psychotherapeutic intervention adapted from IPT for adults (Weissman et al. 2000). IPT is based on the principle that regardless of the underlying cause, depression occurs within an interpersonal context. The goal of treatment, therefore, is to decrease depressive symptoms by focusing on current interpersonal difficulties and helping the individual improve his or her relationships and communication patterns. **(pp. 887–888)**

Mufson L, Dorta KP, Moreau D, et al: Interpersonal Psychotherapy for Depressed Adolescents, 2nd Edition. New York, Guilford, 2004

Weissman MM, Markowitz JC, Klerman GL: Comprehensive Guide to Interpersonal Psychotherapy. New York, Basic Books, 2000

57.2 Which of the following statements regarding the course of treatment using interpersonal psychotherapy for depressed adolescents (IPT-A) is *false?*

    A. IPT-A is usually delivered once a week for 12 weeks.

    B. IPT-A is an individual treatment that requires parental participation.

    C. There are three treatment phases: initial, middle, and termination.

    D. Each session begins with an assessment of the adolescent patient's mood using a 1–10 scale.

    E. The therapist and patient focus on tasks that are specific to the phase of treatment after reviewing of the symptoms.

The correct response is option B.

IPT-A is an individual treatment that recommends, but does not require, parental participation. Parental session attendance can range from none to several, although nonattendance is strongly discouraged.

IPT-A is designed to be delivered once a week for 12 weeks, although the treatment schedule can be more flexible if necessary.

IPT-A is divided into three treatment phases: initial, middle, and termination. Each session begins with the therapist assessing the adolescent's depressive symptoms and asking the adolescent to rate his or her mood using a 1–10 scale. **(p. 888)**

57.3   Which of the following interpersonal problem areas may be identified during interpersonal psychotherapy for depressed adolescents (IPT-A)?

    A. Grief due to death.
    B. Interpersonal role disputes.
    C. Interpersonal role transitions.
    D. Interpersonal deficits.
    E. All of the above.

The correct response is option E.

Based on the interpersonal inventory, the therapist helps the adolescent link the status and quality of his or her relationships to his or her depressive symptoms. The therapist identifies common themes or problems in the adolescent's relationships and together with the adolescent, identifies one of four interpersonal problem areas that will be the focus of treatment: grief due to death, interpersonal role disputes, interpersonal role transitions, or interpersonal deficits. Generally, only one interpersonal problem area is identified, but it is also possible to identify a secondary problem area. **(p. 889)**

57.4   General techniques commonly used in interpersonal psychotherapy for depressed adolescents (IPT-A) include all of the following *except*

    A. Encouragement of affect and linkage with interpersonal events.
    B. Reinforcements of coping skills.
    C. Communication analysis.
    D. Decision analysis.
    E. Role-playing.

The correct response is option B.

Reinforcements of coping are more likely to be used in supportive psychotherapy.

Encouragement of affect and linkage with interpersonal events are used to help the adolescent become aware of, acknowledge, and accept negative emotions about events and relationships and understand how emotions affect relationships (Weissman et al. 2000).

Communication analysis is used to explore the adolescent's patterns of interacting with others in order to identify ways in which his or her communication is problematic and the skills the adolescent needs to master to have more satisfying relationships.

Decision analysis is similar to problem-solving techniques that are used in other models of therapy but is focused more specifically on addressing interpersonal problems.

Role-playing is a way for adolescents to practice the communication and interpersonal problem-solving skills that they have learned in order to feel more comfortable using them in real life. **(pp. 890–891)**

Weissman MM, Markowitz JC, Klerman GL: Comprehensive Guide to Interpersonal Psychotherapy. New York, Basic Books, 2000

57.5   Interpersonal psychotherapy for depressed adolescents (IPT-A) has been examined in a number of randomized, controlled clinical trials. For which of the following target symptoms do the greatest amount of empirical data support the effectiveness of IPT-A?

    A. Anxiety symptoms.
    B. Symptoms related to abusing substances.
    C. Depressive symptoms.
    D. Obsessive-compulsive disorder (OCD)–like symptoms.
    E. Attention-deficit/hyperactivity disorder (ADHD) symptoms.

The correct response is option C.

The efficacy and effectiveness of IPT-A for reducing adolescents' depressive symptoms have been examined in three randomized controlled clinical trials (Mufson et al. 1999; Mufson et al. 2004; Rossello and Bernal 1999). Depressed adolescents treated with IPT-A demonstrated fewer depressive symptoms, better social functioning, and better global functioning at the completion of treatment than adolescents in control conditions. Based on the empirical support for treatment efficacy, IPT-A meets the American Psychological Association Division 12 criteria for a "well-established" psychotherapy for depression in youth.

Depressed adolescents with comorbid anxiety disorders, ADHD, and oppositional defiant disorder have been successfully treated with IPT-A, although IPT-A is most effective when depression is the primary diagnosis and the comorbid diagnoses are limited. **(pp. 888, 894)**

Mufson L, Weissman MM, Moreau D, et al: Efficacy of interpersonal psychotherapy for depressed adolescents. Arch Gen Psychiatry 56:573–579, 1999

Mufson L, Dorta KP, Wickramaratne P, et al: A randomized effectiveness trial of interpersonal psychotherapy for depressed adolescents. Arch Gen Psychiatry 61:577–584, 2004

Rossello J, Bernal G: The efficacy of cognitive-behavioral and interpersonal treatments for depression in Puerto Rican adolescents. J Consult Clin Psychol 67:734–745, 1999

Chapter 58

Cognitive-Behavioral Treatment for Anxiety Disorders

Select the single best response for each question.

58.1 Cognitive-behavioral therapy (CBT) has been shown to be efficacious in treating which of the following childhood disorders?

A. Social phobia/social anxiety disorder.
B. Avoidant disorder.
C. Generalized anxiety disorder.
D. Overanxious disorder.
E. All of the above.

The correct response is option E.

Data from controlled trials support the efficacy of CBT for many childhood anxiety disorders, including generalized anxiety disorder, overanxious disorder, separation anxiety disorder, social phobia/social anxiety disorder, and school refusal (see Table 58–1). **(p. 898 [Table 58–1])**

Barrett PM: Evaluation of cognitive-behavioral group treatments for childhood anxiety disorders. J Clin Child Psychol 27:459–468, 1998

Barrett PM, Rapee RM, Dadds MR, et al: Family enhancement of cognitive style in anxious and aggressive children: threat bias and the FEAR effect. J Abnorm Child Psychol 24:187–203, 1996

Beidel DC, Turner SM, Morris TL: Behavioral treatment of childhood social phobia. J Consult Clin Psychol 68:1072–1080, 2000

Beidel DC, Turner SM, Sallee FR, et al: SET-C vs. fluoxetine in the treatment of childhood social phobia. J Am Acad Child Adolesc Psychiatry 46:1622–1632, 2007

Bernstein GA, Borchardt C, Perwien AR: Imipramine plus cognitive-behavioral therapy in the treatment of school refusal. J Am Acad Child Adolesc Psychiatry 39:276–283, 2000

Dadds MR, Spence SH, Holland DE, et al: Prevention and early intervention for anxiety disorders: a controlled trial. J Consult Clin Psychol 65:627–635, 1997

Flannery-Schroeder EC, Kendall PC: Group and individual cognitive-behavioral treatments for youth with anxiety disorders: a randomized clinical trial. Cognit Ther Res 24:251–278, 2000

Hayward C, Varady S, Albano AM, et al: Cognitive-behavioral group therapy for social phobia in female adolescents: results of a pilot study. J Am Acad Child Adolesc Psychiatry 39:721–726, 2000

Kendall PC: Treating anxiety disorders in children: results of a randomized clinical trial. J Clin Child Psychol 62:100–110, 1994

Kendall PC, Flannery-Schroeder E, Panichelli-Mindel SM: Therapy with youths with anxiety disorders: a second randomized clinical trial. J Consult Clin Psychol 65:366–380, 1997

Shortt AL, Barrett PM, Fox TL: Evaluating the FRIENDS program: a cognitive-behavioral group treatment for anxious children and their parents. J Clin Child Psychol 30:25–535, 2001

Silverman WK, Kurtines WM, Ginsburg GS, et al: Treating anxiety disorders in children with group cognitive-behavioral therapy: a randomized clinical trial. J Consult Clin Psychol 67:995–1003, 1999

Spence SH, Donovan C, Brechman-Toussain M: The treatment of childhood social phobia: the effectiveness of a social skills training-based, cognitive-behavioral intervention, with and without parental involvement. J Child Psychol Psychiatry 41:713–726, 2000

Table 58–1. Randomized controlled trials examining the efficacy of cognitive-behavioral therapy (CBT)

Author	Participants	Active treatment	Control treatment	Results
Barrett et al. 1996	79 children with SAD, OAD, or SP	CBT; CBT plus family management	Waitlist	CBT plus family management > CBT alone > waitlist
Barrett 1998	60 children with SAD, OAD, or SP	Group CBT; group CBT plus family management	Waitlist	Group CBT = group CBT plus family management > waitlist
Beidel et al. 2000	67 children with SP	Group CBT (SET-C)	Nonspecific active condition (Testbusters)	Group CBT > nonspecific active condition
Beidel et al. 2007	139 children/adolescents with primary diagnosis of SP	Group CBT (SET-C) or fluoxetine	Placebo	Group CBT > fluoxetine > placebo
Bernstein et al. 2000	47 adolescents with school refusal plus anxiety or depression	CBT plus imipramine	CBT plus placebo	CBT plus imipramine > CBT plus placebo
Dadds et al. 1997	128 children with DSM-IV anxiety diagnosis	Group CBT (Coping Koala)	Monitoring group	Group CBT = monitoring group posttreatment; group CBT > monitoring group at 6-month follow-up
Flannery-Schroeder and Kendall 2000	37 children with GAD, SAD, or SP	CBT; group CBT (Coping Cat)	Waitlist	CBT = group CBT > waitlist
Hayward et al. 2000	35 female adolescents	Group CBT	Waitlist	Group CBT > waitlist
Kendall 1994	47 children with OAD, SAD, or avoidant disorder	CBT (Coping Cat)	Waitlist	CBT > waitlist
Kendall et al. 1997	94 children with OAD, SAD, or avoidant disorder	CBT (Coping Cat)	Waitlist	CBT > waitlist
Shortt et al. 2001	71 children with SAD, GAD, or SP	Family-based group CBT (FRIENDS)	Waitlist	Family-based group CBT > waitlist
Silverman et al. 1999b	56 children/adolescents with OAD, GAD, or SP	Group CBT	Waitlist	Group CBT > waitlist
Spence et al. 2000	50 children/adolescents with SP	CBT; CBT with parental involvement	Waitlist	CBT with parental involvement > CBT > waitlist

Note. GAD = generalized anxiety disorder; OAD = overanxious disorder; SAD = separation anxiety disorder; SET-C = Social Effectiveness Therapy for Children; SP = social phobia.

58.2   There is widespread agreement that the key ingredient in cognitive-behavioral therapy (CBT) is the behavioral intervention known as

A. Exposure.
B. Cognitive restructuring.
C. Extinction.
D. Within-session habituation.
E. None of the above.

The correct response is option A.

There is now virtually uniform agreement that the key ingredient in CBT is the behavioral intervention commonly known as *exposure*, a procedure whereby the individual is placed in contact with the object or situation that elicits fear or distress. Graduated exposure is based on a classical conditioning paradigm whereby situations that elicit a low level of fear are introduced first, followed over time by situations that elicit more intense fear. As the number of times that the child confronts the situations increases, even former "high-fear" items no longer elicit distress.

In many instances, graduated exposure is combined with cognitive strategies such as *cognitive restructuring* in an attempt to elicit and change negative thoughts that may be part of the fear complex.

Elimination of fearful behavior is based on an *extinction* model, whereby a person is exposed to a feared object or event but escape or avoidance is prohibited. The individual remains in contact with the feared stimulus until physiological arousal and subjective distress extinguish (dissipate), a process known as *within-session habituation*. **(p. 899)**

58.3   A parent comes to you to express her concern about her 10-year-old daughter, Jackie, who is afraid of dogs and runs away whenever she sees one. You schedule a session with Jackie and her mother and arrange to have a well-behaved dog present. Although Jackie is highly fearful at first, you encourage her to remain in the office until her anxiety diminishes. You are employing a model of treatment based on

A. Implosion therapy.
B. Relaxation training.
C. Extinction.
D. Cognitive restructuring.
E. None of the above.

The correct response is option C.

Elimination of fearful behavior is based on an *extinction* model, whereby a person is exposed to a feared object or event but escape or avoidance is prohibited. The individual remains in contact with the feared stimulus until physiological arousal and subjective distress are extinguished (dissipate), a process known as *within-session habituation*.

Exposure strategies have been misunderstood and mistakenly associated with *implosion therapy*, which uses horrific, frightening, and psychodynamic cues in order to maximize anxiety arousal, which in turn was presumed to enhance rapid extinction. Empirical studies demonstrate that such cues are often ineffective and in many instances may even be countertherapeutic.

Another behavioral intervention is *relaxation training*, a procedure in which children learn to decrease their physiological and subjective arousal by engaging in either muscle tension-relaxation sequences or through cognitive meditation.

Cognitive restructuring, which often is used in conjunction with exposure, teaches children first to recognize negative self-thoughts and then to replace those thoughts with less anxiety-provoking self-statements. **(pp. 899–900)**

58.4   Which of the following treatment approaches may not be effective in preadolescent children?

    A. Intensive exposure.
    B. Cognitive restructuring.
    C. Lack of parental involvement in homework assignments.
    D. All of the above.
    E. None of the above.

The correct response is option D.

Exposure to feared stimuli is essential for successful outcome and the exposure paradigm must be developmentally appropriate. Because of cognitive immaturity, younger children often have difficulty understanding the rationale behind intensive exposure, which is therefore typically reserved for adolescents. With younger children, graduated exposure procedures are recommended and are efficacious. Younger patients may also require more parental involvement with exposure tasks to be completed outside of the session (i.e., homework), whereas adolescents may be more autonomous with scheduling and completing homework assignments.

Young children may not have the mental faculties necessary to engage in cognitive restructuring (Alfano et al. 2002). Fortunately, the elimination of this component from some cognitive-behavioral therapy programs, resulting in a program utilizing primarily exposure techniques, does not reduce its efficacy (Spence et al. 2000). **(p. 900)**

Alfano C, Beidel DC, Turner SM: Cognition in childhood anxiety: conceptual, methodological, and developmental issues. Clin Psychol Rev 22:1209–1238, 2002

Spence SH, Donovan C, Brechman Toussaint M: The treatment of childhood social phobia: the effectiveness of a social skills training-based, cognitive-behavioral intervention, with and without parental involvement. J Child Psychol Psychiatry 41:713–726, 2000

58.5   In controlled trials of cognitive-behavioral therapy (CBT) in children and adolescents, which of the following factors was associated with more positive outcomes?

    A. Higher levels of overall family dysfunction.
    B. Symptoms of depression, fear, and hostility in parents.
    C. Massed treatment sessions rather than once weekly.
    D. At least 6–8 weeks of treatment rather than 4 weeks.
    E. Comorbid symptoms of depression and trait anxiety in children.

The correct response is option C.

In addition to duration, frequency of the treatment sessions also affects treatment response. Specifically, massed treatment sessions (frequent and temporally close applications of the intervention, perhaps occurring 2–3 times per week) achieve superior outcome in a shorter period of time than once-weekly sessions.

Few data are available that specifically examine the number of treatment sessions necessary for optimal treatment response. Outcome data from controlled trials indicate that many children demonstrate significant improvement after 12–16 weeks of treatment.

Parental psychopathology may affect successful treatment of the child. Symptoms of depression, fear, hostility, psychoticism, paranoia, and obsessive-compulsive tendencies have all been negatively associated with treatment outcome (Berman et al. 2000; Southam-Gerow et al. 2001). Additionally, higher levels of overall family dysfunction predict poorer prognosis (Barrett et al. 2005). In contrast, sociodemographic variables do not seem to significantly affect treatment outcome. Efficacy appears consistent across ethnicity, gender, and socioeconomic status (Berman et al. 2000; Ferrell et al. 2004; Pina et al. 2003; Southam-Gerow et al. 2001).

Baseline psychopathology also may affect treatment outcome. Comorbid symptoms of depression and trait anxiety in particular, or higher levels of childhood internalizing disorders in general, were negatively associated with treatment efficacy (Berman et al. 2000; Southam-Gerow et al. 2001). **(p. 901)**

Barrett P, Farrell C, Dadds M et al: Cognitive-behavioral family treatment of childhood obsessive-compulsive disorder: long-term follow-up and predictors of outcome. J Am Acad Child Adolesc Psychiatry 44:1005–1014, 2005

Berman SL, Weems CF, Silverman WK, et al: Predictors of outcome in exposure-based cognitive and behavioral treatments for phobic and anxiety disorders in children. Behav Ther 31:713–731, 2000

Ferrell C, Beidel DC, Turner SM: Assessment and treatment of socially phobic children: a cross cultural comparison. J Clin Child Psychol 33:260–268, 2004

Pina AA, Silverman WK, Fuentes RM, et al: Exposure-based cognitive-behavioral treatment for phobic and anxiety disorders: treatment effects and maintenance for Hispanic/Latino relative to European-American youths. J Am Acad Child Adolesc Psychiatry 42:1179–1187, 2003

Southam-Gerow MA, Kendall PC, Weersing VR: Examining outcome variability: correlates of treatment response in a child and adolescent anxiety clinic. J Clin Child Psychol 30:422–436, 2001

Chapter 59

Cognitive-Behavioral Therapy for Depression

Select the single best response for each question.

59.1 Which of the following statements regarding cognitive-behavioral therapy (CBT) is *false?*

A. CBT has been found to be efficacious in treating depressed youth.

B. Early meta-analyses reported low mean effect sizes for CBT with depressed youth compared with more recent meta-analyses, which found higher mean effect sizes.

C. CBT delivered in clinical settings yields smaller effect sizes relative to CBT delivered in research settings.

D. CBT can be effective in reducing suicidal ideation among depressed adolescents.

E. None of the above.

The correct response is option B.

Early meta-analyses reported high mean effect sizes for CBT with depressed youth (Lewinsohn and Clarke 1999; Michael and Crowley 2002; Reinecke et al. 1998). More recent meta-analyses found smaller mean effect sizes but still presented positive evidence for the efficacy of CBT (Klein et al. 2007; Weisz et al. 2006).

Klein et al. (2007) found several moderators of treatment outcome effect sizes. Studies that yielded significantly smaller effect sizes employed intent-to-treat statistical analyses, compared CBT to active treatments rather than controls, and delivered the intervention in clinical rather than research settings.

Current evidence suggests that CBT can be effective for the treatment of major depression among youth, that improvements in mood are associated with improved psychosocial functioning, and that CBT can be effective in reducing suicidal ideation among depressed adolescents. **(p. 907)**

Klein JB, Jacobs RH, Reinecke MA: Cognitive-behavioral therapy for adolescent depression: a meta-analytic investigation of changes in effect-size estimates. J Am Acad Child Adolesc Psychiatry 46:1403-1413, 2007

Lewinsohn P, Clarke G: Psychosocial treatments for adolescent depression. Clin Psychol Rev 19:329–342, 1999

Michael KD, Crowley SL: How effective are treatments for child and adolescent depression? A meta-analytic review. Clin Psychol Rev 22:247–269, 2002

Reinecke MA, Ryan N, DuBois D: Cognitive-behavioral therapy of depression and depressive symptoms during adolescence: a review and meta-analysis. J Am Acad Child Adolesc Psychiatry 37:26–34, 1998

Weisz JR, McCarty CA, Valeri SM: Effects of psychotherapy for children and adolescents: a meta-analysis. Psychol Bull 132:132–149, 2006

59.2 Which of the following cognitive vulnerabilities observed in depressed children and adolescents can be targets of cognitive-behavioral therapy (CBT) interventions?

A. Negative thoughts about self.

B. Anticipation of rejection.

C. Anticipation of failure.

D. Perfectionistic standards.

E. All of the above.

The correct response is option E.

Depressed children and adolescents demonstrate many of the same biases and distortions characteristic of depressed adults. They manifest negative thoughts about themselves, the world, and their future, attending selectively to negative events.

Depressed youth anticipate rejection and tend to ruminate about their problems. Deficits in rational problem-solving and problem-solving motivation also are manifest. Specifically, they anticipate that their attempts to solve life's problems will be unsuccessful, choosing to either avoid addressing problems directly or approach them impulsively. Perfectionistic standards can impede both treatment and overall sense of self-esteem. A negative attributional style includes viewing losses or failures as stemming from personal characteristics that are broad, stable, and unchanging. These proposed cognitive vulnerabilities are all targets of CBT intervention. **(p. 908)**

59.3   Which of the following statements regarding cognitive-behavioral therapy (CBT) is *false?*

   A. CBT is formulation based and prescriptive.
   B. CBT treatment is usually open ended.
   C. An agenda is set up and homework is usually assigned.
   D. Collaboration between the therapist and the patient is needed to work together toward specific goals.
   E. Negative thoughts are seen not as facts, but rather as hypotheses to be explored.

The correct response is option B.

An essential characteristic of CBT is its *time-limited* nature. Treatment is not typically open ended or long term.

CBT is formulation based and prescriptive. Active and focused treatment is organized in accord with an *agenda. Homework* assignments allow for practicing cognitive and behavioral skills during the week. The therapeutic relationship is characterized by *collaboration.* Negative thoughts are seen as hypotheses to be explored rather than facts to be accepted. Working together, therapist and child test the utility and validity of these beliefs. **(p. 908)**

59.4   Which of the following is *not* a specific intervention commonly used in cognitive-behavioral therapy (CBT)?

   A. Rational problem-solving.
   B. Rationally disputing automatic thoughts.
   C. Affect regulation.
   D. Defense interpretation.
   E. Parent training.

The correct response is option D.

Defense interpretation is not a specific intervention commonly used in CBT.

Specific interventions commonly used in CBT are as follows:

   1. Introducing CBT model and treatment rationale
   2. Goal setting
   3. Mood monitoring
   4. Activity scheduling (Pleasant/Social/Mastery)
   5. Rational problem-solving and problem-solving motivation
   6. Rationally disputing automatic thoughts, replacing with adaptive self-statements
   7. Cognitive distortions
   8. Affect regulation
   9. Social skills
   10. Assertiveness

11. Communication and compromise
12. Attachment security
13. Parent training
14. Booster sessions and relapse prevention

(p. 909 [Table 59–2])

59.5 In cognitive-behavioral therapy (CBT), patients are encouraged to test the validity and utility of their negative and upsetting thoughts by asking which of the following questions?

    A. What is the evidence that supports the thought?
    B. Is there any contradicting evidence?
    C. Is there another way to look at the situation?
    D. If the negative thought is true, is it really so big a deal?
    E. All of the above.

The correct response is option E.

Adaptive counterthoughts allow the patient to "talk back" to negative cognitions. Using automatic thoughts the adolescent has identified, the CBT therapist teaches the adolescent specific strategies for rectifying maladaptive thoughts. Upsetting thoughts are seen as questions or hypotheses to be tested, and evidence is sought to ascertain their validity and utility. Specifically, patients are taught to ask the following: 1) What is the evidence that supports the thought? 2) Is there any contradictory evidence? Is there any evidence I have overlooked or anything that might lead me to think that the thought may not be true? 3) Is there another way of looking at the situation? 4) If the negative thought is true, is it really so big a deal? 5) What's the solution? What can be done to handle this? **(p. 910)**

Chapter 60

Motivational Interviewing

Select the single best response for each question.

60.1   What is the major goal of motivational interviewing?

A. Providing insight.
B. Healing conflict.
C. Resolving ambivalence.
D. Improving relationships.
E. Stabilizing affect.

The correct response is option C.

Motivational interviewing is "a client-centered, directive method for enhancing intrinsic motivation for change by exploring and resolving ambivalence" (Miller and Rollnick 2002, p. 25).

Motivational interviewing posits that resistance to behavior change may be due to a lack of awareness or concern about a problem or to a conflict of opposing desires expressed as ambivalence. Ambivalence is viewed as normal rather than pathological, and a primary goal of motivational interviewing is to identify, explore, and resolve ambivalence (Miller and Rollnick 1991). **(pp. 915–916)**

> Miller WR, Rollnick S: Motivational Interviewing: Preparing People to Change Addictive Behavior. New York, Guilford, 1991
> Miller WR, Rollnick S: Motivational Interviewing: Preparing People for Change, 2nd Edition. New York, Guilford, 2002

60.2   Motivational interviewing uses a cluster of counseling skills referred to as OARS. Which of the following letter–skill pairings is correct?

A. O = organization.
B. A = affect resolution.
C. R = resistance awareness.
D. S = symptom relief.
E. None of the above.

The correct response is option E.

Motivational interviewing uses a cluster of counseling skills referred to as OARS: **O**pen-ended questions, **A**ffirmations, **R**eflective listening, and **S**ummaries. Motivational interviewing assumes that client awareness and concern will be facilitated by using these skills while examining an individual's particular values, interests, and concerns in a collaborative, nonjudgmental manner (Miller and Rollnick 2002). **(p. 916)**

> Miller WR, Rollnick S: Motivational Interviewing: Preparing People for Change, 2nd Edition. New York, Guilford, 2002

60.3 In the stages of change model, a patient who has some ambivalence and is willing to consider change, but who has not yet made a commitment, would be considered to be in what stage?

    A. Maintenance.
    B. Preparation.
    C. Precontemplation.
    D. Contemplation.
    E. Action.

The correct response is option D.

The stages of change model (Prochaska and DiClemente 1982) suggests that change is based on a client's level of awareness and concern about a particular problem as well as the degree of commitment for change. These stages include *precontemplation* (is not aware of the need for change or is resistant to change), *contemplation* (has some ambivalence and is willing to consider change but not yet willing to make a commitment), *preparation* (is planning change and willing to plan goal-oriented steps), *action* (is actively taking steps to change), and *maintenance* (has achieved change goals and works to maintain changes). Motivational interviewing suggests that applying different approaches in order to meet people where they are in the change process leads to better therapeutic outcomes (Miller and Rollnick 1991). **(p. 916)**

> Miller WR, Rollnick S: Motivational Interviewing: Preparing People to Change Addictive Behavior. New York, Guilford, 1991
> Prochaska JO, DiClemente CC: Transtheoretical therapy: toward a more integrative model of change. Psychotherapy Theory, Research, and Practice 19:276–288, 1982

60.4 Much of the research literature on the efficacy of motivational interviewing in adolescents has focused on which of the following disorders?

    A. Generalized anxiety disorder.
    B. Alcohol and substance use disorders.
    C. Social phobia.
    D. Panic disorder.
    E. Avoidant disorder.

The correct response is option B.

The literature describing the use of motivational interviewing with adolescents is limited but growing. Studies to date have suggested efficacy while also informing the potential benefit of incorporating motivational interviewing into other standard treatments. Motivational interviewing has primarily been evaluated in studies of brief intervention models for alcohol- and drug-using youth based on motivational interviewing principles and techniques (Feldstein and Ginsburg 2006). These models are very brief (one to five sessions), and although abstinence is an expressed outcome, reduction in harmful alcohol use and drug using patterns is the primary target. The approach in each of these brief intervention programs is raising patient awareness of the problem while eliciting motivation by providing personal feedback about the ways in which the behavior might be interfering with expressed personal goals. Further goal setting is then conducted to modify the behavior in an effort to reduce harm while also informing and encouraging future behavior that might enhance progress toward personal goals. **(p. 917)**

> Feldstein SW, Ginsburg JID: Motivational interviewing with dually diagnosed adolescents in juvenile justice settings. Brief Treatment and Crisis Intervention 6:218–233, 2006

60.5   Motivational interviewing is guided by which of the following principles?

    A. Express empathy.
    B. Develop discrepancy.
    C. Roll with resistance.
    D. Support self-efficacy.
    E. All of the above.

The correct response is option E.

All of the above are principles of motivational interviewing:

- *Express empathy.* Empathy is the ability to view the world through the eyes of another by seeing, feeling, and understanding things as if living the same life experience. Expression of empathy works to reduce defensiveness by reassuring patients that they are understood and not "crazy" for having their particular set of thoughts and feelings.
- *Develop discrepancy.* Motivation for change occurs when clients recognize a faulty connection between their behavior and their self-image, desires, or goals. In motivational interviewing the therapist's task is to gently but directly guide the patient toward evaluating whether or not behavior choices are consistent with personal values and aspirations (develops discrepancy). Motivational interviewing encourages individuals to examine whether they are living with full integrity, and if not, to consider making the changes that would enable a more congruent sense of self.
- *Roll with resistance.* Resistance is common when working with adolescent patients. Rolling with resistance is best accomplished by using a collaborative and friendly style and by not arguing with or provoking the patient. Motivational interviewing techniques that may help in overcoming patient resistance include simple reflections, amplified reflections, double-sided reflections, shifting focus, agreement with a twist, reframing, and siding with the negative (Miller and Rollnick 2002).
- *Support self-efficacy.* The client must come to believe in his or her own capacity for change. The motivational interviewing therapist helps the patient identify his or her assets and strengths by guiding him or her to call up past victories that might inform the patient's ability to handle new challenges (support self-efficacy).

(pp. 916–917)

Miller WR, Rollnick S: Motivational Interviewing: Preparing People for Change, 2nd Edition. New York, Guilford, 2002

Chapter 61

Systems of Care, Wraparound Services, and Home-Based Services

Select the single best response for each question.

61.1 Which of the following statements regarding the historical roots of system of care (SOC) approaches and wraparound services is *false?*

    A. Congress funded the Child and Adolescent Service System Program (CASSP) in 1984.
    B. At the time CASSP was founded, a wide range of services were available to children with significant difficulties.
    C. The guiding principle of the CASSP was the SOC.
    D. The three core values of SOC are child and family centered, community based, and culturally competent.
    E. Wraparound services and intensive home-based services are common features of an SOC approach.

The correct response is option B.

At the time CASSP was funded by Congress in 1984, children who had the most significant difficulties were also those least likely to get the range of services they might need.

The guiding principle of the CASSP was the SOC, a multiagency approach to the delivery of services. The three core values of an SOC are the child and family's needs, community-based services with decision making remaining at the community level, and care that is culturally competent and responsive to the family's cultural, racial, and ethnic characteristics (Stroul 2003).

With the focus on empowering families in forging individualized care plans, wraparound services and intensive home-based services also became common features of an SOC approach (Burns et al. 2000). **(p. 926)**

> Burns BJ, Schoenwald SK, Burchard JD, et al: Comprehensive community-based interventions for youth with severe emotional disorders: multisystemic therapy and the wraparound process. Journal of Child and Family Studies 9:283–314, 2000
> Stroul BA: Systems of care: a framework for children's mental health care, in The Handbook of Child and Adolescent Systems of Care: The New Community Psychiatry. San Francisco, CA, Jossey-Bass, 2003, pp 17–34

61.2 Which of the following is *not* a guiding principle of systems of care?

    A. Services should be individualized for the child and family.
    B. Services should be developmentally appropriate and least restrictive.
    C. Case management should be provided to coordinate care as needed.
    D. A smooth transition to adult services should be ensured.
    E. Caregivers need not be fully integrated in the treatment process.

The correct response is option E.

Systems of care are guided by the following principles (Stroul 2003):

- Children with emotional disturbances should receive services that address their emotional, social, educational, and physical needs.
- Services should be individualized for the child and family.
- Services should be developmentally appropriate and least restrictive.
- Caregivers should be fully integrated in the planning and treatment process.
- Services should be integrated and linked to one another.
- Case management should be provided to coordinate care as needed.
- Early identification and intervention should be promoted to ameliorate outcomes.
- A smooth transition to adult services should be ensured.
- The rights of children with emotional disturbances should be protected and efforts at advocacy promoted.
- All children with emotional disturbances should receive services regardless of race, sex, physical disability, religion, or other characteristics.

(p. 927 [Table 61–2])

Stroul BA: Systems of care: a framework for children's mental health care, in The Handbook of Child and Adolescent Systems of Care: The New Community Psychiatry. San Francisco, CA, Jossey-Bass, 2003, pp 17–34

61.3   Wraparound services are helpful when children and families have significant emotional and behavioral difficulties. Key elements of wraparound services include all of the following *except*

A. The youth and family must be full and active partners at every level in every activity.
B. The wraparound approach must be team driven.
C. The services must encompass both community and inpatient settings.
D. There must be an unconditional commitment to serve children and their families.
E. The wraparound teams must have flexible approaches and adequate funding.

The correct response is option C.

Wraparound services are located in the community (in residential and school settings), not in inpatient environments.

A consensus group of experts (Burns and Goldman 1999) defined the key elements of wraparound services as follows:

- The youth and family must be full and active partners at every level and in every activity of the wraparound process. They must have a voice.
- The wraparound approach must be a team-driven process involving the family, child, natural supports, agencies, and community services working together to develop, implement, and evaluate the individualized plan.
- Wraparound services must be located in the community, with all efforts toward serving the identified youth in community, residential, and school settings.
- The process must be culturally competent, building on the unique values, preferences, and strengths of children and families and their communities.
- Services and supports must be individualized and built on strengths, and must meet the needs of children and families across life domains to promote success, safety, and permanence in home, school, and community.
- Wraparound plans must include a balance of formal services and informal community and family supports.
- There must be an unconditional commitment to serve children and their families.

- Plans of care should be developed and implemented based on an interagency, community-based collaborative process.
- Wraparound child and family teams must have flexible approaches and adequate and flexible funding.
- Outcomes must be determined and measured for the system, for the program, and for the individual child and family.

(p. 928 [Table 61–3])

> Burns BK, Goldman SK: Executive summary, in Promising Practices in Wraparound for Children With Severe Emotional Disorders and Their Families (Systems of Care: Promising Practices in Children's Mental Health series, Vol IV, edited by Burns BK, Goldman SK). Washington, DC, Center for Effective Collaboration and Practice, American Institutes for Research, 1999, pp 11–18

61.4   Home-based services serve children with mental health needs who are involved in the child welfare or juvenile justice systems. Which of the following programs is generally delivered in the office but has also been used as an in-home service?

   A. Brief Strategic Family Therapy.
   B. Multisystemic Therapy.
   C. Intensive In-Home Child and Adolescent Psychiatric Service.
   D. Massachusetts Mental Health Services Program for Youth (MHSPY).
   E. The Nurse-Family Partnership.

The correct response is option A.

Brief Strategic Family Therapy is a 12- to 15-session problem-focused intervention delivered over 3 months. Although generally delivered in the office, it has also been used as an in-home service.

Multisystemic therapy is a home-based, family-focused program, meant to treat youth who have serious behavioral problems. It was developed and refined serving the juvenile justice population and has been available for more than two decades. An adapted model has been applied to populations with primarily mental health needs (Multisystemic Therapy Services 2007).

The Intensive In-Home Child and Adolescent Psychiatric Service (IICAPS) (Woolston et al. 2007), developed at Yale University in 1997, is a home-based intervention for children and adolescents with serious emotional and behavioral problems. Most of the youth served are at risk of requiring institutional care or have exhausted traditional outpatient services.

Although the MHSPY is limited to Massachusetts (Grimes and Mullin 2006), it is an example of services delivered with a system of care and wraparound philosophy and in which clinical data are tracked. The care manager is responsible for direct clinical intervention, which includes home-based work to identify the family's needs, coordination of care among formal and informal supports, and case administration such as payment authorization or creation of new services.

The Nurse-Family Partnership service is delivered in the home as both treatment for the parent and prevention for the child. In this program, nurses visit low-income, first-time mothers weekly or biweekly from the prenatal period until the child reaches the age of 2 years. **(pp. 932–936)**

> Grimes KE, Mullin B: MHSPY: a children's health initiative for maintaining at-risk youth in the community. J Behav Health Serv Res 33:196–212, 2006
> Multisystemic Therapy Services: Complete Overview: Research on Effectiveness. Mt. Pleasant, SC, Multisystemic Therapy Services, 2007. Available at: http://www.mstservices.com/complete_overview.php. Accessed April 29, 2009.
> Woolston JL, Adnopoz J, Berkowitz SJ: IICAPS: A Home-Based Psychiatric Treatment for Children and Adolescents. New Haven, CT, Yale University Press, 2007

61.5 Which of the following interventions has been empirically validated for the treatment of substance abuse and conduct problems?

    A. Intensive In-Home Child and Adolescent Psychiatric Service.
    B. Functional Family Therapy.
    C. Multidimensional Treatment Foster Care.
    D. Brief Strategic Family Therapy.
    E. Nurse-Family Partnership.

The correct response is option D.

Brief Strategic Family Therapy is manualized and has been empirically validated for the treatment of substance abuse and conduct problems and has also been modified to serve the cultural needs of Hispanic youth (Szapocznik et al. 2002). **(p. 935)**

> Szapocznik J, Robbins MS, Mitrani VB, et al: Brief strategic family therapy, in Comprehensive Handbook of Psychotherapy: Integrative/Eclectic, Vol 4. Edited by Kaslow FW. Hoboken, NJ, John Wiley & Sons, 2002, pp 83–109

Chapter 62

Milieu Treatment

Inpatient, Partial Hospitalization, and Residential Programs

Select the single best response for each question.

62.1 Which of the following statements regarding the historical perspective of milieu treatments is *false?*

A. Therapeutic milieus began as orphanages and boarding schools for youth with mental handicaps and psychiatric illness.
B. Later, they evolved into child care institutions and group foster homes.
C. In the past 15 years there has been a marked proliferation of unregulated facilities.
D. Managed care has lessened problems of access to hospital inpatient units (IUs).
E. There was a decreased use of IUs in the 1990s.

The correct response is option D.

Managed care has not lessened problems of access to and appropriate use of IU care across geographical areas but has resulted in decreased use and shortened lengths of stay (Case et al. 2007; Cuellar et al. 2001).

Therapeutic milieus began as orphanages and boarding schools for youngsters with mental handicaps and psychiatric illness and evolved into child care institutions and group foster homes to assist emotionally disturbed and socially deviant children. The past 15 years were marked by a proliferation of unregulated facilities, generating critical media attention concerning lack of community contact and serious abuses (Teich and Ireys 2007). Behavior problems were the predominant focus of IUs that began in the early 1920s. Ascendancy of a managed mental health care model and other forces led to their decreased use in the 1990s. Closing of mostly for-profit programs and publicly funded state and county units has resulted (Parmelee and Nierman 2006). **(pp. 939–940)**

Case BG, Olfson M, Marcus SC, et al: Trends in the inpatient mental health treatment of children and adolescents in US community hospitals. Arch Gen Psychiatry 64:89–96, 2007

Cuellar AE, Libby AM, Snowden LR: How capitated mental health care affects utilization by youth in the juvenile justice and child welfare systems. Ment Health Serv Res 3:61–72, 2001

Parmelee DX, Nierman P: Transitions from institutional to community systems of care, in Community Child and Adolescent Psychiatry: A Manual of Clinical Practice and Consultation. Edited by Petti TA, Salguero C. Washington, DC, American Psychiatric Publishing, 2006, pp 249–257

Teich JL, Ireys HT: A national survey of state licensing, regulating, and monitoring of residential facilities for children with mental illness. Psychiatr Serv 58:991–998, 2007

62.2 Which of the following components is essential for providing effective milieu treatment?

A. Estimation of ability to form therapeutic alliance.
B. Determination of critical factors prior to admission.
C. Consideration of multiple domains in the life of the mentally ill child and family.
D. Availability of aftercare by other services in the continuum of care.
E. All of the above.

The correct response is option E.

All of the factors listed above are essential in providing effective milieu treatments (Table 62–1). **(p. 941 [Table 62–1])**

Table 62–1.   Essential milieu factors for patient assessment, safety monitoring and assurance, and transition to community

Patient assessment

Estimation of ability to form therapeutic alliance

Determination of critical factors prior to admission

    Child and family functioning

    Consistency of discipline within family

    Family perceived stress

    Contact with delinquent peers for those with disruptive disorders

    Extent of drug and/or alcohol use or abuse

Consideration of multiple domains in the life of mentally ill child and family

Safety monitoring and assurance

Protection of vulnerable populations of youth (e.g., autism spectrum, developmentally delayed, prior abuse or neglect)

Monitoring extent of

    Contact with delinquent peers

    Potential harm to self or others

    Adherence of patient and family to program rules and recommendations

    Appropriate assessment of biopsychosocial risk factors (i.e., predisposing, precipitating, perpetuating, and preventive factors)

Transition to community

Interdisciplinary functioning, coordination, and communication

Availability of aftercare by other services in the continuum of care

    Transitional psychosocial services for step-down processes within the mental health system

    Physicians and related professionals for medication management

---

62.3   In determining whether a patient warrants an inpatient admission for suicidality, which of the following factors is considered to be least risky?

    A. Dysfunctional family patterns.

    B. Clearly abnormal mental state in a suicide attempter.

    C. Stated persistent wish to die.

    D. Adequate supervision and support not possible outside therapeutic milieu.

    E. Unresolved biopsychosocial risk factors unlikely to change sufficiently to allow safe return home.

The correct response is option A.

A dysfunctional family pattern is not a critical factor in determining the need to hospitalize a youngster with suicidal behavior.

    Risk factors warranting admission include a clearly abnormal mental state or suicidal ideation in a suicide attempter, a stated persistent wish to die, the absence of adequate supervision and support outside a therapeutic milieu, and unresolved biopsychosocial risk factors unlikely to change sufficiently to allow safe return home. **(pp. 943 [Table 62–3])**

62.4 Some milieu treatment programs are more successful than others in providing effective care. Components of effective milieu treatment include all of the following *except*

    A. Optimization of safety for patient, peers, and staff.
    B. Limitation of dysfunctional family involvement.
    C. Presence of treatment plan addressing factors identified in case formulation.
    D. Availability of financial support for duration of required treatment.
    E. Discharge when lesser level of care will suffice and is appropriate.

The correct response is option B.

Limitation of family involvement is not a recommended component of effective milieu treatment; rather, ongoing family involvement is encouraged. Recommendations for ensuring effective milieu treatment (Leichtman et al. 2001; Lyons and Schaefer 2000; Whittaker 2004) are as follows:

- Optimize safety for patient, peers, and staff.
- Urge family and patient collaboration in treatment plan development.
- Encourage ongoing family involvement (transportation, funding).
- Ensure that treatment plan addresses factors identified in case formulation.
- Arrange for financial support for duration of required treatment.
- Discharge when a lesser level of care will suffice and is appropriate.

(p. 944 [Table 62–4])

Leichtman M, Leichtman ML, Barber CC, et al: Effectiveness of intensive short-term residential treatment with severely disturbed adolescents. Am J Orthopsychiatry 71:227–235, 2001

Lyons JS, Schaefer K: Mental health and dangerousness: characteristics and outcomes of children and adolescents in residential care. J Child Fam Stud 9:67–73, 2000

Whittaker JK: The re-invention of residential treatment: an agenda for research and practice. Child Adolesc Psychiatr Clin North Am 13:267–278, 2004

62.5 According to Pottick et al. (2004), which of the following is the most frequent presenting problem in acute specialty mental health inpatient programs?

    A. Suicidality.
    B. Aggression.
    C. Depressed or anxious mood (including self-harm).
    D. Family problems.
    E. Alcohol or drug use.

The correct response is option C.

The most frequent presenting problem in acute specialty mental health inpatient programs is depression or anxious mood, with a prevalence rate of 65%. Suicidality (55%), aggression (49%), family problems (47%), alcohol or drug use (26%), and delinquent behavior (25%) follow. **(p. 948 [Table 62–6])**

Pottick K, Warner L, Isaacs M, et al: Children and adolescents admitted to specialty mental health care in the United States, 1986 and 1997, in Mental Health in the United States, 2002. DHHS Publ No SMA-3938. Edited by Manderscheid RW, Henderson MJ. Rockville, MD. Center for Mental Health Services, Substance Abuse and Mental Health Services Administration, 2004, pp 314–326

62.6   In regard to future directions in the field of milieu treatment, critical issues to be addressed include which of the following?

    A. Overcoming barriers to translating evidence-based practice into milieu treatment settings.

    B. Improving aftercare services.

    C. Decreasing readmission rates.

    D. Expanding and evaluating use of standardized measures for milieu treatments.

    E. All of the above.

The correct response is option E.

Clinical questions and controversies expected to be addressed in the next 5 years for milieu treatments must include issues of greatest need: 1) overcoming barriers to translating evidence-based practice into milieu treatment settings and incorporating related systematic evaluation; 2) improving aftercare services so that gains made in milieu treatment settings will be maintained; 3) determining modifiable factors related to failed return to home or other placements; 4) decreasing readmission rates; 5) expanding and evaluating use of standardized measures for milieu treatments; 6) moving toward more manualized, time-limited treatments for families and patients; 7) regulating non–mental health residential facilities; 8) reducing impulsive aggression and violence; and 9) eliminating deaths from seclusion and restraint in mental health milieu treatment settings. **(p. 950)**

Chapter 63

School-Based Interventions

Select the single best response for each question.

63.1 Since the mid-twentieth century, mental health consultation and service to schools has undergone significant expansion, stimulated by a number of broad sociocultural movements coincident with that period. Which of the following is *not* one of the major sociocultural movements contributing to the expanded role of mental health in education?

    A. The community mental health movement after the Vietnam War.
    B. The civil rights movement of the 1960s.
    C. The dramatic changes in social norms from the 1960s through the 1980s.
    D. The growth of the school-based health clinic movement in the 1990s.
    E. Recent trends toward greater academic accountability in school settings.

The correct response is option A.

The community mental health movement after World War II, not the Vietnam War, advanced the idea that schools were appropriate community-based sites for the delivery of mental health services.

For more than a century, clinicians have collaborated with school personnel to improve the mental health of students. Since the 1950s, a number of psychiatrists have made seminal contributions to the interface between psychiatry and education, notably Caplan (1970), Berlin (1975), Comer (1992), and Berkovitz (1998, 2001). During this time, mental health consultation and service to schools underwent five major periods of expansion that were stimulated by broad sociocultural movements. First, the community mental health movement after World War II advanced the idea that schools were appropriate community-based sites for the delivery of mental health services. Second, the civil rights movement in the 1960s led to educational rights legislation prohibiting discrimination against and providing services to students with mental disabilities. Third, the dramatic change in social mores in the 1960s through the 1980s led to students' increased involvement in risky behaviors and pressure on schools to intervene with preventive interventions. Fourth, the growth of the school-based health clinic movement in the 1990s led to recognition of the high prevalence of mental health problems among students attending the clinics (Lear et al. 1991; Walter et al. 1995) and the corresponding need for increased mental health services. Most recent is the move toward greater academic accountability in the school setting (as exemplified by the "No Child Left Behind" legislation), which is leading to a call for parallel accountability in the social-emotional domain of education. **(pp. 957–958)**

Berkovitz IH: School consultation, in Handbook of Child and Adolescent Psychiatry, Vol 7. Edited by Noshpitz JD, Adams PL, Bleiberg E. New York, Wiley, 1998

Berkovitz IH (ed): School Consultation/Intervention: Child and Adolescent Psychiatric Clinics of North America Philadelphia, PA, WB Saunders, 2001

Berlin IN: Psychiatry and the school, in Comprehensive Textbook of Psychiatry II. Edited by Freedman AM, Kaplan HI, Sadow BJ. Baltimore, MD, Williams & Wilkins, 1975, pp 2253–2255

Caplan G: The Theory and Practice of Mental Health Consultation. New York, Basic Books, 1970

Comer JP: School consultation, in Psychiatry, Vol 2. Edited by Michels R, Cooper AM, Guze SB. Philadelphia, PA, Lippincott, 1992, pp 1–10

Lear JG, Gleicher HB, St. Germaine A, et al: Reorganizing health care for adolescents: the experience of the school-based adolescent health care program. J Adolesc Health 12:450–458, 1991

Walter HJ, Vaughan RD, Armstrong B, et al: School-based health care for urban minority junior high school students. Arch Pediatr Adolesc Med 149:1221–1225, 1995

63.2 Which of the following statements regarding models of school consultation and clinical care is *false?*

    A. In the case consultation model, the consultation may be direct or indirect.
    B. In the systems consultation model, individual students' needs are specifically addressed.
    C. In the school-based health center model, a broad range of mental health services are provided by mental health practitioners.
    D. In the school-linked health center model, off-site hospitals or community clinics are contracted to provide mental health services to school students.
    E. In the expanded school mental health programs model, schools partner with community organizations to coordinate and integrate the variety of existing programs into a coherent whole.

The correct response is option B.

In the systems consultation model, clinicians are paid by the school to advise school personnel about the creation of a milieu that is conducive to learning. Individual students' needs typically are not addressed in this type of consultation, rather the focus of consultation may include creating a positive school environment, valuing diversity in the school, improving attendance, building school connectedness among students and parents, fostering teacher and staff morale, developing and coordinating mental health programs, and planning for crisis situations.

In the consultation model, clinicians advise school personnel about appropriate educational and/or therapeutic approaches to and/or services for students with developmental, cognitive, emotional, behavioral, or social problems. The consultation may be direct or indirect.

School-based health centers typically are staffed by a multidisciplinary team of providers and are funded by a variety of mechanisms (e.g., grants, contracts, state and local allocations, fee-for-service). Centers with mental health practitioners can provide a broad range of mental health services, including assessment; individual, group, and family psychotherapy; pharmacotherapy; and prevention and health promotion activities.

In school-linked health centers, schools are linked with hospitals or community clinics that are contracted to provide medical and mental health services to students at convenient locations off-site from the school.

Proponents of expanded school mental health (Weist and Albus 2004) espouse the belief that all students should have access to a broad range of preventive, early intervention, and clinical treatment services. To achieve this goal, schools must partner with community organizations to coordinate and integrate the variety of existing programs and funding streams into a coherent whole. **(pp. 958–959)**

Weist MD, Albus KE: Expanded school mental health: exploring program details and developing the research base. Behav Mod 28:463–471, 2004

63.3 School climate greatly influences the desirability and effectiveness of mental health interventions. Key components of a positive school climate include all of the following *except*

    A. A supportive, welcoming atmosphere.
    B. A variety of learning experiences.
    C. Low expectations for achievement and self-regulation.
    D. Fair and effective discipline.
    E. Opportunities for participation in extracurricular activities.

The correct response is option C.

The milieu of a school is a key factor influencing the desirability and effectiveness of mental health interventions. The school climate literature supports several key components of a positive climate, including a supportive, welcoming atmosphere; respectful peer and adult relationships; a variety of learning experiences; high expectations for achievement and self-regulation; fair and effective discipline; participation in extracurricular activities; and parent/community involvement (Libbey 2004). **(p. 959)**

> Libbey HP: Measuring student relationship to school: attachment, bonding, connectedness, and engagement. J Sch Health 74:274–283, 2004

63.4   Classroom accommodations provided for students with attention-deficit/hyperactivity disorder (ADHD) include all of the following *except*

    A. Provide verbal and visual cues to stay on task.
    B. Use small-group instruction.
    C. Simplify and repeat directions.
    D. Provide duplicate materials.
    E. Allow student to observe others before performing tasks.

The correct response is option E.

All of the above accommodations are appropriate for students with ADHD, with the exception of option E, which is recommended for students with social anxiety.

The Americans With Disabilities Act prohibits the denial of educational services to students with disabilities and prohibits discrimination against all such students once enrolled. If parents suspect their child has a disability, they can request an evaluation to see what accommodations might be helpful. Accommodations are environmental changes designed to overcome impediments to learning posed by the disability. Accommodations can be formalized in a written 504 Plan. This type of plan derives from Section 504 of the Rehabilitation Act of 1973, which mandates inclusion without discrimination for any person who has a "physical or mental impairment that substantially limits a major life activity." **(p. 961; see also Table 63–1)**

> Rehabilitation Act of 1973. P.L. 93–112 93rd Congress, H. R. 8070 September 26, 1973

63.5   A child with a suspected disability should undergo a special education evaluation to determine eligibility for special education services. All of the following statements concerning Individualized Education Programs (IEPs) are correct *except*

    A. IEPs can include specific accommodations.
    B. IEPs can include curriculum modification.
    C. IEPs are reviewed and revised annually.
    D. Every year a comprehensive reevaluation is conducted to determine continued eligibility for an IEP.
    E. Children in an IEP are afforded special disciplinary consideration.

The correct response is option D.

Every 3 years, a comprehensive reevaluation is conducted by a school-based team to determine whether the child continues to meet eligibility criteria for special education services and what services should be provided.

In addition to special education (i.e., instructional) services, the IEP may specify relevant modifications, accommodations and/or related services, and the setting in which they will be provided.

Specific accommodations (i.e., environmental changes designed to overcome impediments to learning posed by the disability) and/or related services (i.e., noninstructional services required to assist a child with a disability to benefit from special education) may be recommended for inclusion in the IEP. Modifications (i.e., curricular changes that can reduce learning expectations) should be recommended only with caution, as they may have the unintended consequence of reducing the child's opportunity to learn critical instructional content. The IEP is reviewed and revised annually.

Children with an IEP are afforded special disciplinary considerations. For example, children with an attention or tic disorder may not be able to sit still or quietly. **(pp. 961–963)**

Chapter 64

Collaborating With Primary Care

Select the single best response for each question.

64.1 Optimal mental health care requires collaboration between the primary care physician and mental health specialists. Collaborative mental health care can be considered along a spectrum encompassing all of the following levels *except*

    A. Primarily primary care.
    B. Primarily primary care with consultation.
    C. Shared care.
    D. Shared care and lower levels of care.
    E. Primarily mental health care.

The correct response is option D.

Collaborative mental health care can be considered along a spectrum of five levels:

    1. *Primarily primary care:* The pediatrician or family physician identifies and treats the child with a mental illness with a mild level of acuity.
    2. *Primarily primary care with consultation:* The primary care provider consults with a child psychiatrist or a psychologist regarding approaches to assessment, diagnosis, and treatment.
    3. *Shared care:* The primary care physician identifies, assesses, and then refers for an emergency consultation with a child and adolescent psychiatrist but then shares in the ongoing care of the patient.
    4. *Shared care and higher levels of care:* The patient may require a higher level of care such as more frequent follow-up visits, closer monitoring, and even hospitalization, partial hospitalization, or day treatment.
    5. *Primarily mental health care:* The patient is referred to mental health specialty care for ongoing treatment and management.

(pp. 980–981)

64.2 For the physician treating a child with attention-deficit/hyperactivity disorder (ADHD) who has been unresponsive to ADHD medications or who experiences exacerbation of a previously controlled depression, which level of collaborative mental health care is warranted?

    A. Primarily primary care.
    B. Primarily primary care with consultation.
    C. Shared care.
    D. Shared care and higher levels of care.
    E. Primarily mental health care.

The correct response is option B.

In the treatment of a child with ADHD unresponsive to stimulants, atomoxetine, clonidine, or guanfacine, or of a child with exacerbation of a previously controlled depression, the primary care physician should continue to follow the patient and seek consultation from a child psychiatrist.

Collaborative mental health care can be considered along a spectrum of five levels:

1. *Primarily primary care:* The pediatrician or family physician identifies and treats the child with a mental illness with a mild level of acuity.
2. *Primarily primary care with consultation:* The primary care provider consults with a child psychiatrist or a psychologist regarding approaches to assessment, diagnosis, and treatment.
3. *Shared care:* The primary care physician identifies, assesses, and then refers for an emergency consultation with a child and adolescent psychiatrist but then shares in the ongoing care of the patient.
4. *Shared care and higher levels of care:* The patient may require a higher level of care such as more frequent follow-up visits, closer monitoring, and even hospitalization, partial hospitalization, or day treatment.
5. *Primarily mental health care:* The patient is referred to mental health specialty care for ongoing treatment and management.

(pp. 980–981)

64.3   What kind of "primary" mental health care services can primary care physicians provide?

    A. Anticipatory guidance.
    B. Mental health screening.
    C. Earlier identification.
    D. Earlier intervention.
    E. All of the above.

The correct response is option E.

Primary care physicians can provide "primary" mental health care services such as anticipatory guidance, mental health screening, earlier identification, and earlier intervention (Jellinek 1997). **(p. 978)**

> Jellinek MS: DSM-PC: bridging pediatric primary care and mental health services. J Dev Behav Pediatr 18:173–174, 1997

64.4   The resources available to assist the primary care physician vary across communities. Which of the following resources is *least* required by pediatricians or family physicians who provide collaborative health care in the primary care clinic?

    A. Local or regional connections with mental health professionals.
    B. Clear and regular communication.
    C. A mental health professional in the clinic.
    D. Onsite structured interviews and psychological testing.
    E. Continuing education.

The correct response is option D.

Onsite structured interviews and psychological testing are not a required resource for provision of collaborative health care in the primary care clinic.

The resources available to assist the primary care physician vary across communities. Providing the mental health care in the primary care clinic requires that the pediatrician or family physician 1) establish local or regional connections with mental health professionals who may be needed to participate as team members in the patient's care; 2) establish clear and regular communication, preferably via a common electronic chart, so that information is available to the emergency room, psychologist, and primary care physician on a timely basis; 3) establish a mental health professional in the clinic to provide triage assessments, crisis counseling, case management services, and patient and family education; 4) establish screening protocols, mechanisms, and treatment and evaluation pathways so that all providers are on the same track, providing similar standards of care; and 5) have continuing education, in either lecture or case discussion format, as a continuing point of connection between psychiatry, psychology, and the primary physician. **(pp. 982–983)**

64.5   What information should be documented in the patient's chart by the primary care physician after consulting a child and adolescent psychiatrist?

      A. Name of the consultant.
      B. The reason for the consultation.
      C. Reference to the case being summarized.
      D. Discussion of the diagnosis and recommendations for treatment.
      E. All of the above.

The correct response is option E.

When a consultation occurs, the primary care physician documents in the patient's chart the results of a consultation with a child and adolescent psychiatrist or psychologist. The notation includes the professional consulted, the reason for the consultation, a reference to the case being summarized, and the resulting discussion of the diagnosis and recommendations for treatment. **(p. 983)**

Chapter 65

Juvenile Justice

Select the single best response for each question.

65.1   Which of the following Supreme Court rulings made the execution of juveniles illegal?

    A. *Kent v. United States* (1966).
    B. *Roper v. Simmons* (2005).
    C. *In re Gault* (1967).
    D. All of the above.
    E. None of the above.

The correct response is option B.

Executing juveniles was legally permissible in the United States until the U.S. Supreme Court ruling in *Roper v. Simmons* in 2005. The Court applied a "standards of decency" test and looked at state and federal trends in sentencing and executing minors, noting that many states had made it unconstitutional to execute minors and that federal law excluded defendants younger than 18 years from execution.

Juvenile courts have undergone considerable change over the past century. The courts have moved away from a model of *parens patriae* to a more adversarial system as a result of a series of cases that recognized juvenile rights during the adjudicatory process. The first of these cases was *Kent v United States* (1966), which established that juveniles have certain rights during a juvenile court proceeding, including the right to have a lawyer present during interrogation and the right to be present during the waiver proceeding. This was followed by *In re Gault* (1967), in which a 15-year-old juvenile was brought before the court on a petition stating that he was a delinquent minor in need of care. On appeal, the U.S. Supreme Court held that all juveniles were entitled to certain due process rights, including notice of charges being brought against them, right to counsel, right to confront witnesses, and the privilege against self-incrimination. **(pp. 987–988, 989)**

> Kent v United States, 383 U.S. 541 (1966)
> In re Gault, 387 U.S. 1 (1967)
> Roper v Simmons, 543 U.S. 551 (2005)

65.2   According to a study by the Northwestern Juvenile Project (Teplin et al. 2002), which of the following are the most common psychiatric disorders/conditions among both male and female juvenile detainees?

    A. Substance abuse.
    B. Disruptive behaviors (oppositional defiant disorder and conduct disorder).
    C. Posttraumatic stress disorder (PTSD).
    D. Mood disorders.
    E. Other anxiety disorders.

The correct response is option A.

A study by the Northwestern Juvenile Project (Teplin et al. 2002) surveyed juvenile detainees within the Cook County Juvenile Detention Center. The most common disorders among both males and females were substance abuse (51% for males and 47% for females) and disruptive behaviors (oppositional defiant disorder and conduct disorder, 41% of males and 46% of females); 93% of all respondents reported at least one trauma, with 11% of participants meeting criteria for PTSD within the last year. Females were significantly more likely to be diagnosed with a mood or anxiety disorder; 22% of females met criteria for major depressive disorder (13% of males) and 31% met criteria for an anxiety disorder, with separation anxiety being the most common. **(p. 990)**

Teplin LA, Abram KM, McClelland GM, et al: Psychiatric disorders in youth in juvenile detention. Arch Gen Psychiatry 59:1133–1143, 2002

65.3   Several medical conditions predispose children to violent and aggressive behavior. For example, youth in juvenile justice are more likely than members of the general population to have been exposed during the postnatal period to which of the following?

A. Lead.
B. Alcohol.
C. Other illicit substances.
D. Head trauma.
E. Verbal abuse.

The correct response is option D.

Youth in juvenile justice are more likely than members of the general population to have experienced head trauma during the postnatal period (Otnow-Lewis 1998).

There are unique considerations for the medical needs of youth in juvenile justice (Morris 2007). Several medical conditions predispose children to violent and aggressive behavior, and testing or further investigation may be warranted. During the prenatal period, exposure to lead (Needleman et al. 1990), alcohol (Fast et al. 1999), or other illicit substances (Lester et al. 1998) has been associated with increased levels of aggression and impulsive behavior in children. Juvenile delinquents are more likely than members of the general population to have a history of head trauma during the postnatal period (Otnow-Lewis 1998). Similarly, a history of physical abuse has also been associated with delinquency, which may extend beyond the effects of the assault to more subtle neurobiological findings that impair social and emotional adjustment (Otnow-Lewis 1998). Finally, temporal-limbic epilepsy has also been associated with violent and aggressive behavior. **(p. 992)**

Fast DK, Conry J, Loock CA: Identifying fetal alcohol syndrome among youths in the criminal justice system. J Dev Behav Pediatr 29:370–372, 1999

Lester BM, LaGasse LL, Seifer R: Cocaine exposure and children: the meaning of subtle effects. Science 282:633–644, 1998

Morris R: Medical issues regarding incarcerated youth, in The Mental Health Needs of Young Offenders: Forging Paths Toward Reintegration and Rehabilitation. Edited by Kessler L, Kraus L. Cambridge, United Kingdom, Cambridge University Press, 2007, pp 256–270

Needleman HL, Schell A, Bellinger D, et al: The long-term effects of exposure to low doses of lead in childhood: an 11-year follow-up report. N Engl J Med 322:83–88, 1990

Otnow-Lewis D: Guilt by Reason of Insanity: A Psychiatrist Probes the Minds of Killers. New York, Fawcett Columbine, 1998

65.4   When did the zero-tolerance policy become mandated by the federal government?

A. 1989.
B. 1993.
C. 1994.
D. 2002.
E. 2004.

The correct response is option C.

In 1989, school districts across the United States began adopting a zero-tolerance policy, which mandated expulsion from school for drugs, fighting, and gang-related activities (Skiba and Noam 2002). By 1993, most schools had adopted such policies, and many had broadened them to include smoking and classroom disruption. In 1994, zero tolerance became mandated by the federal government with the adoption of the Gun-Free Schools Act, which required a 1-year expulsion for any child bringing a firearm onto school property. **(p. 992)**

> Skiba RJ, Noam GG: Zero tolerance, zero evidence: an analysis of school disciplinary practices. New Dir Youth Dev 92:17–43, 2002

65.5   Which of the following factors increases suicide risk among incarcerated youth?

   A. Depression.
   B. History of impulsivity and drug abuse.
   C. History of abuse.
   D. Separation from biological parents.
   E. All of the above.

The correct response is option E.

From 1950 to 2002, the suicide rate for young people (ages 15–24 years) tripled, increasing from 2.7 per 100,000 to 9.9 per 100,000 (Arias et al. 2003; Kochanek et al. 2002). Among this group, children and adolescents who are incarcerated are at the highest risk for serious suicide attempts (Gray et al. 2002). Several risk factors have been identified that place incarcerated youth at increased risk for suicide attempts: depression, history of impulsivity and drug abuse (Sanislow et al. 2003), history of abuse (Morris et al. 1995), and not living with a biological parent before incarceration (Rohde et al. 1997). **(p. 990)**

> Arias E, Anderson R, Kung H, et al: Deaths: Final Data for 2001. Natl Vital Stat Rep 53:1–115, 2003
> Gray D, Achilles J, Keller T, et al: Utah Youth Suicide Study, phase I: government agency contact before death. J Am Acad Child Adolesc Psychiatry 41:427–434, 2002
> Kochanek KD, Murphy SL, Anderson RN, et al: Deaths: Final Data for 2002. Natl Vital Stat Rep 53:1–115, 2004 Hyattsville, MD, National Center for Health Statistics, 2002
> Morris R, Harrison E, Knox G, et al: Health risk behavioral survey from 39 juvenile correctional facilities in the United States. J Adolesc Health 17:334–344, 1995
> Rohde P, Seeley JR, Mace DE: Correlates of suicidal behavior in a juvenile detention population. Suicide Life Threat Behav 27:164–175, 1997
> Sanislow C, Grilo C, Fehon D, et al: Correlates of suicide risk in juvenile detainees and adolescent in-patients. J Am Acad Child Adolesc Psychiatry 42:234–240, 2003